T0226557

Hepatocellular Cancer, Cholangiocarcinoma, and Metastatic Tumors of the Liver

Editor

LAWRENCE D. WAGMAN

SURGICAL ONCOLOGY CLINICS OF NORTH AMERICA

www.surgonc.theclinics.com

Consulting Editor
NICHOLAS J. PETRELLI

January 2015 • Volume 24 • Number 1

ELSEVIER

1600 John F. Kennedy Boulevard • Suite 1800 • Philadelphia, Pennsylvania, 19103-2899

http://www.theclinics.com

SURGICAL ONCOLOGY CLINICS OF NORTH AMERICA Volume 24, Number 1
January 2015 ISSN 1055-3207, ISBN-13: 978-0-323-34186-8

Editor: Jessica McCool
Developmental Editor: Stephanie Carter

Surgical Oncology Clinics of North America (ISSN 1055-3207) is published quarterly by Elsevier Inc., 360 Park Avenue South, New York, NY 10010-1710. Months of publication are January, April, July, and October. Business and Editorial Offices: 1600 John F. Kennedy Blvd., Ste. 1800, Philadelphia, PA 19103-2899. Customer Service Office: 3251 Riverport Lane, Maryland Heights, MO 63043. Periodicals postage paid at New York, NY and additional mailing offices. Subscription prices are $290.00 per year (US individuals), $421.00 (US institutions) $140.00 (US student/resident), $330.00 (Canadian individuals), $533.00 (Canadian institutions), $205.00 (Canadian student/resident), $410.00 (foreign individuals), $533.00 (foreign institutions), and $205.00 (foreign student/resident). Foreign air speed delivery is included in all *Clinics* subscription prices. All prices are subject to change without notice. **POSTMASTER:** Send address changes to *Surgical Oncology Clinics of North America*, Elsevier Health Science Division, Subscription Customer Service, 3251 Riverport Lane, Maryland Heights, MO 63043. **Customer Service: 1-800-654-2452 (US and Canada). 314-447-8871 (outside US and Canada). Fax: 314-447-8029. E-mail: journalscustomerservice-usa@elsevier.com** (for print support); **journalsonline support-usa@elsevier.com** (for online support).

Reprints. For copies of 100 or more, of articles in this publication, please contact the Commercial Reprints Department, Elsevier Inc., 360 Park Avenue South, New York, New York 10010-1710. Tel. 212-633-3874; Fax: 212-633-3820; E-mail: reprints@elsevier.com.

Surgical Oncology Clinics of North America is covered in *MEDLINE/PubMed (Index Medicus)* and *EMBASE/ Excerpta Medica, Current Contents/Clinical Medicine, and ISI/BIOMED.*

Contributors

CONSULTING EDITOR

NICHOLAS J. PETRELLI, MD, FACS
Bank of America Endowed Medical Director, Helen F. Graham Cancer Center & Research Institute, Christiana Care Health System, Newark, Delaware; Professor of Surgery, Thomas Jefferson University, Philadelphia, Pennsylvania

EDITOR

LAWRENCE D. WAGMAN, MD, FACS
Executive Medical Director and Director Liver, Bile Duct and Pancreas Tumor Program, The Center for Cancer Prevention and Treatment, St Joseph Hospital, Orange, California

AUTHORS

KEVIN G. BILLINGSLEY, MD
Chief, Division of Surgical Oncology; Professor, Department of Surgery, Oregon Health and Science University, Portland, Oregon

MARIA A. CASSERA, BSc
Research Fellow, Providence Cancer Center, Providence Portland Medical Center, Portland, Oregon

CLIFFORD S. CHO, MD, FACS
Associate Professor; Chief, Section of Surgical Oncology, Department of Surgery, University of Wisconsin School of Medicine and Public Health, Madison, Wisconsin

VINCENT CHUNG, MD, FACP
Clinical Associate Professor; Clinical Director Phase 1 Program, Department of Medical Oncology and Therapeutics Research, City of Hope, Duarte, California

ARAM N. DEMIRJIAN, MD
Assistant Professor, Department of Surgery, University of California-Irvine, Orange, California

KATHRYN J. FOWLER, MD
Assistant Professor of Radiology, Washington University, St Louis, Missouri

T. CLARK GAMBLIN, MD, MS
Division of Surgical Oncology, Department of Surgery, Medical College of Wisconsin, Milwaukee, Wisconsin

PAUL D. HANSEN, MD, FACS
Medical Director, Surgical Oncology; Medical Co-Director, Liver and Pancreas Surgery, Providence Cancer Center, Providence Portland Medical Center, Portland, Oregon

MATTHEW F. KALADY, MD
Digestive Disease Institute, Cleveland Clinic Foundation, Cleveland, Ohio

ALOK A. KHORANA, MD
Taussig Cancer Institute, Cleveland Clinic Foundation, Cleveland, Ohio

T. PETER KINGHAM, MD, FACS
Assistant Attending, Department of Surgery, Division of Hepatopancreatobiliary Surgery, Memorial Sloan Kettering Cancer Center, New York, New York

KELLY J. LAFARO, MD, MPH
Postdoctoral Fellow, Department of Surgery, Johns Hopkins Hospital, The Johns Hopkins University School of Medicine, Baltimore, Maryland

JULIE N. LEAL, MD, FRCSC
Department of Surgery, Division of Hepatopancreatobiliary Surgery, Memorial Sloan Kettering Cancer Center, New York, New York

EDWARD W. LEE, MD, PhD
Interventional Radiology, Department of Radiology, University of California-Los Angeles Medical Center, David Geffen School of Medicine, Los Angeles, California

DAVID LINEHAN, MD
Professor of Surgery, Washington University, St Louis, Missouri

DAVID M. LIU, MD
Interventional Radiology, Department of Radiology, University of British Columbia Medical Center, Vancouver, British Columbia, Canada

KAIHONG MI, MD, PhD
Taussig Cancer Institute, Cleveland Clinic Foundation, Cleveland, Ohio

CHRISTOPH W. MICHALSKI, MD
Division of Surgical Oncology, Oregon Health and Science University, Portland, Oregon

JOHN T. MIURA, MD
Division of Surgical Oncology, Medical College of Wisconsin, Milwaukee, Wisconsin

TIMOTHY M. PAWLIK, MD, MPH, PhD, FACS
Professor of Surgery and Oncology; Chief, Division of Surgical Oncology; John L. Cameron Professor of Alimentary Surgery, Department of Surgery, Johns Hopkins Hospital, Baltimore, Maryland

CRISTIANO QUINTINI, MD
Digestive Disease Institute, Cleveland Clinic Foundation, Cleveland, Ohio

MARIA C. RUSSELL, MD
Assistant Professor of Surgery, Emory University Hospital, Atlanta, Georgia

NAEL E. SAAD, MD
Assistant Professor of Interventional Radiology, Washington University, St Louis, Missouri

BASHIR A. TAFTI, MD
Interventional Radiology, Department of Radiology, University of California-Los Angeles Medical Center, David Geffen School of Medicine, Los Angeles, California

AVNESH S. THAKOR, MD, PhD
Interventional Radiology, Department of Radiology, University of British Columbia Medical Center, Vancouver, British Columbia, Canada

RONALD F. WOLF, MD, FACS
Medical Co-Director, Liver and Pancreas Surgery, Providence Cancer Center, Providence Portland Medical Center, Portland, Oregon

Contents

Hepatocellular carcinoma (HCC) is the most common histologic type of primary liver cancer, accounting for between 85% and 90% of these malignancies. The overall prognosis of patients with liver cancer is poor, and an understanding of this disease and its risk factors is crucial for screening at-risk individuals, early recognition, and timely diagnosis. Most HCCs arise in the background of chronic liver disease caused by hepatitis B virus, hepatitis C virus, and chronic excessive alcohol intake. These underlying causes are characterized by marked variations in geography, gender, and other well-documented risk factors, some of which are potentially preventable.

Liver imaging is a highly evolving field with new imaging contrast agents and modalities. Knowledge of the different imaging options and what they have to offer in primary and metastatic liver disease is essential for appropriate diagnosis, staging, and prognosis in patients. This review summarizes the major imaging modalities in liver neoplasms and provides specific discussion of imaging hepatocellular carcinoma, cholangiocarcinoma, and colorectal liver metastases. The final sections provide an overview of presurgical imaging relevant to planning hepatectomies and ablative procedures.

Staging systems are an attempt to incorporate the biology and therapy for cancer in a way that enables categorization and prediction of oncologic outcomes. Because of unusual disease biology and complexities related to treatment intervention, efforts to develop reliable staging systems for hepatic malignancies have been challenging. This article discusses the ways in which improved understanding of these diseases has informed the evolution of prognostication systems as applied to hepatocellular carcinoma, cholangiocarcinoma, and hepatic colorectal adenocarcinoma.

> Techniques in liver surgery have improved considerably during the last decades, allowing for liver resections with low morbidity and mortality. Preoperative patient selection, perioperative management, and intraoperative blood-sparing techniques are the cornerstones of modern liver surgery. Multimodal treatment of colorectal liver metastases has expanded the group of patients who are potential candidates for liver resection. Adjunctive techniques, including preoperative portal vein embolization and staged hepatectomy, have facilitated the safe performance of extensive liver resection. This article provides an overview of indications for liver resection and a systematic description of the technical approach to the most commonly performed resections.

> As the number of liver resections in the United States has increased, operations are more commonly performed on older patients with multiple comorbidities. The advent of effective chemotherapy and techniques such as portal vein embolization, have compounded the number of increasingly complex resections taking up to 75% of healthy livers. Four potentially devastating complications of liver resection include postoperative hemorrhage, venous thromboembolism, bile leak, and post-hepatectomy liver failure. The risk factors and management of these complications are herein explored, stressing the importance of identifying preoperative factors that can decrease the risk for these potentially fatal complications.

> A wide array of ablation technologies, in addition to the progressive sophistication of imaging technologies and percutaneous, laparoscopic, and open surgical techniques, have allowed us to expand treatment options for patients with liver tumors. In this article, technical considerations of chemical and thermal ablations and their application in hepatic oncology are reviewed.

> To date, hepatic artery infusion (HAI) chemotherapy has primarily been investigated in the setting of colorectal cancer liver metastases (CRLM). Few studies have been conducted in North America regarding HAI chemotherapy for primary liver cancers (PLC) or noncolorectal liver metastases (non-CRLM). Despite decades of evaluation, controversy surrounding the use of HAI chemotherapy still exists. In this article the methods of HAI chemotherapy delivery, technical aspects of catheter and pump insertion, and specific complications of HAI chemotherapy are discussed. Outcomes of clinical trials and reviews of HAI chemotherapy in the setting of CRLM, PLC, and non-CRLM are evaluated.

John T. Miura and T. Clark Gamblin

Management of liver malignancies, both primary and metastatic, requires a host of treatment modalities when attempting to prolong survival. Although surgical resection and transplantation continue to offer the best chance for a cure, most patients are not amenable to these therapies because of their advanced disease at presentation. Taking advantage of the unique blood supply of the liver, transarterial chemoembolization has emerged as an alternative and effective therapy for unresectable tumors. In this article, the current role along with future perspectives of transarterial chemoembolization for hepatocellular carcinoma, intrahepatic cholangio-carcinoma, and colorectal liver metastasis are discussed.

Edward W. Lee, Avnesh S. Thakor, Bashir A. Tafti, and David M. Liu

Primary liver malignancies and liver metastases are affecting millions of individuals worldwide. Because of their late and advanced stage presen-tation, only 10% of patients can receive curative surgical treatment, including transplant or resection. Alternative treatments, such as systemic chemotherapy, ablative therapy, and chemoembolization, have been used with marginal survival benefits. Selective internal radiation therapy (SIRT), also known as radioembolization, is a compelling alternative treatment option for primary and metastatic liver malignancies with a growing body of evidence. In this article, an introduction to SIRT including background, techniques, clinical outcomes, and complications is reviewed.

Vincent Chung

Understanding core signaling pathways in hepatic carcinogenesis has brought about a new era in the management of hepatocellular carcinoma. Sorafenib was the first molecular targeted therapy to be approved for advanced hepatocellular carcinoma and is the benchmark for all other therapies. Cytotoxic chemotherapy remains the mainstay treatment of advanced cholangiocarcinoma and there are no US Food and Drug Administration–approved molecular targeted therapies. If clinicians are able to minimize the toxicity of therapy by targeting the driving mechanism of cell proliferation, they will be able to significantly improve the survival and quality of life of patients.

Kaihong Mi, Matthew F. Kalady, Cristiano Quintini, and Alok A. Khorana

Multiple new treatment options for metastatic colorectal cancer have been developed over the past 2 decades, including conventional chemotherapy and agents directed against vascular endothelial growth factor and epidermal growth factor receptor. Combination regimens, integrated with surgical approaches, have led to an increase in median survival, and a minority of patients with resectable disease can survive for years.

Clinical decision-making therefore requires a strategic, biomarker-based multidisciplinary approach to maximize life expectancy and quality of life. This review describes systemic approaches to the treatment of patients with metastatic colorectal cancer, including integration with liver resection, other liver-directed therapies, and primary resection.

SURGICAL ONCOLOGY
CLINICS OF NORTH AMERICA

FORTHCOMING ISSUES

April 2015
Melanoma
Adam Berger, *Editor*

July 2015
Head and Neck Cancer
John Ridge, *Editor*

October 2015
Genetic Testing and its Surgical Oncology
Implications
Thomas Weber, *Editor*

RECENT ISSUES

October 2014
Imaging in Oncology
Vijay Khatri, *Editor*

July 2014
Breast Cancer
Lisa A. Newman, *Editor*

April 2014
Biliary Tract and Primary Liver Tumors
Timothy M. Pawlik, *Editor*

RELATED INTEREST

Clinics in Liver Disease, May 2013 (Vol. 18, Issue 4)
Interventional Procedures in Hepatobiliary Diseases
Andres Cardenas and Paul J. Thuluvath, *Editors*
Available at: http://www.liver.theclinics.com

NOW AVAILABLE FOR YOUR iPhone and iPad

Foreword

Hepatocellular Cancer, Cholangiocarcinoma, and Metastatic Tumors of the Liver

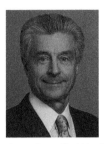

Nicholas J. Petrelli, MD, FACS
Consulting Editor

This issue of the *Surgical Oncology Clinics of North America* discusses hepatocellular cancer, cholangiocarcinoma, and metastatic tumors of the liver. The guest editor is Lawrence D. Wagman, MD, Executive Medical Director of the Center for Cancer Prevention and Treatment at St. Joseph's Hospital, Orange, California. Dr Wagman completed his general surgery residency at the Medical College of Virginia and also a fellowship at the National Institutes of Health at the National Cancer Institute Surgery Branch. He is an outstanding surgical oncologist with experience in liver, bile duct, and pancreatic surgery. Dr Wagman is an advocate for clinical trials and has spent his entire career developing national protocols and accruing patients to National Cancer Institute clinical trials.

One would think that taking on hepatocellular cancer, cholangiocarcinoma, and metastatic tumors of the liver would be too much information to put into eleven articles. However, Dr Wagman and his colleagues have made an outstanding effort in describing these cancer entities. Dr Pawlik and his colleagues from Johns Hopkins have an excellent discussion on the epidemiology of hepatocellular carcinoma. David Linehan, MD, Chief of the Section of Hepatobiliary-Pancreatic and Gastrointestinal Surgery at Washington University and the Siteman Cancer Center in St. Louis, has an excellent article on imaging approaches to hepatocellular carcinoma, cholangiocarcinoma, and liver metastasis from colorectal cancer. Other articles deal with complications following hepatic resection and hepatic artery infusion chemotherapy for liver malignancy, among other topics.

Surg Oncol Clin N Am 24 (2015) xi–xii
http://dx.doi.org/10.1016/j.soc.2014.10.002
1055-3207/15/$ – see front matter © 2015 Elsevier Inc. All rights reserved.
surgonc.theclinics.com

I'd like to take this opportunity to thank Dr Wagman and his colleagues for this outstanding issue of the *Surgical Oncology Clinics of North America*. I encourage our readers to share this information with all of their trainees.

Nicholas J. Petrelli, MD, FACS
Helen F. Graham Cancer Center & Research Institute
Christiana Care Health System
4701 Ogletown-Stanton Road, Suite 1213
Newark, DE 19713, USA

E-mail address:
npetrelli@christianacare.org

Preface

Hepatocellular Cancer, Cholangiocarcinoma, and Metastatic Tumors of the Liver

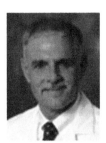

Lawrence D. Wagman, MD, FACS
Editor

Development of an issue for the *Surgical Oncology Clinics of North America* is initiated by defining an area of need and interest. Interest in the treatment of liver tumors has expanded logarithmically in the past ten years. The current needs are exemplified by what was a rare presentation at a specialty society meeting two decades ago and has morphed into a highly sought-after section at virtually every meeting in oncology. To identify the most timely and knowledgeable authors for each article, I reviewed the prior year's literature and specialty society meetings, seeking those with recognized expertise and high-quality presentations and writing skills.

While liver tumors, primary and metastatic, are approached in multidisciplinary motifs, the wide variety of treatments, procedures, and operations further increases the variability of the potential therapeutic plans. Several features of the liver play strongly into the approaches: its association of viral-induced carcinogenesis, dual inflow blood supply, central role in drug metabolism, critical synthetic functions, large functional reserve, and, most remarkably, the unique function of cellular regeneration.

This issue guides the reader through several aspects of primary (hepatocellular and cholangiocarcinoma) and metastatic tumors to the liver (directed mostly at colorectal cancer as the primary with a nod to selected other primary sites). The issue starts with the epidemiology of hepatocellular carcinoma with special emphasis on viral induction. It then moves to imaging with a description of the imaging modality, contrast agents utilized, technique, and cancer-specific interpretive methodology. The introductory articles conclude with a prognostic and risk assessment article to provide prospective for the following articles on specific interventions and techniques.

Leaving no stone unturned, the balance of the issue reviews the discreet surgical, interventional radiologic, and chemotherapeutic modalities. While each and every individual article discussing a therapeutic intervention delineates the indications and

Surg Oncol Clin N Am 24 (2015) xiii–xiv
http://dx.doi.org/10.1016/j.soc.2014.10.001
1055-3207/15/$ – see front matter © 2015 Elsevier Inc. All rights reserved.

surgonc.theclinics.com

anticipated outcomes, risks, and benefits, one article is devoted to the potential surgical complications that accompany liver surgery. The issue is designed to provide the full spectrum of needed information with minimal redundancy, as the reader moves from article to article.

To conclude, let me first thank Dr Petrelli for the invitation to guest edit and second thank the authors for their willingness to focus their unique expertise. As the guest editor, my vision for succinct and comprehensive coverage of the subject material was realized. The authors wrote within the confines of the overall goal of the issue by adhering to the need for data-based recounting as well as their personal clinical sense of the field. Finally, I wish to thank the editorial team at Elsevier, who guided, prodded, proofed, and committed our work to paper.

Lawrence D. Wagman, MD, FACS
Bile Duct and Pancreas Tumor Program
The Center for Cancer Prevention and Treatment
St Joseph Hospital
Orange, California 92868, USA

E-mail address:
Lawrence.Wagman@stjoe.org

Epidemiology of Hepatocellular Carcinoma

Kelly J. Lafaro, MD, MPH[a], Aram N. Demirjian, MD[b],
Timothy M. Pawlik, MD, MPH, PhD[c],*

KEYWORDS

- Hepatocellular carcinoma • Chronic liver disease • Cirrhosis • Hepatitis B
- Hepatitis C • Incidence • Risk factors • Aflatoxin

KEY POINTS

- HCC is a common malignancy worldwide with nearly equal numbers of new cases and cancer-related death each year.
- Most HCCs arise in the background of chronic liver disease caused by hepatitis B virus, hepatitis C virus, and chronic excessive alcohol intake.
- A detailed understanding of these risk factors and how they lead to cancer development is necessary to improve the screaming, prevention, early identification and management of HCC.

INTRODUCTION

Primary liver cancer is the fifth most common cancer worldwide and the second leading cause of cancer mortality. In 2008, there were 749,000 new cases and 695,000 deaths from liver cancer, which increased to an estimated 782,000 new cases in 2012.[1] Hepatocellular carcinoma (HCC) is the most common histologic type of primary liver cancer, and it accounts for between 85% and 90% of these malignancies. HCC arises from hepatocytes that comprise the parenchymal cells of the liver. The overall prognosis of patients with liver cancer is poor (ratio of mortality to incidence 0.95), and thus, a detailed understanding of this disease and its risk factors is crucial for screening at-risk individuals, early recognition, and timely diagnosis, and therefore,

Funding sources: none (Dr T.M. Pawlik, Dr K.J. Lafaro); Speaker's Bureau – Bayer, Speaker's Bureau – Aptalis (Dr A.N. Demirjian).
Conflicts of interest: none.
[a] Department of Surgery, Johns Hopkins Hospital, The Johns Hopkins University School of Medicine, 600 North Wolfe Street, Blalock 688, Baltimore, MD 21287, USA; [b] Department of Surgery, University of California-Irvine, 333 City Boulevard West, Suite 1205, Orange, CA 92868, USA; [c] Division of Surgical Oncology, Department of Surgery, Johns Hopkins Hospital, 600 North Wolfe Street, Blalock 688, Baltimore, MD 21287, USA
* Corresponding author.
E-mail address: tpawlik1@jhmi.edu

it is hoped, more effective and successful intervention.[1] Most HCCs arise in the background of chronic liver disease, and these underlying causes are characterized by marked variations in geography, gender, and other well-documented risk factors, some of which have become potentially preventable in recent years.

INCIDENCE

The incidence of HCC is not evenly distributed throughout the globe. A great preponderance of cases occur in sub-Saharan Africa and Eastern Asia (>80%), and China is believed to account for approximately 50% of all cases of HCC worldwide. Conversely, North and South America, as well as Europe, have a comparatively low incidence of HCC. These marked differences can be attributed to several specific factors.

Asia

More than half of HCCs occur in China alone, where in 2008, the age-standardized incidence rate was 37.4 per 100,000 individuals for males and 13.7 per 100,000 individuals for females.[1] The incidence of HCC in Mongolia and Korea are also high, with 99 and 49 cases per 100,000 persons, respectively.[1] The high incidence of HCC in these areas is related to the high hepatitis B virus (HBV) infection rates in Asia, and especially in China, where HBV has traditionally been acquired via vertical transmission from mother to child.[2,3] Widespread HBV vaccination programs introduced in the 1980s have brought hope that reduction of the HBV burden might be achieved, thereby decreasing the HCC rates in these endemic areas. In a recent 20-year follow-up study[4] after the introduction of the vaccine in Taiwan, hepatitis B surface antigen (HBsAg) seropositivity rates decreased from 10% to 17% to 0.7% to 1.7%. These studies in Taiwan also showed a decrease in the incidence of HCC among children aged 6 to 19 years (from 0.51 to 0.15/100,000 person-years in children aged 6–9 years, from 0.6 to 0.19/100,000 person-years in children aged 10–14 years, and from 0.52 to 0.16/100,000 person-years in children aged 15–19 years).[4]

Japan also has a high incidence of HCC with a case index of approximately 40 per 100,000 population. Unlike other Asian countries where HBV predominates, hepatitis C virus (HCV) is the dominant hepatitis virus in Japan, accounting for 80% of HCC cases.[5] The prevalence of HCV increased in Japan after World War II secondary to intravenous (IV) drug use, as well as contaminated blood transfusions, which led to quickly increasing rates of infection in the 1970s.[5,6] It is estimated that the peak in HCV-related HCC rates will occur in approximately 2015. The HCC incidence associated with HCV in Japan is 2-fold higher than that in Europe or the United States, with 5-year cumulative incidences of 30% and 17%, respectively.[7] This incidence may be attributed to the increased incidence of HCV genotype 1b in Japan, which has been shown to have decreased response to antiviral therapy compared with genotype 1 a, which is prevalent in the United States and Europe.[8]

Africa

The first case of HCC in Africa was reported in 1879.[9] Although the true incidence of HCC in Africa is likely underestimated, because of lack of screening and access to medical care in rural areas, it is a major cause of death in the black African population. Within Africa, Mozambique has the highest incidence of recorded HCC, with an age-standardized incidence of 41.2/100,000 persons each year. Most of these cases are found in rural areas. Cirrhosis coexists with HCC in about 60% of patients in this region. Whites living in the subcontinent have a low incidence of HCC. Chronic HBV infection is the major cause of HCC in Africa, where infection occurs early in childhood through horizontal transmission of the virus from sibling to sibling, differing from the vertical transmission commonly seen in Asia (**Fig. 1**).

United States and Europe

Although the overall incidence of HCC in the United States is lower than in other parts of the world, the age-adjusted incidence rate tripled from 1975 to 2005 from 1.6/100,000 to 4.9/100,000.[10] This increase is likely a result of the increasing prevalence of HCV from unscreened blood transfusions and IV drug use in the 1960s and 1970s, although there are other likely contributing factors. The incidence of HCC in the United States is expected to continue to increase over the next decade, because of peak HCV infection rates in the 1980s and the 20-year to 40-year lag time observed between HCV acquisition and HCC development. HCC is believed to be most associated with HCV, because widespread HBV vaccination programs have been implemented, and HBV accounts for only 10% to 15% of HCC cases in the United States.[11] The mean age of diagnosis of HCC in the United States is 65 years; 74% of cases occur in men. The racial distribution is 48% white, 13% African American, 15% Hispanic, and 24% other/Asian.[5] The highest incidence of HCC is seen in the Asian/Pacific Islander population (11.7/100,000), and the lowest is among whites (3.9/100,000).[10]

Europe has a slightly higher incidence (2–4 times) of HCC than the United States. The Mediterranean countries (Italy, Spain, and Greece) have incidence rates ranging from 10 to 20 per 100,000 individuals. These countries also attribute approximately two-thirds of their cases to chronic HCV infection.[12] The greatest gender disparity has been reported by countries in central Europe, where the male/female ratio is greater than 4:1.[1]

RISK FACTORS

HCC is a genetically heterogeneous tumor. Hepatocarcinogenesis is complex, requiring multiple genetic and epigenetic alterations and the involvement of several

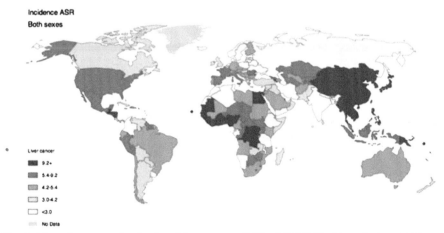

Fig. 1. Map of age-standardized incidence rates (ASR) of HCC/100. (*From* Ferlay J, Shin H, Bray F, et al. GLOBOCAN 2008 v2.0, Cancer incidence and mortality worldwide: IARC Cancer-Base No. 10. Lyon (France): International Agency for Research on Cancer; 2010.)

signal transduction pathways, including p53, Ras, MAPK, JAK/STAT, Wnt/β-catenin, and hedgehog.[13,14] Multiple predisposing causes of HCC have been defined, including HBV, HCV, excessive alcohol consumption, obesity, and aflatoxins, and the prevalence/contribution of these risk factors vary by region (**Fig. 2**).

Hepatitis B Virus

HBV is a DNA virus with a circular genome that encodes structural and replicative viral proteins. The now widely recognized association of chronic HBV infection and HCC was first elucidated in 1981 by Beasely and colleagues[15] in Taiwanese HBsAg-positive patients. Serum HBsAg, the marker of HBV infection, without the presence of any additional risk factors is found in 70% of patients with HCC in China, 41% of patients with HCC in the United States, and 24% to 27% of patients with HCC in Japan.[16] In Asia, HBV infection is acquired through vertical transmission from mother to child, whereas in Africa, horizontal transmission early in childhood from sibling to sibling, likely via saliva and open wounds, is more common. In low-risk areas, the pattern of transmission is horizontal, through blood from needlesticks with IV drug use, as well as sexual exposure occurring in adulthood (**Fig. 3**).

There are 8 genotypes of HBV, classified using the letters A to H. The viral genome of each genotype differs by greater than 8%. Genotype A is found in sub-Saharan Africa, Western Africa, and Northern Europe. Genotype B is found primarily in Japan and East Asia. Genotype C is more commonly associated with severe liver disease and an increased risk of HCC than other genotypes and is found in China, Korea, Japan, Southeast Asia, and several South Pacific Island countries. Genotype D is widely distributed throughout Eastern Europe, North Africa, the Mediterranean region, Russia, the Middle East, India, and the Arctic. Genotype E is primarily found in West Africa. Genotypes F and H are found in Central and South America. Genotype C is the most widely studied of these genotypes. Most studies[17–21] have shown an association between genotype C and an increased risk of liver fibrosis and HCC.

HBV, unlike other risk factors, increases the risk of HCC in cirrhotic as well as non-cirrhotic patients. In the setting of cirrhosis, HBV infection causes a chronic

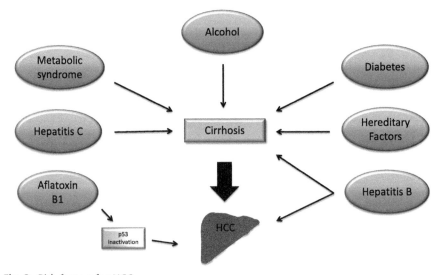

Fig. 2. Risk factors for HCC.

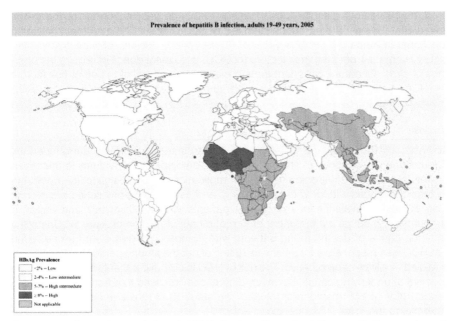

Fig. 3. MAP of prevalence of chronic HBV infection. (*From* Ott J, Stevens G, Groeger J, et al. Global epidemiology of hepatitis B virus infection: new estimates of age-specific HBsAg seroprevalence and endemicity. Vaccine 2012;30(12):2215; with permission.)

necroinflammatory process with fibrosis and hepatocyte proliferation, similar to that seen with other risk factors. Independent from cirrhosis, HBV is capable of hepatocarcinogenesis secondary to virus-specific factors. HBV is a DNA virus with a circular genome that encodes structural and replicative proteins. It also contains DNA regulatory elements. The virus enters hepatocytes, viral messenger RNAs are transcribed and translated into viral proteins, and viral DNA is synthesized. Viral DNA is then able to integrate into the genome of the host in infected hepatocytes. This process may facilitate carcinogenesis in multiple ways, including rapid cell cycling of hepatocytes[22] and integration of viral DNA into the genome, causing instability,[23] and it may insert into, or adjacent to, genes encoding proteins necessary for carcinogenesis.[24,25] In addition, HBV overexpression alone has been shown to lead to malignant transformation in mice.[26] An increased risk of HCC development correlates with HBV viral load greater than 13 pg/mL.[27–29]

Vaccination is the most effective intervention to prevent HBV infection and is one of the first examples of a vaccination that significantly reduces the risk of developing cancer. Although the vaccine has been shown to be ineffective in as many as 5% to 10% of people because of hepatitis B surface antibody levels less than 10 U/mL, there have been drastic decreases in the incidence of HBV after vaccination campaigns. In a 20-year follow-up study after the introduction of the vaccine, HBsAg seropositivity rates decreased from 10% to 17% to 0.7% to 1.7% in Taiwan, where transmission of HBV occurs by both horizontal as well as perinatal vertical transmission in approximately equal rates.[4] Twenty-year follow-up studies in Taiwan also showed a decrease in the incidence of HCC among children aged 6 to 19 years (from 0.51 to 0.15/100,000 person-years in children aged 6–9 years, from 0.6 to 0.19/100,000 person-years in children aged 10–14 years, and from 0.52 to 0.16/100,000 person-years in children aged 15–19 years).[4] Despite these findings, although vaccination is routine in the United States and Europe, vaccination is still not routine in all countries, including sub-Saharan Africa.

HBV is unique from other risk factors for HCC, because it does not require the presence of cirrhosis before malignant transformation. Virtually all of the other risk factors for HCC typically are associated with cirrhosis, which is required for HCC development.

Cirrhosis

Cirrhosis, or the histologic development of regenerative nodules surrounded by fibrous bands in response to chronic liver injury, predisposes individuals to the development of HCC.[7,30] In addition to HCC, complications of cirrhosis include portal hypertension, varices with or without bleeding, and ascites. Autopsy series suggest an 80% to 90% prevalence of cirrhosis in patients with HCC in Italy and Japan.[31] Although the medical management of cirrhotic patients has improved, HCC is still a common cause of death among patients with cirrhosis. Studies from Europe found that HCC was responsible for 54%[32] to 70%[33] of deaths among persons with cirrhosis who died of a liver-related cause. The risk of HCC in cirrhotic patients is increased irrespective of underlying cause; however, different causes lead to different rates of incidence: HCV >HBV >hemochromatosis. The stage of cirrhosis is also significant in determining the risk of HCC development.[7,34]

Hepatitis C Virus

HCV is an RNA virus belonging to the Flaviviridae family and was first identified in 1989.[10,35,36] Greater than 200 million people are estimated to be infected with HCV worldwide,[6] and it is a major risk factor for HCC development. HCV infection rates in patients with HCC are variable, ranging from 44% to 66% in Italy to 80% to 90% in Japan.[6] A meta-analysis of 21 studies[37] showed a 17-fold increased risk of HCC in HCV-infected patients compared with HCV negative controls.

There have been 6 major genotypes identified (genotypes HCV-1–HCV-6), each with multiple subtypes (distinguished by lowercase letters). These genotypes have different geographic as well as virulence patterns. Genotype 1 (a and b) is the most common worldwide. Genotype 1b predominates in Asia, whereas 1a and 1b are most common in Europe and North and South America. Genotype 4 is predominant in Africa.[38]

Mechanism of increased HCC risk

The increased risk of HCC development in HCV-infected patients comes from the development of liver fibrosis and cirrhosis as a result of chronic inflammation. This inflammation leads to the distortion of hepatic architecture and impairment of cellular functions as well as the microcirculation of the liver. Unlike HBV, HCV is unable to integrate into the host genome. Instead, in HCV, viral proteins such as HCV core protein and their evoked host response have been implicated in apoptosis, signal transduction, reactive oxygen species (ROS) formation, transcriptional activation, and immune modulation through upregulation of interleukin 1 (IL-1), IL-6, and tumor necrosis factor α (TNF-α), contributing to malignant transformation.[14]

Twenty-five to 30 years after HCV infection, rates of cirrhosis range between 12% and 35%.[5,39] Chronic HCV infection is the leading cause of cirrhosis, and the most common indication for liver transplantation in North and South America, Europe, Australia, and Japan.[38,40] Environmental factors such as age greater than 40 years at time of infection,[41] degree of alcohol intake (greater than 40–50 g daily), male sex, obesity, presence of an increased alanine transaminase level[42,43] and coinfection with HBV or HIV seem to have a greater impact than genotype or viral load in the progression to cirrhosis.[39]

Effect of treatment on incidence of hepatocellular carcinoma

Unlike other viral infections, antiviral treatment of HCV can eradicate the virus with sustained virologic response (SVR) and the absence of detectable HCV RNA after successful treatment. SVR has been associated with a 54% reduction in all-cause mortality,[44] including HCC-related and liver-related death.[45] A recent meta-analysis showed that HCC developed at a rate of 0.33% per person year (95% confidence interval [CI] 0.22%–0.5%) among individuals who achieved SVR compared with 1.67% per person year (95% CI 1.15%–2.42%) among nonresponders.[46]

Alcohol

Excessive alcohol consumption has been linked with a variety of disorders. Approximately 8% to 20% of chronic alcoholics develop liver cirrhosis.[47] The International Agency for Research on Cancer working group (IARC) suggested a causal relationship between alcohol consumption and liver cancer in 1988[48] and has since deemed beverages containing alcohol as carcinogenic to humans. The initial causal relationship between alcohol and HCC was subsequently confirmed by multiple studies, with odds ratios (ORs) between 2.4 and 7.[37,49] Chronic excessive alcohol use (>80 g/d) for greater than 10 years has been shown to increase HCC risk 5-fold.[37,50] A dose-dependent risk effect was shown by researchers at the University of Michigan,[51] in which 1500 gram-years of alcohol exposure (60 g/d for >25 years) increased the risk of HCC 6-fold (OR 5.7; 95% CI 2.4–13.7). Data from the European Prospective Investigation into Cancer and Nutrition,[52] including 4,409,809 person-years from 1992 to 2006, showed an association between heavy (>40 g/d for men and >20 g/d for women) alcohol intake (OR 1.77; 95% CI 0.73–4.27) and development of HCC. Although there has never been a safety limit set for the hepatotoxic effects of alcohol, a meta-analysis[53] showed a dose-response relationship between alcohol intake and HCC with relative risks (RRs) of 1.19 (95% CI 1.12–1.27), 1.40 (95% CI 1.25–1.56), and 1.81 (95% CI 1.50–2.19) for 25 g/d, 50 g/d and 100 g/d, respectively.

Conversely, a cessation of alcohol consumption has been shown to decrease the risk of liver cancer. A meta-analysis showed that the risk of HCC decreases after abstinence by 6% to 7% per year compared with ongoing drinkers. The same study estimated that a period of 23 years is required after alcohol cessation for the risk of HCC development to return to that of nondrinkers regardless of cirrhotic status.[54]

Mechanism of hepatocellular carcinoma development

Alcohol is metabolized in hepatocytes via oxidation of alcohol to acetaldehyde and subsequently from acetaldehyde to acetate. This reaction is catalyzed by multiple enzymatic pathways, including alcohol dehydrogenase, cytochrome P4502E1, and catalase. The mechanism of alcohol-induced liver damage resulting in HCC is believed to stem from 2 separate processes studied in animal models. First, alcoholic fatty liver that predisposes to cirrhosis with continued chronic alcohol intake results from the oxidative metabolism of alcohol. The oxidative metabolism generates excess of reduced nicotinamide adenine dinucleotide (NADH), resulting in an increased ratio of NADH to NAD+ in hepatocytes, leading to the inhibition of fatty acid oxidation and promotion of lipogenesis.[47] The second mechanism that contributes to hepatocarcinogenesis is the generation of ROS as well as other free radical species in hepatocytes during metabolism of alcohol in the liver. This process results in increased levels of NADH, which provide electrons for the mitochondrial electron transport chain, leading to increased 1-electron reduction of oxygen to superoxide as well as reduction of antioxidants.[47,55,56]

Synergism between ethanol and other risk factors

Alcohol has a synergistic effect with preexisting chronic liver disease on HCC risk, including HCV, HBV, fatty liver disease, tobacco use, and obesity.[37,49,57] Poynard and colleagues,[41] in their study on the natural history of liver fibrosis progression in patients with HCV, found that daily alcohol consumption greater than 50 g was one of 3 independent factors associated with an increased rate of fibrosis progression. Another retrospective cohort study[58] showed that patients with cirrhosis caused by a combination of HCV and alcohol had a significantly increased risk of HCC compared with those individuals with cirrhosis caused by alcohol alone (hazard ratio [HR] 11.2; 95%, CI 2.3–55.0). It has been suggested that HCC development in patients with HCV and alcohol may differ biologically from patients with HCV alone. When histology was studied after resection of HCC in 80 patients with HCV infection, the proportion of well-differentiated HCC was lower (2/38 [5%]) in those who had consumed greater than 86 g/d of alcohol than those who were nondrinkers (19/42 [45%], P<.0001).[59] Also, patients with HCV and alcohol as risk factors had reduced tumor-free survival compared with those with HCV alone (P<.05).[59]

A prospective case-control study of 210 patients in the United States[51] showed that the risk of HCC increased 6-fold for patients with lifetime alcohol exposure greater than 1500 gram-years; 5-fold with greater than 20 pack-years of smoking, and 4-fold with body mass index (BMI, calculated as weight in kilograms divided by the square of height in meters) greater than 30. There were synergistic indices for the interaction between alcohol and tobacco, tobacco and obesity, and alcohol and obesity of 3.3, 2.9 and 2.5, respectively.

Aflatoxin

Aflatoxin is a mycotoxin produced by molds *Aspergillus flavus* and *Apsergillus parasiticus*, which can contaminate grains, legumes, tree nuts, maize, and ground nuts. In addition, when dairy-producing animals consume aflatoxin-contaminated feed, a metabolite, aflatoxin M1, is excreted in the milk. Countries with high risk of dietary aflatoxin intake include Mozambique, Vietnam, China, and India, because of their warm and humid climate, favoring growth of aflatoxin-producing molds. Aflatoxin has been classified as a hepatic carcinogen by the International Agency for Research on Cancer.[60] A risk assessment from 2010[61] found that aflatoxin is associated with 4.6% to 28.2% of HCC worldwide. There are 4 aflatoxins: B1, B2, G1, and G2. Aflatoxin B1 (AFB1) has been shown to be the most potent hepatic carcinogen of the 4. According to an estimate from 2006,[61] greater than 55 million people worldwide suffer from uncontrolled exposure to aflatoxin. AFB1 is metabolized to the active intermediate AFB1 exo-8,9-epoxide, which can bind to DNA. Detection of a signature aflatoxin mutation was found at codon 249 in the tumor suppressor gene p53, causing a G >T transversion in 30% to 60% of tumors from persons in aflatoxin-rich environments.[62–64]

AFB1 has a synergistic effect with chronic HBV infection and alcohol on HCC risk. A prospective study in China[65] showed that urinary excretion of AFB1 metabolites was associated with a 4-fold increased risk of HCC, whereas those who excreted AFB1 metabolites and were HBV positive had a 60-fold increase in HCC risk.

PATIENT FACTORS
Metabolic Syndromes

Although worldwide, most HCC is related to hepatitis viral infection and alcoholic liver disease, many patients (5%–20%) with HCC are negative for both HBV and HCV. Nonalcoholic fatty liver disease (NAFLD) and the more severe form, biopsy proven nonalcoholic steatohepatitis (NASH), are characterized by liver disease in the absence of a history of significant alcohol use, or liver disease of unknown cause, and have become the most common cause of cryptogenic chronic liver disease in the United States and Western countries. NAFLD is the hepatic manifestation of a metabolic syndrome including hypertension, insulin resistance, central obesity, and dyslipidemia. Up to 90% of obese individuals have some degree of chronic fatty liver disease, and the degree of hepatic steatosis correlates with increasing BMI.[66] NASH has been reported in 1% to 3% of the adult Japanese population and approximately 6% in Western countries.[67–69]

There is increasing evidence to support the fact that NASH and NAFLD can progress to cirrhosis and HCC, and recently, a SEER (Surveillance Epidemiology and End Results)-Medicare–based database study showed an association between the metabolic syndrome and HCC (HR 2.13; 95% CI 1.96–2.31).[70] Also, cohort studies from Denmark and Sweden have identified an increase in HCC risk in obese males compared with those with a normal BMI.[71,72]

There are few data regarding the natural history and prognosis of NASH. A Japanese cohort study[73] followed 137 patients with NASH (biopsy proven) advanced fibrosis and found a 5-year cumulative HCC incidence of 7.6%. In a slightly larger study, Ascha and colleagues[74] found a yearly cumulative incidence rate of HCC to be 2.6% in patients with cirrhosis related to NASH. This finding was compared with 4% in patients with HCV-related cirrhosis. Obesity has also been implicated in increased mortality in patients with HCC. A large 16-year prospective cohort study in the United States showed HCC mortality 5 times greater among men with a BMI of 35 to 40 compared with men who had a normal BMI.[75] These studies are important, because the obesity epidemic increases, most notably in the United States, and this may translate into significant increases in HCC incidence (**Fig. 4**).

Mechanism of increased risk of hepatocellular carcinoma

The hepatocarcinogenesis rate in NASH-related cirrhosis is lower than that of HCV-related cirrhosis. Insulin resistance and fatty liver disease lead to inflammatory and angiogenic changes in the liver. Adipose tissue expresses the proinflammatory cytokines TNF-α and IL-6, both of which are dysregulated in obesity. These cytokines are essential cancer promoters in carcinogenesis stemming from inflammation.[76] In addition, like many other HCC risk factors, NASH and NAFLD promote malignant transformation to HCC through cirrhosis.

Diabetes Type 2 (Diabetes Mellitus)

Insulin resistance as a part of a metabolic syndrome has been linked to HCC, likely because of the inflammatory and angiogenic changes seen. As a result, the risk of HCC associated with diabetes mellitus (DM) has been examined. Similar to obesity, a large percentage ($\geq$70%) of patients with DM have some degree of fatty liver disease.[66] Although there have been some small controversial studies,[77] DM has been associated with HCC risk. El-Serag and colleagues[78] conducted a longitudinal study looking at 173,643 patients with DM and 650,620 without DM (98% male) to elucidate an association between DM and HCC. These investigators reported that DM was associated with an HR of 1.98 (95% CI 1.88–2.09) for chronic nonalcoholic liver

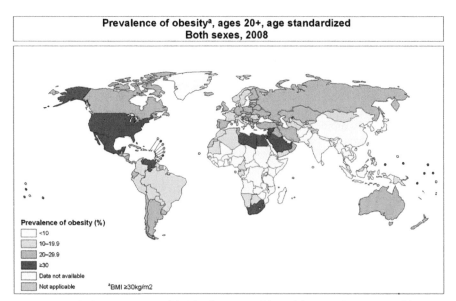

**Prevalence of obesity[a], ages 20+, age standardized
Both sexes, 2008**

Prevalence of obesity (%)

- <10
- 10–19.9
- 20–29.9
- ≥30
- Data not available
- Not applicable   [a]BMI ≥30kg/m2

Fig. 4. Map of obesity rates worldwide. (*From* World Health Organization. World: prevalence of obesity, ages 20+, age standardized: both sexes, 2008. 2011. Available at: http://www.who.int/gho/ncd/risk_factors/obesity_text/en/. Accessed February 10, 2014.)

disease and an HR of 2.16 (95% CI 1.86–2.52) for HCC development. A case-control study from the United States that compared 420 HCC cases with 1104 healthy controls[79] found DM to increase the risk of HCC (adjusted OR 4.2; 95% CI 3.0–5.9) in a duration-dependent manner. Compared with patients with diabetes for 2 to 5 years, the estimated adjusted ORs for those with a diabetes duration of 6 to 10 years and those with a diabetes duration greater than 10 years were 1.8 (95% CI, 0.8–4.1) and 2.2 (95% CI, 1.2–4.8), respectively. A retrospective case-control study in China[80] showed an increased risk of HCC for patients with DM using a stepwise linear regression model (OR 2.35; 95% CI 1.36–4.05). Polesel and colleagues[81] published a case-control study in Italy looking at 185 cases of HCC and found that DM was associated with HCC risk among patients without HBV or HCV (OR 3.5; 95% CI 1.3–9.2). Although most of these studies have small numbers, Wang and colleagues[82] recently conducted a meta-analysis including a total of 25 cohort studies to examine the relationship between DM and HCC. The investigators reported that DM was associated with an increased incidence of HCC (HR 2.01; 95% CI 1.61–2.51), compared with individuals without DM, and that it was also associated with HCC mortality (HR 1.56; 95% CI 1.30–1.87). Thus, DM was concluded to be an independent risk factor for progression of chronic liver disease and HCC development.

Mechanism of increased risk of hepatocellular carcinoma

DM induces liver cell damage though insulin resistance and hyperinsulinemia.[83,84] Hyperinsulinemia leads to HCC through inflammation, cellular proliferation, and inhibition of apoptosis. In addition, the increased insulin levels can cause decreased liver synthesis of insulin growth factor binding protein 1, which is believed to lead to increased bioavailability of insulin like growth factor 1, as well as increased cellular proliferation and inhibition of apoptosis.[85] Insulin has also been associated with an increase in oxidative stress and the generation of ROS, contributing to DNA mutation.[86]

Treatment of DM with metformin, an oral antihyperglycemic agent that increases insulin sensitivity, has been shown to decrease the risk of HCC development. Donadon and colleagues[87] showed in a multivariate analysis that metformin treatment was associated with a strong and statistically significant reduction of the risk of HCC, compared with the use of sulfonylureas or insulin, in diabetic patients with HCC versus controls (OR 0.15; CI 0.04–0.50; $P = .005$). These investigators also found increased risk for HCC in patients with DM treated with insulin or other antidiabetic oral agents that enhance insulin secretion, such as sulfonylureas, caused by the resulting hyperinsulinism, which has been implicated in HCC development.[87]

Hereditary Hemochromatosis

Hereditary hemochromatosis (HH) is an autosomal-recessive genetically mediated disorder caused by a single missense mutation (C282Y and H63D) in the HFE gene located on chromosome 6. The disease is characterized by excessive absorption of iron by the gastrointestinal tract, causing iron overload. A population-based cohort study of 1847 Swedish patients with HH and 5973 of their first-degree relatives in Sweden[88] found that patients with HH were at a 20-fold increased risk of developing liver cancer (standardized incidence ratio 21; 95% CI 16–22). A large study from the US National Center for Health Statistics found that patients previously diagnosed with HH were 23-fold more likely to have liver cancer compared with those without a diagnosis of HH at time of death (proportionate mortality ratio (PMR) 22.5; 95% CI 20.6–24.6).[89] The iron overload caused by HH may stimulate hepatic fibrogenesis through oxygen free radical production and the production of cytokines, including tumor growth factor β.[90]

Tobacco

Multiple studies have been published regarding the relationship between tobacco use and HCC; however, the results are inconsistent. A prospective cohort study in Japan[91] that followed 4050 men older than 40 years for a mean of 9 years found a 3-fold increased risk of primary liver cancer in current smokers compared with nonsmokers, in a non–dose-dependent manner. A 2005 study from Korea[92] that looked at 733,134 men followed over a 4-year period found an adjusted RR of 1.53 (95% CI 1.30–1.79) for former smokers and 1.50 (95% CI 1.29–1.74) for current smokers, although this study did not take into account hepatitis status. A prospective case-control study from Michigan[51] looking at 210 patients with HCC found an increased risk of HCC in tobacco smokers with greater than 20 pack-years compared with cirrhotic patients without HCC (OR 4.9; 95% CI 2.2–10.6) as well as compared with patients with no underlying liver disease (OR 63.7; 95% CI 16.7–144.2). However, a US study using case-control data from the Selected Cancers Study[93] found no increase in risk of primary liver cancer in current smokers. The investigators did find a statistically significant increase in risk (1.85; 95% CI, 1.05–3.25) of primary liver cancer in former smokers. The results of this study may suggest that there is a time-dependent risk associated with tobacco use. A synergistic effect between tobacco smoking, alcohol consumption, and obesity on the risk of HCC has been reported.[51]

Although the association between tobacco smoking and development of HCC is still unclear, studies have shown an increased risk of mortality in patients with HCC with tobacco use. A 2004 Korean study found that current smoking was associated with increased risk of mortality from HCC in men (RR 1.4; 95% CI 1.3–1.6).[94] A prospective study of 12,008 men in Taiwan showed that tobacco interacted additively with anti-HCV positivity; however, the synergistic indices were not statistically significant.[95]

Gender

Men have higher rates of HCC than women in almost all countries, with the highest discrepancies existing in Europe (>4:1).[2] Although likely multifactorial, there are sex-specific differences in exposure to risk factors. Men are more likely to be infected with HBV, consume alcohol, and smoke tobacco. However, this increased risk may also be conferred by nonmodifiable factors as well. An early prospective study of 613 cirrhotic patients from London showed male gender as a significant independent risk factor for the progression of cirrhosis to HCC.[96] Yuan and colleagues[97] showed a correlation between testosterone levels and HCC risk, suggesting an inherently higher risk for men. In addition, mouse models using carcinogens to induce HCC showed a propensity for male mice to develop tumors over female mice. IL-6, a cytokine largely responsible for the hepatic response to infection and inflammation, has also been linked to hepatocarcinogenesis. Naugler and colleagues[98] found that estrogens, at concentrations present in females, suppressed IL-6 production in murine models and decreased chemically induced liver carcinogenesis.

ECONOMIC/PUBLIC HEALTH ASPECT

The burden of HCC on the health systems of Western countries will likely increase in the coming years as a result of disease progression of HCV-positive baby boomers, and the 20-year to 40-year lag time between viral infection and development of HCC. Because of HCV, as well as other risk factors discussed earlier, it is projected that both compensated cirrhosis and HCC will increase by more than 80% from 2000 to 2020 in the United States.[99] Although the figure is dated, the total cost of primary liver cancer in the United States in 1998 was estimated to be 988 million dollars, with 978 million dollars in direct costs and 10 million dollars in indirect costs defined as the cost of forgone earnings as a result of hospitalization, ambulatory care, and premature death. The direct costs can further be broken down by service, with 548 million dollars spent on inpatient hospital costs, 89 million dollars on outpatient hospital costs, 139 million dollars on office visits, and 80 million dollars in medications.[100] As new medications are found to treat HCV and HCC, these medication costs will continue to soar. HCC exacts heavy economic and social costs on the United States, as well as the rest of the world, where it has a higher prevalence.

SUMMARY

HCC is a common malignancy worldwide, with nearly equal numbers of new cases and cancer-related death each year. Most HCCs develop in the setting of chronic underlying liver disease, the cause of which can differ widely based on multiple factors. The principal causal factors for carcinogenesis in HCC are HBV, HCV, and alcohol abuse, although there seems to be an increasing incidence of NASH-associated HCC in Western countries. A detailed understanding of these risk factors and how they lead to cancer development is necessary to improve the screening, prevention, early identification, and management of HCC.

REFERENCES

1. Ferlay J, Shin H, Bray F, et al. GLOBOCAN 2008 v2.0, Cancer incidence and mortality worldwide: IARC CancerBase No. 10 [Internet]. Lyon (France): International Agency for Research on Cancer; 2010.

2. Shariff M, Cox I, Gomaa A, et al. Hepatocellular carcinoma: current trends in worldwide epidemiology, risk factors, diagnosis and therapeutics. Expert Rev Gastroenterol Hepatol 2009;3(4):353–67.
3. Custer B, Sullivan S, Hazlet T, et al. Global epidemiology of hepatitis B virus. J Clin Gastroenterol 2004;38(10):S158–68.
4. Chang M, You S, Chen C, et al. Decreased incidence of hepatocellular carcinoma in hepatitis B vaccinees: a 20-year follow-up study. J Natl Cancer Inst 2009;101(19):1348–55.
5. El-Serag H, Rudolph K. Hepatocellular carcinoma: epidemiology and molecular carcinogenesis. Gastroenterology 2007;132(7):2557–76.
6. Yoshizawa H. Hepatocellular carcinoma associated with hepatitis C virus infection in Japan: projection to other countries in the foreseeable future. Oncology 2002;62(S1):8–17.
7. Fattovich G, Stroffolini T, Zagni I, et al. Hepatocellular carcinoma in cirrhosis: incidence and risk factors. Gastroenterology 2004;127(5):35–S50.
8. Pellicelli A, Romano M, Stroffolini T, et al. HCV genotype 1a shows a better virologic response to antiviral therapy than HCV genotype 1b. BMC Gastroenterol 2012;12(162):1–7.
9. Kew M. Epidemiology of hepatocellular carcinoma in sub-Saharan Africa. Ann Hepatol 2013;12(2):173–82.
10. Altekruse S, McGlynn K, Reichman M. Hepatocellular carcinoma incidence, mortality, and survival trends in the United States from 1975 to 2005. J Clin Oncol 2009;27(9):1485–91.
11. Mittal S, El-Serag H. Epidemiology of hepatocellular carcinoma: consider the population. J Clin Gastroenterol 2013;47:S2–6.
12. Bosch F, Ribes J, Cléries R, et al. Epidemiology of hepatocellular carcinoma. Clin Liver Dis 2005;9(2):191–211.
13. Branda M, Wands J. Signal transduction cascades and hepatitis B and C related hepatocellular carcinoma. Hepatology 2006;43(5):891–902.
14. Tsai W, Chung R. Viral hepatocarcinogenesis. Oncogene 2010;29(16):2309–24.
15. Beasley R, Hwang L, Lin C, et al. Hepatocellular carcinoma and hepatitis B virus: a prospective study of 22,707 men in Taiwan. Lancet 1981;2(8256):1129–33.
16. Tabor E. Hepatocellular carcinoma: global epidemiology. Dig Liver Dis 2001; 33(2):115–7.
17. McMahon B. The influence of hepatitis B virus genotype and subgenotype on the natural history of chronic hepatitis B. Hepatol Int 2009;3(2):334–42.
18. Chan H, Hui A, Wong M, et al. Genotype C hepatitis B virus infection is associated with an increased risk of hepatocellular carcinoma. Gut 2004;53(10): 1494–8.
19. Kao J, Chen P, Lai M, et al. Hepatitis B genotypes correlate with clinical outcomes in patients with chronic hepatitis B. Gastroenterology 2000;118(3):554–9.
20. Lee C, Chen C, Lu S, et al. Prevalence and clinical implications of hepatitis B virus genotypes in southern Taiwan. Scand J Gastroenterol 2003;38(1):95–101.
21. Tangkijvanich P, Mahachai V, Komolmit P, et al. Hepatitis B virus genotypes and hepatocellular carcinoma in Thailand. World J Gastroenterol 2005;11(15): 2238–43.
22. Chisari F. Rous-Whipple award lecture. Viruses, immunity, and cancer: lessons from hepatitis B. Am J Pathol 2000;156(4):1117–32.
23. Dandri M, Burda M, Bürkle A, et al. Increase in de novo HBV DNA integrations in response to oxidative DNA damage or inhibition of poly(ADP-ribosyl)ation. Hepatology 2002;35(1):217–23.

24. Bonilla Guerrero R, Roberts L. The role of hepatitis B virus integrations in the pathogenesis of human hepatocellular carcinoma. J Hepatol 2005;42(5):760–77.
25. Ferber M, Montoya D, Yu C, et al. Integrations of the hepatitis B virus (HBV) and human papillomavirus (HPV) into the human telomerase reverse transcriptase (hTERT) gene in liver and cervical cancers. Oncogene 2003;22(24): 3813–20.
26. Wu B, Li C, Chen H, et al. Blocking of G1/S transition and cell death in the regenerating liver of hepatitis B virus X protein transgenic mice. Biochem Biophys Res Commun 2006;340(3):916–28.
27. Yang H, Lu S, Liaw Y, et al. Hepatitis B e antigen and the risk of hepatocellular carcinoma. N Engl J Med 2002;347(3):168–74.
28. Yuen M, Tanaka Y, Fong D, et al. Independent risk factors and predictive score for the development of hepatocellular carcinoma in chronic hepatitis B. J Hepatol 2009;10(1):80–8.
29. Chen C, Yang H, Su J, et al. Risk of hepatocellular carcinoma across a biological gradient of serum hepatitis B virus DNA level. JAMA 2006;295(1):65–73.
30. Simonietti R, Camma C, Fiorello F, et al. Hepatocellular carcinoma. A worldwide problem and the major risk factors. Dig Dis Sci 1991;36:962–72.
31. Tiribelli C, Melato M, Croce L, et al. Prevalence of hepatocellular carcinoma and relation to cirrhosis: comparison of two different cities in the world–Trieste, Italy and China, Japan. Hepatology 1989;10:998–1002.
32. Sangiovanni A, Del Ninno E, Fasani P, et al. Increased survival of cirrhotic patients with a hepatocellular carcinoma detected during surveillance. Gastroenterology 2004;126:1005–14.
33. Benvegnu L, Gios M, Boccato S, et al. Natural history of compensated viral cirrhosis: a prospective study on the incidence and hierarchy of major complications. Gut 2004;53:744–9.
34. Tsai J, Jeng J, Ho M, et al. Effect of hepatitis C and B virus infection on risk of hepatocellular carcinoma: a prospective study. Br J Cancer 1997;76:968–74.
35. McGlynn K, London W. The global epidemiology of hepatocellular carcinoma: present and future. Clin Liver Dis 2011;15(2):223–43.
36. Choo Q, Kuo G, Weiner A, et al. Isolation of a cDNA clone derived from a blood-borne non-A, non-B viral hepatitis genome. Science 1989;244(4902):359–62.
37. Donato F, Tagger A, Gelatti U, et al. Alcohol and hepatocellular carcinoma: the effect of lifetime intake and hepatitis virus infections in men and women. Am J Epidemiol 2002;155(4):323–31.
38. Zaltron S, Spinetti A, Biasi L, et al. Chronic HCV infection: epidemiological and clinical relevance. BMC Infect Dis 2012;12(Suppl 2):S2–7.
39. Freeman A, Dore G, Law M, et al. Estimating progression to cirrhosis in chronic hepatitis C virus infection. Hepatology 2001;34(4):809–16.
40. Seeff L. Natural history of chronic hepatitis C. Hepatology 2002;36(5 Suppl 1): S35–46.
41. Poynard T, Bedossa P, Opolon P. Natural history of liver fibrosis progression in patients with chronic hepatitis C. The OBSVIRC, METAVIR, CLINIVIR, and DOSVIRC groups. Lancet 1997;349(9055):825–32.
42. Shindo M, Arai K, Sokawa Y, et al. The virological and histological states of anti-hepatitis C virus-positive subjects with normal liver biochemical values. Hepatology 1995;22(2):418–25.
43. Mathurin P, Moussalli J, Cadranel J, et al. Slow progression rate of fibrosis in hepatitis C virus patients with persistently normal alanine transaminase activity. Hepatology 1998;27(3):868–72.

44. Backus L, Boothroyd D, Phillips B, et al. A sustained virologic response reduces risk of all-cause mortality in patients with hepatitis C. Clin Gastroenterol Hepatol 2011;9(6):509–16.

45. Singal A, Volk M, Jensen D, et al. A sustained viral response is associated with reduced liver-related morbidity and mortality in patients with hepatitis C virus. Clin Gastroenterol Hepatol 2010;8(3):280–8.

46. Morgan R, Baack B, Smith B, et al. Eradication of hepatitis C virus infection and the development of hepatocellular carcinoma: a meta-analysis of observational studies. Ann Intern Med 2013;158(5 Pt 1):329–37.

47. Zhu H, Jia Z, Misra H, et al. Oxidative stress and redox signaling mechanisms of alcoholic liver disease: updated experimental and clinical evidence. J Dig Dis 2012;13(3):133–42.

48. IARC Working Group. Alcohol drinking. IARC Monogr Eval Carcinog Risks Hum 1988;44:1–378.

49. Yuan J, Govindarajan S, Arakawa K, et al. Synergism of alcohol, diabetes, and viral hepatitis on the risk of hepatocellular carcinoma in blacks and whites in the US. Cancer 2004;101(5):1009–17.

50. Grewal P, Viswanathen V. Liver cancer and alcohol. Clin Liver Dis 2012;16(4): 839–50.

51. Marrero J, Fontana R, Fu S, et al. Alcohol, tobacco and obesity are synergistic risk factors for hepatocellular carcinoma. J Hepatol 2005;42(2):218–24.

52. Trichopoulos D, Bamia C, Lagiou P, et al. Hepatocellular carcinoma risk factors and disease burden in a European cohort: a nested case-control study. J Natl Cancer Inst 2011;103(22):1686–95.

53. Corrao G, Bagnardi V, Zambon A, et al. A meta-analysis of alcohol consumption and the risk of 15 diseases. Prev Med 2004;38(5):613–9.

54. Heckley G, Jarl J, Asamoah B, et al. How the risk of liver cancer changes after alcohol cessation: a review and meta-analysis of the current literature. BMC Cancer 2011;11(446):1–10.

55. Boveris A, Fraga C, Varsavsky A, et al. Increased chemiluminescence and superoxide production in the liver of chronically ethanol-treated rats. Arch Biochem Biophys 1983;227(2):534–41.

56. Kukiełka E, Dicker E, Cederbaum A. Increased production of reactive oxygen species by rat liver mitochondria after chronic ethanol treatment. Arch Biochem Biophys 1994;309(2):377–86.

57. Kuper H, Tzonou A, Kaklamani E, et al. Tobacco smoking, alcohol consumption and their interaction in the causation of hepatocellular carcinoma. Int J Cancer 2000;85(4):498–502.

58. Berman K, Tandra S, Vuppalanchi R, et al. Hepatic and extrahepatic cancer in cirrhosis: a longitudinal cohort study. Am J Gastroenterol 2011;106(5):899–906.

59. Kubo S, Kinoshita H, Hirohashi K, et al. High malignancy of hepatocellular carcinoma in alcoholic patients with hepatitis C virus. Surgery 1997;121(4): 425–9.

60. IARC Working Group. Aflatoxins. IARC Monogr Eval Carcinog Risks Hum 2002; 82:171–300.

61. Liu Y, Wu F. Global burden of aflatoxin-induced hepatocellular carcinoma: a risk assessment. Environ Health Perspect 2010;118(6):818–24.

62. Hsu I, Metcalf R, Sun T, et al. Mutational hotspot in the p53 gene in human hepatocellular carcinomas. Nature 1991;350(6317):427–8.

63. Bressac B, Kew M, Wands J, et al. Selective G to T mutations of p53 gene in hepatocellular carcinoma from southern Africa. Nature 1991;350(6317):429–31.

64. Ozturk M. p53 mutation in hepatocellular carcinoma after aflatoxin exposure. Lancet 1991;338(8779):1356–9.
65. Qian G, Ross R, Yu M, et al. A follow-up study of urinary markers of aflatoxin exposure and liver cancer risk in Shanghai, People's Republic of China. Cancer Epidemiol Biomarkers Prev 1994;3(1):3–10.
66. Neuschwander-Tetri B, Caldwell S. Nonalcoholic steatohepatitis: summary of an AASLD Single Topic Conference. Hepatology 2003;37(5):1202–19.
67. Nishikawa H, Osaki Y. Non-B, non-C hepatocellular carcinoma (review). Int J Oncol 2013;43(5):1333–42.
68. Tokushige K, Hashimoto E, Horie Y, et al. Hepatocellular carcinoma in Japanese patients with nonalcoholic fatty liver disease, alcoholic liver disease, and chronic liver disease of unknown etiology: report of the nationwide survey. J Gastroenterol 2011;46(10):1230–7.
69. Torres D, Harrison S. Nonalcoholic steatohepatitis and noncirrhotic hepatocellular carcinoma: fertile soil. Semin Liver Dis 2012;32(1):30–8.
70. Welzel T, Graubard B, Zeuzem S, et al. Metabolic syndrome increases the risk of primary liver cancer in the United States: a study in the SEER-Medicare database. Hepatology 2011;54(2):463–71.
71. Wolk A, Gridley G, Svensson M, et al. A prospective study of obesity and cancer risk (Sweden). Cancer Causes Control 2001;12(1):13–21.
72. Attner B, Landin-Olsson M, Lithman T, et al. Cancer among patients with diabetes, obesity and abnormal blood lipids: a population-based register study in Sweden. Cancer Causes Control 2012;23(5):769–77.
73. Hashimoto E, Yatsuji S, Tobari M, et al. Hepatocellular carcinoma in patients with nonalcoholic steatohepatitis. J Gastroenterol 2009;44(Suppl 19):89–95.
74. Ascha M, Hanouneh I, Lopez R, et al. The incidence and risk factors of hepatocellular carcinoma in patients with nonalcoholic steatohepatitis. Hepatology 2010;51(6):1972–8.
75. Calle E, Rodriguez C, Walker-Thurmond K, et al. Overweight, obesity, and mortality from cancer in a prospectively studied cohort of US adults. N Engl J Med 2003;348(17):1625–38.
76. Shimizu M, Tanaka T, Moriwaki H. Obesity and hepatocellular carcinoma: targeting obesity-related inflammation for chemoprevention of liver carcinogenesis. Semin Immunopathol 2013;35(2):191–202.
77. Tung H, Wang J, Tseng P, et al. Neither diabetes mellitus nor overweight is a risk factor for hepatocellular carcinoma in a dual HBV and HCV endemic area: community cross-sectional and case-control studies. Am J Gastroenterol 2010; 105(3):624–31.
78. El-Serag H, Tran T, Everhart J. Diabetes increases the risk of chronic liver disease and hepatocellular carcinoma. Gastroenterology 2004;126(2):460–8.
79. Hassan M, Curley S, Li D, et al. Association of diabetes duration and diabetes treatment with the risk of hepatocellular carcinoma. Cancer 2010;116(8): 1938–46.
80. Zheng Z, Zhang C, Yan J, et al. Diabetes mellitus is associated with hepatocellular carcinoma: a retrospective case-control study in hepatitis endemic area. PLoS One 2013;8(12):e84776.
81. Polesel J, Zucchetto A, Montella M, et al. The impact of obesity and diabetes mellitus on the risk of hepatocellular carcinoma. Ann Oncol 2009;20(2):353–7.
82. Wang C, Wang X, Gong G, et al. Increased risk of hepatocellular carcinoma in patients with diabetes mellitus: a systematic review and meta-analysis of cohort studies. Int J Cancer 2012;130(7):1639–48.

83. Hassan M, Kaseb A. Hepatocellular carcinoma. In: McMasters K, Vauthey JN, editors. Targeted therapy and multidisciplinary care, vol. 1. New York (NY): Springer; 2011. p. 1–19.
84. Harrison S. Liver disease in patients with diabetes mellitus. J Clin Gastroenterol 2006;40(1):68–76.
85. Alexia C, Fallot G, Lasfer M, et al. An evaluation of the role of insulin-like growth factors (IGF) and of type-I IGF receptor signalling in hepatocarcinogenesis and in the resistance of hepatocarcinoma cells against drug-induced apoptosis. Biochem Pharmacol 2004;68(6):1003–15.
86. Hu W, Feng Z, Eveleigh J, et al. The major lipid peroxidation product, trans-4-hydroxy-2-nonenal, preferentially forms DNA adducts at codon 249 of human p53 gene, a unique mutational hotspot in hepatocellular carcinoma. Carcinogenesis 2002;23(11):1781–9.
87. Donadon V, Balbi M, Dal Mas M, et al. Metformin and reduced risk of hepatocellular carcinoma in diabetic patients with chronic liver disease. Liver Int 2010; 30(5):750–8.
88. Elmberg M, Hultcrantz R, Ekbom A, et al. Cancer risk in patients with hereditary hemochromatosis and in their first-degree relatives. Gastroenterology 2003; 125(6):1733–41.
89. Yang Q, McDonnell S, Khoury M, et al. Hemochromatosis-associated mortality in the United States from 1979 to 1992: an analysis of multiple-cause mortality data. Ann Intern Med 1998;129(11):946–53.
90. Lata J. Chronic liver diseases as liver tumor precursors. Dig Dis 2010;28(4–5): 596–9.
91. Mizoue T, Tokui N, Nishisaka K, et al. Prospective study on the relation of cigarette smoking with cancer of the liver and stomach in an endemic region. Int J Epidemiol 2000;29(2):232–7.
92. Yun Y, Jung K, Bae J, et al. Cigarette smoking and cancer incidence risk in adult men: National Health Insurance Corporation Study. Cancer Detect Prev 2005; 29(1):15–24.
93. Zhu K, Moriarty C, Caplan L, et al. Cigarette smoking and primary liver cancer: a population-based case-control study in US men. Cancer Causes Control 2007; 18(3):315–21.
94. Jee S, Ohrr H, Sull J, et al. Cigarette smoking, alcohol drinking, hepatitis B, and risk for hepatocellular carcinoma in Korea. J Natl Cancer Inst 2004;96(24): 1851–6.
95. Sun C, Wu D, Lin C, et al. Incidence and cofactors of hepatitis C virus-related hepatocellular carcinoma: a prospective study of 12,008 men in Taiwan. Am J Epidemiol 2003;157(8):674–82.
96. Zaman S, Melia W, Johnson R, et al. Risk factors in development of hepatocellular carcinoma in cirrhosis: prospective study of 613 patients. Lancet 1985; 1(8442):1357–60.
97. Yuan J, Ross R, Stanczyk F, et al. A cohort study of serum testosterone and hepatocellular carcinoma in Shanghai, China. Int J Cancer 1995;63(4):491–3.
98. Naugler W, Sakurai T, Kim S, et al. Gender disparity in liver cancer due to sex differences in MyD88-dependent IL-6 production. Science 2007;317(5834):121–4.
99. Davis G, Albright J, Cook S, et al. Projecting future complications of chronic hepatitis C in the United States. Liver Transpl 2003;9(4):331–8.
100. Sandler R, Everhart J, Donowitz M, et al. The burden of selected digestive diseases in the United States. Gastroenterology 2002;122(5):1500–11.

Imaging Approach to Hepatocellular Carcinoma, Cholangiocarcinoma, and Metastatic Colorectal Cancer

 CrossMark

Kathryn J. Fowler, MD[a],*, Nael E. Saad, MD[b], David Linehan, MD[c]

KEYWORDS

- Liver imaging • Metastatic liver disease • Hepatocellular carcinoma
- Cholangiocarcinoma • Colorectal liver metastases

KEY POINTS

- Hepatocellular carcinoma (HCC) diagnostic criteria allow imaging diagnosis to supplant pathology.
- Determination of resectability is the main goal of imaging cholangiocarcinoma.
- MRI provides the best sensitivity for detecting colorectal metastases.

INTRODUCTION

Imaging has become an integral component of managing patients with suspected liver diseases and tumors. Options have evolved along with technology to provide important information and at times supplant pathology for diagnosis of liver lesions. This article provides an overview of the most common liver imaging modalities and their use in HCC, intrahepatic cholangiocarcinoma (ICC), and colorectal cancer (CRC) liver metastatic disease.

LIVER IMAGING MODALITIES

Ultrasound

Ultrasound basics

Ultrasound (US) is one of the oldest modalities in radiology. Transducers (probes) create sound waves that transmit through tissues and are variably impeded and reflected back to the transducer. Structures appear of varying echogenicity (brightness) based on their acoustic impedance/density. When performing transcutaneous US, transducers of

[a] Department of Radiology, Washington University, 510 S. Kingshighway Blvd, St. Louis, MO 63110, USA; [b] Department of Interventional Radiology, Washington University, 510 S. Kingshighway Blvd, St. Louis, MO 63110, USA; [c] Department of Surgery, Washington University, 510 S. Kingshighway Blvd, St. Louis, MO 63110, USA
* Corresponding author.
E-mail address: fowlerk@mir.wustl.edu

Surg Oncol Clin N Am 24 (2015) 19–40
http://dx.doi.org/10.1016/j.soc.2014.09.002
1055-3207/15/$ – see front matter © 2015 Elsevier Inc. All rights reserved.

different frequencies (lower frequencies of 3–5 MHz penetrate deeper than higher frequencies) are chosen based on the depth of the region of interest and tissues being penetrated. US gel is required to establish good acoustic contact because air acts as a reflector. Gray-scale and Doppler US have been used to evaluate focal liver lesions based on differences in echogenicity and vascularity; however, definitive diagnosis is often difficult. Transcutaneous US and in some instances endoscopic US can be used to guide percutaneous biopsies when imaging fails to provide definitive diagnosis.

Contrast-enhanced ultrasound

Diagnostic accuracy of US is greatly improved with the addition of contrast; however, to date, the use of contrast-enhanced US (CEUS) has been limited in the United States due to lack of Food and Drug Administration (FDA) approval. There are 3 contrast agents currently used worldwide: SonoVue (Bracco, Milan, Italy), Definity (Bristol-Myers Squibb, New York, NY, USA), and Sonazoid (GE Healthcare, Oslo, Norway). The first 2 act as vascular agents only, providing information regarding the early dynamic appearance of lesions with no diffusivity outside of the vessels (which is slightly different from computerized tomography (CT) and magnetic resonance [MR] agents). Sonazoid is taken up by the Kupffer cells and exhibits a hepatobiliary phase for approximately 1 hour after injection, which has been likened to the hepatobiliary phase on MRI and may be useful for lesion detection, as in metastatic work-ups. The main role of CEUS has been in focal liver lesion characterization and monitoring local ablative treatments.[1] The benefits of CEUS are the real-time visualization of contrast enhancement, lack of nephrotoxicity, lack of ionizing radiation, and decreased cost compared with CT or MRI. The main disadvantage of CEUS is the relative lack of availability in the United States. Additionally, CEUS was dropped from the most recent American Association for the Study of Liver Disease (AASLD) guidelines due to the potential risk of misdiagnosis of ICC as HCC.[2]

Computerized Tomography

Computerized tomography basics

CT is rapidly available, demonstrates high diagnostic accuracy for many indications, and is well known to radiologists and clinicians alike. Image creation on CT is the result of an ionizing radiation (x-ray) source, which rotates around the patient with detectors opposite the source that measure the degree of attenuation of the x-ray beam. The end result is a cross-sectional image with different attenuation values (brightness) assigned to different structures based on their relative attenuation coefficient (degree to which they impede the x-ray beam). Most soft tissues have similar attenuation properties; hence, intravenous contrast is used to improve conspicuity of organs, lesions, and vasculature.

CT contrast is composed of iodinated medium, which causes greater absorption and scatter of x-ray radiation, yielding increased attenuation (brighter appearance) of structures. The relative enhancement of organs is complex and related to an organ's perfusion rate, tissue volume, composition, and permeability throughout the microvasculature. The initial enhancement is most influenced by the vascular supply and cardiac output, with later enhancement more dependent on intravascular dilution and redistribution of contrast within the extracellular space.[3] Because iodinated contrast medium does not cross into the intracellular compartment, it can be assumed to distribute within the intravascular and extracellular compartments by way of diffusion or transcapillary exchange.[4] A basic understanding of contrast pharmacokinetics allows greater appreciation for the different enhancement patterns (described later).

In the liver, there are well-defined postcontrast phases, during which the parenchyma follows a predictable pattern of enhancement. These phases consist of the late arterial, portal venous, equilibrium, and delayed phases.[5] Most tumors within the liver (especially hypervascular lesions like HCC) receive preferential hepatic arterial blood supply compared with normal hepatic parenchyma, which is supplied predominately by portal venous blood.[6–8] This differential blood supply allows for greatest lesion:background conspicuity of hypervascular tumors during the late arterial phase. Hypovascular tumors (many metastatic tumors) are generally seen most easily on the portal venous or equilibrium phases of contrast. A routine CT with contrast is usually timed for the portal venous phase; hence, arterially enhancing lesions may not be readily seen (**Fig. 1**). In addition to improved conspicuity of lesions, the pattern of enhancement on the different phases of contrast helps narrow the differential diagnosis and in some instances is pathognomonic, such as in hemangiomas (**Fig. 2**). Therefore, when assessing a liver tumor, multiple phases of contrast or a liver protocol CT should be obtained (**Table 1**).[9]

Nephrotoxicity of computerized tomography contrast

Although CT contrast is essential to liver tumor characterization, it should be avoided in patients with poor renal function because it is potentially nephrotoxic. The American College of Radiology defines contrast-induced nephrotoxicity (CIN) as sudden deterioration in renal function after recent administration of iodinated contrast in the absence of another nephrotoxic event.[10] Controversy exists as to the diagnostic criteria for CIN with variable definitions in the literature leading to a lack of consensus as to the actual incidence, risk factors, and diagnosis. The Acute Kidney Injury Network in a consensus group suggested the diagnosis of acute kidney injury could be made if one of the following criteria is met within 48 hours of a nephrotoxic event: absolute serum creatinine increase of greater than or equal to 0.3 mg/dL; percentage

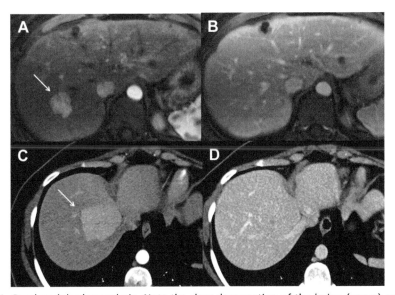

Fig. 1. Focal nodular hyperplasia. Note the clear demarcation of the lesion (*arrow*) on the arterial phase postcontrast MRI (*A*) and the near stealth appearance on the portal venous phase MRI (*B*). This demonstrates the importance of acquiring multiple phases for adequate lesion characterization. C-arterial, D-portal venous phase. Demonstrating the same phenomenon in a second patient with focal nodular hyperplasia on CT (*arrow*) during the arterial (*C*) and portal venous phases (*D*).

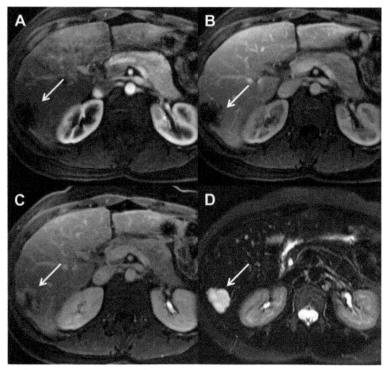

Fig. 2. Pathognomic appearance of a hemangioma. *A*-arterial, *B*-portal venous, *C*-delayed phase. Dynamic postcontrast MRI (*A–C*) and fat-suppressed T2 image (*D*) show the pathognomic appearance of a hemangioma (*arrows*). Confident characterization requires multiple phases of contrast to show the classic centripetal filling pattern.

Table 1
Liver protocol CT

Contrast Phases	Comments	Technical Specifications
Noncontrast	Provides information of lesion density (calcification, blood products, fat) • Optional for lesion characterization • Mandatory in post-TACE setting to evaluate enhancement relative to dense Lipiodol/Ethiodol uptake	• Multidetector row scanner (minimum 8 detectors) • Power injection for contrast (at least 3 mL/s) • Minimum of 5 mm reconstructed section thickness (slice thickness)
Late arterial phase	Artery fully enhanced, some contrast in portal vein, no contrast in hepatic veins • Optimal timing essential (bolus tracking)	
Portal venous phase	Peak liver parenchymal enhancement, beginning contrast enhancement of hepatic veins	
Delayed phase	>120 s After injection, variable appearance	

Abbreviation: TACE, transarterial chemoembolization.

increase in serum creatinine of greater than or equal to 50%; or urine output reduced to less than or equal to 0.5 mL/kg/hour for at least 6 hours.[11] Given that these creatinine changes are small, it remains controversial and difficult to apply these strict cutoffs in practice. In a retrospective study, including 8826 contrast-enhanced CT studies, administration of iodinated contrast was identified as a nephrotoxic risk factor in patients with estimated glomerular filtration rate (eGFR) less than 30 mL/min/1.73 m^2 and a trend toward significance in patients with eGFR 30 to 44 mL/min/1.73 m^2.[12] Clinical risk factors may also contribute to development of contrast-induced nephropathy, including diabetes, liver disease, chronic kidney disease, hypertension, low hematocrit, and heart failure.[13] Policies for administration of contrast to patients with borderline function vary from institution to institution and screening patients who are potentially at risk is advised. See **Table 2** for our institutional policy. Although there is abundant literature on the use of normal saline, bicarbonate drips, and other measures to reduce risk of nephrotoxicity, no clearly superior method exists and the best mitigation is avoidance of exposure in at-risk patients. In patients who cannot undergo a contrast-enhanced CT, MRI may be an option with a wider range of creatinine acceptance due to the lack of nephrotoxicity of gadolinium agents.

In addition to CIN, allergy to iodinated contrast presents a challenge. Premedication for prior mild reactions (hives, itching, and so forth) can be performed with steroids and antihistamines; however, avoidance of contrast in patients with prior severe reactions (laryngeal edema, dyspnea, and shock) is recommended. Although a prior reaction indicates a degree of predisposition/atopia, there is insufficient evidence to support cross-reactivity between CT contrast and MR contrast. Therefore, depending on institutional policy, a contrast MRI examination may be an alternative in patients with prior severe reaction to CT contrast.

Table 2 Washington University CT contrast policy	
Renal Function	**Guideline**
Serum Cr <1.4	Contrast permitted
Chronic serum Cr <2	Contrast permitted
Chronicity unknown, serum Cr >1.4	Calculate eGFR; if >30, then contrast permitted
Acute elevation in serum Cr	Contrast should be avoided if possible
Patient on dialysis	Contrast may be permitted (allowing preservation of residual renal function is not a goal) Arrangement of dialysis after contrast administration is advised

When to check serum Cr
- During current admission for any acutely ill or hospitalized patient
- Adult patients <70 y old, a Cr value within 30–90 d is sufficient

How to reduce risk of nephrotoxicity
- For patients with elevated GFR who require contrast, hydration prior to and after CT is recommended

Risk factors for kidney disease
- Family history, diabetes, paraproteneimia syndromes, collagen vascular diseases, medications, renal surgery, chronic use of nonsteroidal anti-inflammatory drugs, inpatient status

Abbreviation: Cr, creatinine.

Policies vary by institution and some use eGFR instead of creatinine cutoff values. Consult the policy at the institution for guidelines specific to a practice.

MRI

Basics of magnetic resonance

MRIs are created by combining strong magnetic fields, radiofrequency pulses, and weaker magnetic fields (gradients), all of which have an impact on the hydrogen protons within the body that become energized and spin at a resonant frequency. This frequency information is decoded by complex mathematical equations (Fourier transform) to produce images. The brightness and darkness of an image are described as signal intensity, either hyperintense or hypointense, respectively. As part of a routine liver MRI, several sequences are obtained. These give different information about the organs and tumors being imaged. **Table 3** shows the routine liver MRI sequences.[9,14]

Similar to CT, contrast is often used to characterize liver lesions and improve visualization. MR contrast agents consist of gadolinium-containing medium. Gadolinium interacts with the water molecules in the blood to produce T1 shortening (bright signal). A majority of MR contrast agents behave in an extracellular fashion, similar to CT contrast, providing dynamic enhancement information during the late arterial, portal venous, and equilibrium/delayed phases. In addition, there are 2 commonly used hepatobiliary contrast agents: gadobenate dimeglumine (MultiHance, Bracco) and gadoxetic acid (Eovist, Bayer Healthcare Pharmaceuticals, Whippany, NJ, USA). Approximately 4% of gadobenate dimeglumine is excreted in the bile, with peak parenchymal enhancement (hepatobiliary phase timing) occurring at approximately 1 hour after injection. Up to 50% of gadoxetic acid is excreted in the bile, with peak enhancement occurring approximately 20 minutes after injection. The mechanism of uptake in the hepatocytes is thought primarily related to active

Table 3 Routine liver MR protocol		
MR Pulse Sequence	**Comments**	**Technical Specifications**
T1-weighted chemical shift (in- and opposed phase, dual-echo gradient-recall echo)	Provides information on iron and fat content within the liver and lesions • Fat-containing lesions may lose signal on opposed-phase images	• 1.5-T or higher field strength • Phased-array coil plus body coil • Power injection for contrast
T2-weighted (TSE T2, ssFSE) T2-weighted fat suppressed (inversion recovery, T2 TSE FS)	Fluid-sensitive sequence • Bile ducts • T2 signal intensity of lesions	• Identical image parameters for pre- and postcontrast images to allow subtraction • 5 mm or Less slice thickness
T1-weighted fat suppressed (VIBE, THRIVE, LAVA, GRE)	Provides precontrast baseline signal intensity to help determine enhancement postcontrast	for postcontrast images and 8 mm or less for other sequences
Dynamic postcontrast (VIBE, THRIVE, LAVA, GRE)	Similar dynamic phases to CT (see **Table 1**)	• Maximum breath-hold length of 20 s • Minimum resolution
Diffusion-weighted images	Optional but recommended • Helps guide differential for benign vs malignant lesions • Improves detection of metastases	128 × 256

Abbreviations: FS, fat suppressed; GRE, gradient recall echo; LAVA, liver acquisition with volume acceleration; ssFSE, steady state fast spin echo; TSE, turbo spin echo; THRIVE, T1 high resolution isotropic volume excitation; VIBE, volumetric interpolated breath held examination.

The names in parentheses under the pulse sequences are commonly encountered vendor acronyms for these sequences.

transport by liver specific multidrug organic anion-transporting polypeptides (OATP1B1 and OATP1B3) on the hepatocyte cell surface.[15–17] The degree of uptake and diagnostic reliability may be diminished in patients with underlying severe fibrosis, cirrhosis, and cholestasis due to reduced transporter function.[18] Hepatobiliary contrast agents are generally suggested for focal liver lesion characterization and gadoxetic acid has been shown to add value in the setting of metastatic tumor detection. Gadoxetic acid has also shown promise in depicting the ductal anatomy due to its relatively high excretion into the bile. The role of hepatobiliary agents in HCC remains controversial and is discussed in greater depth later.

The main advantages of MRI in liver evaluation hinge on the high diagnostic accuracy, improved contrast resolution, noninvasive imaging of the biliary tree, and lack of ionizing radiation. An additional advantage is the lack of nephrotoxicity of gadolinium contrast agents. The main disadvantage of MRI relates to patient suitability. The most common reasons for nonsuitability are certain contraindicated implanted ferromagnetic devices, claustrophobia, severe ascites, and inability to comply with breath-holding commands. Patients with large-volume ascites should have paracentesis prior to MRI. In addition, for optimal image quality, patients must be able to lie very still and hold their breath for at least 15 to 18 seconds. Motion due to patient discomfort and inability to hold the breath is a common cause of image artifact and may be severe enough to render an examination nondiagnostic.

Nephrogenic systemic fibrosis and MRI contrast agents
Although initially reported as a disease in 1997, nephrogenic systemic fibrosis (NSF) has more recently been linked with gadolinium contrast administration in patients with severe acute or chronic renal insufficiency. The FDA first issued an advisory in 2006 regarding the safety concerns of gadolinium use in renal failure, followed by a black box warning on gadolinium contrast in 2010. NSF is a progressive skin condition in which the skin eventually becomes thickened and hardened and may lead to joint contractures. A vast majority of NSF cases have occurred in patients with a glomerular filtration rate (GFR) less than 15 mL/min in combination with hemodialysis or peritoneal dialysis.[19] No reports of NSF in normal renal function patients exist. The American College of Radiology advises against use of high-risk gadolinium agents in patients with GFR less than 45 mL/min. Most hospitals have institutional policies that emphasize screening for at-risk patients and avoidance of administration of gadolinium in the setting of severe dysfunction. **Table 4** discusses the institutional policy at Washington University on gadolinium contrast and renal dysfunction as well as some special considerations for MRI contrast.

PET/Computerized Tomography
PET/CT is an imaging study in which a radioactive tracer, commonly fluorodeoxyglucose F 18 (FDG), is injected intravenously and the radioactivity within local tissue distributions is imaged tomographically and fused with CT images. The CT images provide not only anatomic information but also attenuation correction for the PET data, allowing for accurate quantitative estimates of uptake within tissues of varying densities (soft tissue, fat, and bone). FDG is a glucose analog that distributes to regions of high cellular glucose utilization, such as are seen in malignancies. Glucose metabolism is often up-regulated in inflammatory conditions as well, which can be problematic for differentiating tumor from inflammation. The radiation dose to a patient is a combination of the injected radiopharmaceutical and that obtained from the CT scan. The radiopharmaceutical is typically excreted in the urine; however, there are often physiologically significant levels of uptake within the liver and bowel. The uptake

Table 4	
Washington University MRI contrast policy	
Renal Function	Guideline
GFR>30	Contrast ok
GFR <30	Assess risk benefit for patient to determine whether a viable alternative exists
Dialysis (hemodialysis or peritoneal)[a]	No contrast

Special considerations for MRI contrast:
  Allergy to CT contrast: patients may be at higher risk for reaction to gadolinium, although cross-reactivity is not supported by literature. No premedication is required.
  Allergies to MR contrast: severe reactions to gadolinium agents are rare. Avoidance of contrast and/or use of a different gadolinium agent recommended. Premedication is advised.
  Pregnancy: gadolinium is category C and only to be administered if benefit outweighs risk. Noncontrast MRI is deemed safe during pregnancy.

[a] Some institutions allow for contrast administration to patients on hemodialysis, allowing patients are dialyzed after administration.
  Contrast policies vary by institution and reference to institution's policy is advised.

in the liver can be heterogeneous and may make discrimination of focal liver lesions difficult, especially if the lesions are small. An additional challenge related to PET imaging of the liver is the effects of respiratory motion. The PET data are acquired from free-breathing images due to the length of acquisition required to obtain sufficient PET counts and image quality (typically 90–120 seconds per bed position). As a result of the free-breathing acquisition, motion of the diaphragm and liver results in significant loss of resolution and blurring (reducing the intrinsic spatial resolution from 4 mm to closer to 11 mm).[20–22] The end result is that small liver lesions (less than 1 cm) may not be easily seen.

IMAGING LIVER LESIONS
Hepatocellular Carcinoma

HCC is the most common primary hepatic malignancy and typically arises in the setting of chronic liver disease. Although controversy exists as to the appropriate combination of imaging and laboratory surveillance for HCC, there is strong support for screening an at-risk population because the early treatment of HCC provides much improved survival.[2,23–26] **Fig. 3** shows the updated AASLD guidelines for screening and diagnosis of HCC.[2]

The hallmark imaging features of HCC are well known and consist of arterial enhancement, washout, and pseudocapsule (**Fig. 4**). When present in combination, a diagnosis of HCC can be made without need for pathologic confirmation. Several national and international organizations have issued guidelines for the imaging diagnosis of HCC. The American College of Radiology has developed a lexicon system for the diagnosis of HCC, called the Liver Imaging Reporting and Data System (LI-RADS).[27] **Table 5** shows the major features for diagnosis of HCC using the LI-RADS system. LI-RADS is intended for use in all at-risk patients, not just the transplant population; hence, the system presents a risk stratification algorithm ranging from definitely benign to probably HCC for lesions that do not meet criteria for definitive diagnosis of HCC (**Table 6**).

In addition to LI-RADS, the United Network for Organ Sharing (UNOS) and Organ Procurement Transplantation Network (OPTN) provided specific guidelines for diagnostic criteria for HCC in 2013. UNOS/OPTN have historically focused on allocation

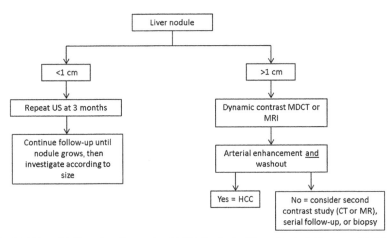

Fig. 3. AASLD guidelines for diagnosis of HCC. (*Adapted from* Bruix J, Sherman M. Management of hepatocellular carcinoma: an update. Hepatology 2011;53(3):1021; with permission.)

guidelines related to the T stage of tumor (within Milan or outside of Milan criteria, T2 stage).[28] Historically, radiology reports that HCC is present were sufficient without strict requirements for how the diagnosis was made. Retrospective reviews, however, of the UNOS database comparing radiology reporting to explant pathology have shown disappointing accuracies and high false-positive rates.[29–31] Given the importance of accurate allocation and the high priority that HCC patients receive as a result

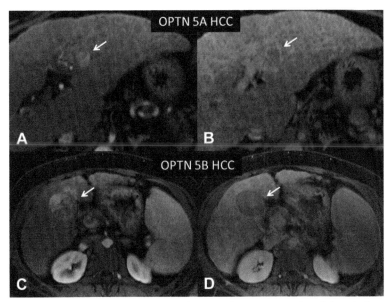

Fig. 4. Classic features of HCC. *A*-arterial, *B*-delayed phase; *C*-arterial, *D*-delayed phase. Arterial and delayed-phase postcontrast images (*A, B*) in patient 1 show a 1.8-cm lesion that demonstrates arterial enhancement, washout, and capsule appearance (*arrows*). Arterial and delayed-phase images (*C, D*) in patient 2 show a 3-cm lesion that demonstrates arterial enhancement and washout (*arrows*).

Table 5
OPTN and LI-RADS classification of HCC. The newest version of LI-RADS v2014 recognizes the OPTN growth criteria and make the LR-5 category congruent with OPTN 5 categorization

Classification	Features	Comments
OPTN 5B	Diameter $\geq$2 and $\leq$5 cm Late arterial hyperenhancement *and one of the following:* washout, capsule appearance, and growth $\geq$50% on study $\leq$6 m apart[a]	Qualifies for automatic exception points for transplantation
OPTN 5A	Diameter $\geq$1 and <2 cm Late arterial hyperenhancement *and both of the following:* washout and capsule appearance	Qualifies as diagnosis of HCC, which can be applied toward exception points (if patient meets T2 stage)
OPTN 5A-g	Diameter $\geq$1 and <2 cm Late arterial hyperenhancement *and* growth $\geq$50% on study $\leq$6 mo apart[a]	Qualifies as diagnosis of HCC, which can be applied toward exception points (if patient meets T2 stage)
LI-RADS 5	Same as for OPTN5A/B**	Although not recognized by UNOS/ OPTN for transplantation, the criteria are identical

[a] Defines threshold growth.
** LI-RADS v2014 achieves congruence with OPTN for growth criteria.
Data from Wald C, Russo MW, Heimbach JK, et al. New OPTN/UNOS policy for liver transplant allocation: standardization of liver imaging, diagnosis, classification, and reporting of hepatocellular carcinoma. Radiology 2013;266(2):376–82.

Table 6
LI-RADS classification system for non-HCC lesions

LI-RADS Category	Comments	Potential Management
LR-1 (definitely benign)	Imaging features diagnostic of a benign entity • Hemangiomas, cysts, fibrosis	Continue routine surveillance
LR-2 (probably benign)	Imaging features suggestive of a benign entity • Focal fat, hypertrophic pseudo- masses, focal scars	Continue routine surveillance
LR-3 (intermediate probability HCC)	Imaging features that are neither definite nor probably benign • Nodular arterial portal shunting, some cirrhotic nodules	Variable follow-up depending on clinical considerations
LR-4 (high probability HCC)	Imaging features suggestive of HCC but that do not meet criteria	Close follow-up imaging, consideration for biopsy or treatment
LR-M (probably malignant but not specific for HCC)	Imaging features may suggest a non-HCC malignancy • Cholangiocarcinoma, bipheno- typic tumor	Discussion at multidisciplinary meeting, correlation with serum tumor markers, consideration for biopsy

Data from American College of Radiology. Liver imaging reporting and data system version 2013.1. Available at: http://www.acr.org/Quality-Safety/Resources/LIRADS/. Accessed August 2014.

of automatic Model for End-Stage Liver Disease exception points, OPTN/UNOS issued a new policy that focuses on the imaging criteria for diagnosis of HCC in transplant patients.[9] If a lesion meets criteria for HCC on MRI or CT, it does not require pathologic confirmation and the patient receives automatic exception points for transplant organ allocation if it meets T2 stage size criteria (single lesion <5 cm or up to 3 lesions 1–3 cm). There is currently an open trial to determine the prospective accuracy of the OPTN classification for lesions in the setting of transplantation (ACRIN 6690).

Although these systems are in near congruence, the OPTN system presents a binary approach to lesion classification (HCC or not) given it is aimed at determining transplant candidacy and automatic exception point status. LI-RADS is meant for use in all at-risk patients and provides a more comprehensive overview of lesion categorization and risk assessment to guide clinical practice.

Although several imaging and surveillance algorithms exist for HCC, the choice between CT and MRI is left to the practitioner and remains controversial, often dictated by the local practice patterns of radiologists. A majority of literature supports improved diagnostic accuracy and sensitivity of MRI over CT; however, many of these studies have been small single-center retrospective reviews.[32–34] A meta-analysis of 15 studies comparing CT to MRI with hepatobiliary contrast demonstrated that MRI has improved sensitivity and specificity over CT (91% and 81%, respectively, for CT vs 95% and 93%, respectively, for MRI), especially in detecting and diagnosing small HCC lesions (<2 cm).[35] In a prospective trial comparing CT, US, and MRI in 140 patients with pathologically proved lesions, dynamic contrast-enhanced MRI demonstrated the highest accuracy of 83%, compared with 80% and 72% for CT and US, respectively ($P<.001$ for all comparisons).[36] The accuracy of MRI increased to 90% when hepatobiliary phase imaging was used. The accuracies for all modalities were lower for small lesions, dropping off significantly for lesions less than 1 cm.

Hepatobiliary contrast-enhanced MRI is of great interest but also controversial in the diagnostic evaluation of HCC. A majority of HCCs lack transporters for gadoxetic acid and hence demonstrate hypointensity during hepatobiliary phase imaging. Early HCCs and small HCCs may demonstrate hepatobiliary phase hypointensity before they develop hypervascularity.[37,38] This is the basis for improved sensitivity of HCC compared with traditional contrast agents. There are pitfalls, however, related to gadoxetic acid–enhanced MRI. There is overlap in appearance between early HCC and cirrhosis-related benign nodules, which can lead to false-positive diagnoses, and a small percentage of HCC may show uptake of contrast and appear hyperintense during the hepatobiliary phase imaging.[39–41] In light of these potential pitfalls and with the emphasis on specificity over sensitivity, the current OPTN imaging algorithm is described for use with extracellular (traditional) MRI contrast agents. The role of hepatobiliary agents for HCC imaging is controversial and varies between imaging centers. At our institution (where transplant candidacy is often the question), use of hepatobiliary agents is reserved for problem solving rather than routine use for HCC imaging.

Cholangiocarcinoma

ICC arises from the biliary epithelium and presents in 3 classic morphologic patterns: periductal infiltrative, papillary (intraductal), and intrahepatic mass forming. The most common risk factor for development of cholangiocarcinoma in the United States is primary sclerosing cholangitis (PSC); however, any chronic inflammatory state (such as infections, hepatolithiasis, viral hepatitis, and choledochal cysts) increases risk.[42] Unlike HCC, there is less evidence and no official guidelines governing screening for ICC in at-risk patients.[43,44] Serial serum CA 19-9 levels have been proposed, demonstrating a sensitivity of 53% and negative predictive value ranging from 76% to 92% if a cutoff of greater than 100 U/mL was used.[45] In a single-center study of 230 patients with PSC who were prospectively followed using a combination of imaging and CA 19-9 screening, 23 developed ICC and a combination of imaging and tumor markers was thought a useful strategy in these patients; however, there were no data to support a survival advantage or cost-effectiveness of routine surveillance.[46] In the absence of overwhelming evidence, many clinicians opt for annual screening with MRI/MR cholangiopancreatography (MRCP) or US as noninvasive surveillance strategies. Once a new dominant stricture or mass is identified, directed endoscopic retrograde cholangiopancreatography (ERCP) with brushing and potentially fluorescence in situ hybdrization analysis may be undertaken to make a diagnosis of ICC.[47]

MRCP provides the best noninvasive imaging option for the biliary system, allowing identification of malignant strictures, staging information regarding ductal and vascular involvement, and accurate lesion characterization for intrahepatic masses. **Fig. 5** shows a classic hilar ICC with an associated mass-forming component. The peripheral arterial enhancement, with progressive central enhancement, diffusion restriction, and ductal obstruction, are all classic features.[48,49] Additionally, ICC may demonstrate findings on MRI secondary to the often fibrotic stroma of the tumor, including capsular retraction and T2 signal hypointensity. Although these classic imaging features often suggest the diagnosis of ICC, biopsy is still required in most cases.

The main role of imaging in ICC is to stage patients for possible resection. Perihilar location is most common and further divided by the Bismuth classification according to the length of involvement of the right and left hepatic ducts.[50] The relationship of the tumor to the hepatic artery and portal vein also dictates resectability.[51,52] A good-quality MRI can provide this detailed information; however, in cases where motion

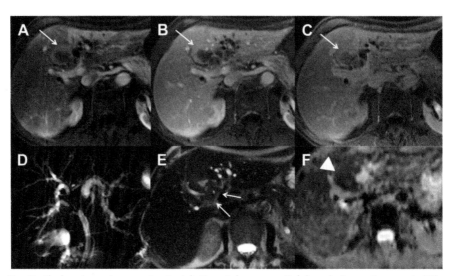

Fig. 5. Cholangiocarcinoma. A-arterial, B-portal venous, C-delayed phase. Apparent diffusion coefficient (ADC) image shows that this lesion is dark on the ADC map compatible with restricted diffusion (*arrowhead*). Arterial, portal venous, and delayed postcontrast images (*A–C*) show an intrahepatic mass component (*arrows*) associated with this hilar cholangiocarcinoma. The MRCP (*D*) nicely depicts the involvement of the right anterior and posterior ducts and left lateral section ducts. T2-weighted image (*E*) shows infiltrative soft tissue along the ducts in the hepatic hilum (*arrows*). Diffusion ADC image (*F*) shows that this lesion restricts diffusion (*arrowhead*), which is a feature of cholangiocarcinoma.

or spatial resolution limit evaluation, a second study, such as thin-slice contrast-enhanced CT or focused Doppler/gray-scale US, may be of value to clear the vessels. The accuracy of MRCP for staging ranges from 81% to 96% and, when inaccurate, seems to underestimate the extent of ductal involvement.[53–58] The negative predictive value of nonresectability on CT is high, ranging from 85% to 100%.[59–62] The goal of surgical intervention is to achieve an R0 resection, because reported 5-year survival rates for margin-positive resections are dismal.[51]

Although noninvasive measures like CT and MRCP generally offer accurate depiction of the biliary system, the extent of involvement may be difficult to appreciate in patients who have undergone stenting and have inflammation involving their ducts. High-quality imaging before intervention and stenting is recommended. Patients with significant biliary duct dilation are often decompressed by ERCP-placed stents. The injection of contrast into an obstructed system, however, places patients at risk for cholangitis; hence, the imaging of the ducts beyond the level of stricture may be suboptimal. If detailed depiction of the secondary bile ducts is required for surgical planning, a percutaneous transhepatic cholangiogram and stent placement can be done in cases where MRCP fails to give a confident depiction.

In addition to determining resectability of the primary tumor, evaluation of peritoneal disease, intrahepatic satellite nodules, and regional lymph nodes is of prognostic importance. CT and MRI have limited specificity and sensitivity in detecting positive lymph nodes. Patients with PSC often have chronically enlarged nodes and size alone is a poor predictor of metastatic involvement. Some studies suggest that PET/CT may improve nodal staging and identify distant metastases, resulting in a change in management in up to 17% to 30% of patients.[63,64] In a prospective study of 123 patients with ICC deemed resectable by conventional imaging, PET/CT altered management in 15.9% of patients, primarily due to improved accuracy in detecting regional lymph node metastases (76% vs 61% on CT and verified with histologic analysis of surgical specimen) and distant metastases (88% vs 79% on CT).[65] PET/CT may be of value in excluding extrahepatic disease prior to surgical intent to cure in patients with relatively advanced disease, but we do not use it routinely. In the setting of mildly enlarged, indeterminate periportal lymph nodes, endoscopic US–guided biopsy can provide definitive diagnosis. Despite high-resolution preoperative imaging, staging laparoscopy may still be warranted in patients with higher-stage tumors (T2 or T3 lesions).[66] Findings at staging laparoscopy alter management in patients deemed resectable by conventional imaging in a high percentage of patients. The yield has declined in recent years, however, with improvements in imaging technology.[67]

Metastatic Disease: Colorectal Carcinoma

Accurate staging of liver-limited disease is essential to management. Dynamic contrast-enhanced CT and MRI are the most frequently used modalities in initial staging of liver disease and both have high sensitivities and specificities (sensitivity 73% and 82% and specificity 97% and 93%, respectively).[68] **Fig. 6** shows colorectal liver metastases in a patient with multifocal disease. The lesions are best seen on MRI with hepatobiliary phase due to background liver steatosis. In the setting of known primary colorectal malignancy, a diagnosis of metastases can be made with high specificity. When incidentally encountered, however, the imaging appearance is nonspecific and overlaps with other adenocarcinoma lesions, such as ICC and metastases from other primaries.

The use of appropriate CT imaging parameters, multiphase dynamic postcontrast imaging, and multidetector CT is essential to achieve the high accuracies reported in the literature.[69,70] There is a lack of good comparative studies, making it difficult

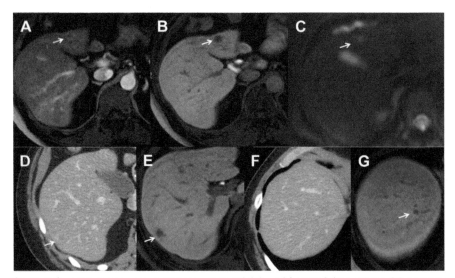

Fig. 6. Colorectal carcinoma metastases. Arterial (*A*) and hepatobiliary phase (*B*) postcontrast images show a metastasis (*arrows*) with early rim enhancement and hypointensity on hepatobiliary phase. The lesion is conspicuous on diffusion-weighted imaging (*C*). CT images (*D, F*) are limited in visualizing 2 additional metastases (*arrows*) in this patient with hepatic steatosis, which are clearly identified on hepatobiliary phase MRI (*E, G*).

to determine which imaging modality is best for patients with CRC liver metastases. Evidence supports, however, that MRI provides superior diagnostic accuracy in the setting of hepatic steatosis and when hepatobiliary phase imaging and diffusion-weighted imaging are incorporated into the protocol.[71–76] In a retrospective study of 242 patients undergoing surgical resection for colorectal liver metastases, patients who had a hepatobiliary MRI prior to surgery had lower rates of intrahepatic recurrence (48 vs 65%; P = .04; n = 92 hepatobiliary MRI and n = 150 without) suggesting improved preoperative staging accuracy.[75] Higher cost may be an argument against routine use of MRI. Yet in patients who often have coexisting hepatic steatosis related to prior chemotherapy and who are being staged for complex intent to cure surgical procedures, MRI is the study of choice at our institution. It provides the highest level of sensitivity for metastatic lesion detection in this population along with information regarding background liver steatosis. When performed correctly, multiphase CT can provide similar results and is used primarily in other large cancer centers for staging and following liver metastases.[77]

The use of PET/CT in staging CRC is controversial. The accuracy of identifying liver lesions on a lesion-by-lesion basis is low compared with contrast-enhanced CT and MRI; however, the value of PET/CT is in identifying extrahepatic disease that precludes hepatic resection. Findings of PET/CT may result in a change in management in 8% to 11% of patients.[78–80] Caution is advised in these cases, because the findings of PET may be nonspecific and potentially result in a negative impact on patient care in up to 9% of patients.[78] In light of the added expense and potentially confusing results, routine PET/CT is not likely to add benefit in all patients. In select patients, where the pretest probability for extrahepatic uptake is balanced by the high stakes of complex hepatic resection, PET/CT is of value in preventing futile surgery. In our practice, PET/CT is obtained when staged or complex hepatic resections are considered in patients with multifocal bilobar disease who are at substantial risk for extrahepatic disease.

A challenge in imaging CRC metastases that has evolved in recent years is the concept of the disappearing lesion, a condition made more prevalent with improved systemic therapies. Some studies performed with PET/CT demonstrated that up to 64% of patients with complete imaging response (resolution of FDG uptake) had correlative complete microscopic response or complete pathologic response.[81–83] Other studies have shown poor correlation between imaging disappearance and pathologic response.[84,85] With improvements in imaging sensitivity, namely hepatobiliary MRI, the definition of a disappearing metastasis may require revision. A meta-analysis by van Kessel and colleagues[86] examined the diagnostic performance of MRI, CT, and PET/CT in detecting metastatic lesions after chemotherapy. The pooled sensitivity for MRI was 85.7% compared with 69.9% for CT and 51.7% for PET/CT. In a study by Auer and colleagues,[82] lesions that had disappeared on CT were later found on MRI and lack of preoperative MRI was associated with a higher rate of intraoperative discovery of lesions that were considered to have disappeared. A useful discussion of the current controversy regarding disappearing metastases is in a recent review article by Bischof and colleagues.[87] Despite controversy regarding management, the evidence is compelling that MRI with hepatobiliary contrast may be the best option for imaging patients who have undergone chemotherapy and are considered for possible surgical resection.

Imaging for Presurgical and Ablative Planning

Assessing the future liver remnant

A major function of presurgical imaging is to predict the future liver remnant (FLR) adequacy/function. Liver failure eventually develops in approximately one-third of patients with postoperative hepatic insufficiency after hepatectomy and is greatest in patients with underlying cirrhosis.[88–90] Both CT and MRI can detect hepatic steatosis, which is important for predicting FLR function and hypertrophy potential in patients requiring hemihepatectomies. Calculation of total and segmental liver volume can be accomplished with either modality and is best performed using images acquired during the portal venous phase, during which there is good enhancement of both the portal veins and hepatic veins. There is consensus that a safe FLR in patients with normal liver function is 20%; the safe volume in the setting of liver disease, including damage related to chemotherapy, is less well understood and minimums of 30% to 40% are suggested.[91,92] In patients with borderline or inadequate FLR volumes, portal vein embolization (PVE) can be performed to induce hypertrophy of the remnant liver in anticipation for hepatectomy. Although the most widely accepted standard for determining adequacy of the FLR is the percentage relative to the total liver volume, a recent article by Shindoh and colleagues[90] demonstrated that the kinetic growth rate (KGR) better predicted postoperative hepatic insufficiency. The investigators calculated the KGR as the degree of hypertrophy at the first postportal vein embolization assessment divided by the time elapsed since PVE. They found that a KGR of at least 2% per week was protective against hepatic complications and liver failure–related death. Presurgical volumetrics should be obtained in all patients considered for major hepatectomy and hypertrophy procedures performed in those with borderline FLR volumes and/or with concern for underlying liver disease. Several studies have suggested utility in performing gadoxetic acid–enhanced MRI, technetium Tc 99m mebrofenin (HIDA) scans, and indocyanine green clearance tests to provide direct functional data to support FLR volumetrics. At our institution, biopsy is obtained if there is concern for fibrosis or functional reserve prior to PVE and/or resection to avoid performing a resection or embolization that may lead to liver failure.

Special considerations for ablation planning

Surgical excision is preferred to ablation when feasible; however, ablation may be a better choice in some cases due to patient comorbidities, prior surgical resection, or inadequate functional reserve. When local ablation is considered for malignant liver tumors, it is essential to have adequate imaging to assess lesion location relative to bile ducts, blood vessels, adjacent organs (diaphragm, bowel, and subcutaneous tissue), and lesion size to determine if adequate margins can be achieved. CT and MRI both provide reasonable image quality for assessing relationship of lesions to adjacent structures. MRI can delineate with higher contrast the location of the bile ducts; however, portal venous phase imaging can do the same given the anatomic location of bile ducts to the portal triads (bile ducts travel next to the portal vein branches). Thermal techniques, such as microwave ablation and radiofrequency ablation, are prone to heat sink, which is the loss of heat and hence effectiveness, when a lesion is adjacent

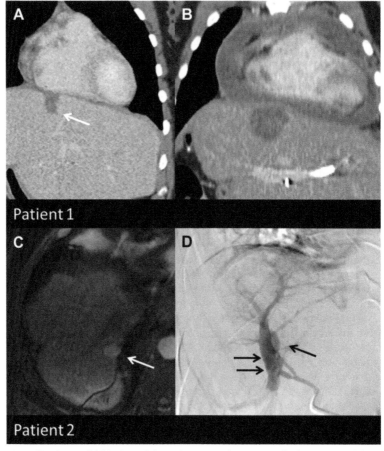

Fig. 7. Complications of ablation. (*A*) Patient 1 underwent radiofrequency ablation of a lesion in segment 2 (recurrent CCA metastasis [*arrow*]). (*B*) Due to the proximity to the heart, there was breach in the pericardium and a resultant hemopericardium requiring pericardiocentesis. (*C*) Patient 2 underwent cryoablation of a segment 7 HCC (*arrow*) and (*D*) subsequently developed hemobilia from a hepatic artery pseudoaneurysm (angiographic image [*black arrow*]) and fistulization with the bile duct (*double black arrows*) requiring coiling.

to a large blood vessel.[93,94] This is more pertinent to radiofrequency ablation than microwave ablation. The appropriate choice of ablation technique is often dictated by lesion size, location, proximity to adjacent structures, and local expertise. Preablation imaging should focus on determining the spatial relationship between the lesion and adjacent structures; both CT and MRI are viable options. **Fig. 7** shows examples of complications after ablation procedures.

SUMMARY

With advances in imaging technology, surgeons and clinicians have more options than ever before to determine the cause and resectability of liver masses. Understanding the relative strengths and weaknesses of the different imaging modalities is essential. A multidisciplinary relationship with diagnostic and interventional radiology allows for confident diagnosis, staging, and planning for these often complex liver cases.

REFERENCES

1. Claudon M, Dietrich CF, Choi BI, et al. Guidelines and good clinical practice recommendations for contrast enhanced ultrasound (CEUS) in the liver–update 2012: a WFUMB-EFSUMB initiative in cooperation with representatives of AFSUMB, AIUM, ASUM, FLAUS and ICUS. Ultraschall Med 2013;34(1):11–29.
2. Bruix J, Dietrich CF, Choi B, et al. Management of hepatocellular carcinoma: an update. Hepatology 2011;53(3):1020–2.
3. Bae KT. Intravenous contrast medium administration and scan timing at CT: considerations and approaches. Radiology 2010;256(1):32–61.
4. Bae KT, Heiken JP, Brink JA. Aortic and hepatic contrast medium enhancement at CT. Part I. Prediction with a computer model. Radiology 1998; 207(3):647–55.
5. Pomfret EA, Washburn K, Wald C, et al. Report of a national conference on liver allocation in patients with hepatocellular carcinoma in the United States. Liver Transpl 2010;16(3):262–78.
6. Archer SG, Gray BN. Vascularization of small liver metastases. Br J Surg 1989; 76(6):545–8.
7. Ackerman NB, Lien WM, Kondi ES, et al. The blood supply of experimental liver metastases. I. The distribution of hepatic artery and portal vein blood to "small" and "large" tumors. Surgery 1969;66(6):1067–72.
8. Lien WM, Ackerman NB. The blood supply of experimental liver metastases. II. A microcirculatory study of the normal and tumor vessels of the liver with the use of perfused silicone rubber. Surgery 1970;68(2):334–40.
9. Wald C, Russo MW, Heimbach JK, et al. New OPTN/UNOS policy for liver transplant allocation: standardization of liver imaging, diagnosis, classification, and reporting of hepatocellular carcinoma. Radiology 2013;266(2):376–82.
10. JSN, JRS and JCS Joint Working Group. Guidelines on the use of iodinated contrast media in patients with kidney disease 2012. Jpn J Radiol 2013;31(8): 546–84.
11. Mehta RL, Kellum JA, Shah SV, et al. Acute Kidney Injury Network: report of an initiative to improve outcomes in acute kidney injury. Crit Care 2007;11(2):R31.
12. Davenport MS, Khalatbari S, Cohan RH, et al. Contrast material-induced nephrotoxicity and intravenous low-osmolality iodinated contrast material: risk stratification by using estimated glomerular filtration rate. Radiology 2013;268(3): 719–28.

13. Traub S. Risk factors for radiocontrast nephropathy after emergency department contrast-enhanced computerized tomography. Acad Emerg Med 2013; 20(1):40–5.

14. Wile GE, Leyendecker JR. Magnetic resonance imaging of the liver: sequence optimization and artifacts. Magn Reson Imaging Clin N Am 2010;18(3): 525–47, xi.

15. van Montfoort JE, Stieger B, Meijer DK, et al. Hepatic uptake of the magnetic resonance imaging contrast agent gadoxetate by the organic anion transporting polypeptide Oatp1. J Pharmacol Exp Ther 1999;290(1):153–7.

16. Leonhardt M, Keiser M, Oswald S, et al. Hepatic uptake of the magnetic resonance imaging contrast agent Gd-EOB-DTPA: role of human organic anion transporters. Drug Metab Dispos 2010;38(7):1024–8.

17. Nassif A, Jia J, Keiser M, et al. Visualization of hepatic uptake transporter function in healthy subjects by using gadoxetic acid-enhanced MR imaging. Radiology 2012;264(3):741–50.

18. Lee NK, Kim S, Kim GH, et al. Significance of the "delayed hyperintense portal vein sign" in the hepatobiliary phase MRI obtained with Gd-EOB-DTPA. J Magn Reson Imaging 2012;36(3):678–85.

19. Cowper SE, Rabach M, Girardi M. Clinical and histological findings in nephrogenic systemic fibrosis. Eur J Radiol 2008;66(2):191–9.

20. Mawlawi O, Townsend DW. Multimodality imaging: an update on PET/CT technology. Eur J Nucl Med Mol Imaging 2009;36(Suppl 1):S15–29.

21. Alessio AM, Stearns CW, Tong S, et al. Application and evaluation of a measured spatially variant system model for PET image reconstruction. IEEE Trans Med Imaging 2010;29(3):938–49.

22. Daou D. Respiratory motion handling is mandatory to accomplish the high-resolution PET destiny. Eur J Nucl Med Mol Imaging 2008;35(11): 1961–70.

23. Garcia-Tsao G, Lim JK. Management and treatment of patients with cirrhosis and portal hypertension: recommendations from the Department of Veterans Affairs Hepatitis C Resource Center Program and the National Hepatitis C Program. Am J Gastroenterol 2009;104(7):1802–29.

24. Ferenci P, Fried M, Labrecque D, et al. World Gastroenterology Organisation Guideline. Hepatocellular carcinoma (HCC): a global perspective. J Gastrointestin Liver Dis 2010;19(3):311–7.

25. Kudo M, Izumi N, Kokudo N, et al. Management of hepatocellular carcinoma in Japan: Consensus-Based Clinical Practice Guidelines proposed by the Japan Society of Hepatology (JSH) 2010 updated version. Dig Dis 2011; 29(3):339–64.

26. Omata M, Lesmana LA, Tateishi R, et al. Asian Pacific Association for the Study of the Liver consensus recommendations on hepatocellular carcinoma. Hepatol Int 2010;4(2):439–74.

27. Radiology, A.C.O. Liver Imaging Reporting and Data System (LI-RADS). 2013. Available at: www.acr.org/quality-safety/Resources/LIRADS. Accessed July 1, 2013.

28. Mazzaferro V, Regalia E, Doci R, et al. Liver transplantation for the treatment of small hepatocellular carcinomas in patients with cirrhosis. N Engl J Med 1996; 334(11):693–9.

29. Freeman RB, Mithoefer A, Ruthazer R, et al. Optimizing staging for hepatocellular carcinoma before liver transplantation: a retrospective analysis of the UNOS/OPTN database. Liver Transpl 2006;12(10):1504–11.

30. Compagnon P, Grandadam S, Lorho R, et al. Liver transplantation for hepatocellular carcinoma without preoperative tumor biopsy. Transplantation 2008;86(8): 1068–76.

31. Hayashi PH, Trotter JF, Forman L, et al. Impact of pretransplant diagnosis of hepatocellular carcinoma on cadveric liver allocation in the era of MELD. Liver Transpl 2004;10(1):42–8.

32. Quaia E, De Paoli L, Angileri R, et al. Evidence of diagnostic enhancement pattern in hepatocellular carcinoma nodules </=2 cm according to the AASLD/EASL revised criteria. Abdom Imaging 2013;38(6):1245–53.

33. Onishi H, Kim T, Imai Y, et al. Hypervascular hepatocellular carcinomas: detection with gadoxetate disodium-enhanced MR imaging and multiphasic multidetector CT. Eur Radiol 2012;22(4):845–54.

34. Pitton MB, Kloeckner R, Herber S, et al. MRI versus 64-row MDCT for diagnosis of hepatocellular carcinoma. World J Gastroenterol 2009;15(48):6044–51.

35. Chen L, Zhang L, Bao J, et al. Comparison of MRI with liver-specific contrast agents and multidetector row CT for the detection of hepatocellular carcinoma: a meta-analysis of 15 direct comparative studies. Gut 2013;62(10):1520–1.

36. Di Martino M, De Filippis G, De Santis A, et al. Hepatocellular carcinoma in cirrhotic patients: prospective comparison of US, CT and MR imaging. Eur Radiol 2013;23(4):887–96.

37. Rhee H, Kim MJ, Park MS, et al. Differentiation of early hepatocellular carcinoma from benign hepatocellular nodules on gadoxetic acid-enhanced MRI. Br J Radiol 2012;85(1018):e837–44.

38. Sun HY, Lee JM, Shin CI, et al. Gadoxetic acid-enhanced magnetic resonance imaging for differentiating small hepatocellular carcinomas (< or =2 cm in diameter) from arterial enhancing pseudolesions: special emphasis on hepatobiliary phase imaging. Invest Radiol 2010;45(2):96–103.

39. Kitao A, Zen Y, Matsui O, et al. Hepatocellular carcinoma: signal intensity at gadoxetic acid-enhanced MR Imaging–correlation with molecular transporters and histopathologic features. Radiology 2010;256(3):817–26.

40. Saito K, Kotake F, Ito N, et al. Gd-EOB-DTPA enhanced MRI for hepatocellular carcinoma: quantitative evaluation of tumor enhancement in hepatobiliary phase. Magn Reson Med Sci 2005;4(1):1–9.

41. Kogita S, Imai Y, Okada M, et al. Gd-EOB-DTPA-enhanced magnetic resonance images of hepatocellular carcinoma: correlation with histological grading and portal blood flow. Eur Radiol 2010;20(10):2405–13.

42. Yazici C, Niemeyer DJ, Iannitti DA, et al. Hepatocellular carcinoma and cholangiocarcinoma: an update. Expert Rev Gastroenterol Hepatol 2014;8(1):63–82.

43. Chapman R, Fevery J, Kalloo A, et al. Diagnosis and management of primary sclerosing cholangitis. Hepatology 2010;51(2):660–78.

44. European Association for the Study of the Liver. EASL Clinical Practice Guidelines: management of cholestatic liver diseases. J Hepatol 2009;51(2):237–67.

45. Patel AH, Harnois DM, Klee GG, et al. The utility of CA 19-9 in the diagnoses of cholangiocarcinoma in patients without primary sclerosing cholangitis. Am J Gastroenterol 2000;95(1):204–7.

46. Charatcharoenwitthaya P, Enders FB, Halling KC, et al. Utility of serum tumor markers, imaging, and biliary cytology for detecting cholangiocarcinoma in primary sclerosing cholangitis. Hepatology 2008;48(4):1106–17.

47. Barr Fritcher EG, Voss JS, Jenkins SM, et al. Primary sclerosing cholangitis with equivocal cytology: fluorescence in situ hybridization and serum CA 19-9 predict risk of malignancy. Cancer Cytopathol 2013;121(12):708–17.

48. Chung YE, Kim MJ, Park YN, et al. Varying appearances of cholangiocarcinoma: radiologic-pathologic correlation. Radiographics 2009;29(3):683–700.

49. Maetani Y, Itoh K, Watanabe C, et al. MR imaging of intrahepatic cholangiocarcinoma with pathologic correlation. AJR Am J Roentgenol 2001;176(6): 1499–507.

50. Bismuth H, Corlette MB. Intrahepatic cholangioenteric anastomosis in carcinoma of the hilus of the liver. Surg Gynecol Obstet 1975;140(2):170–8.

51. Jarnagin WR, Fong Y, DeMatteo RP, et al. Staging, resectability, and outcome in 225 patients with hilar cholangiocarcinoma. Ann Surg 2001;234(4):507–17 [discussion: 517–9].

52. Ruys AT, Busch OR, Rauws EA, et al. Prognostic impact of preoperative imaging parameters on resectability of hilar cholangiocarcinoma. HPB Surg 2013;2013: 657309.

53. Vogl TJ, Schwarz WO, Heller M, et al. Staging of Klatskin tumours (hilar cholangiocarcinomas): comparison of MR cholangiography, MR imaging, and endoscopic retrograde cholangiography. Eur Radiol 2006;16(10):2317–25.

54. Lopera JE, Soto JA, Munera F. Malignant hilar and perihilar biliary obstruction: use of MR cholangiography to define the extent of biliary ductal involvement and plan percutaneous interventions. Radiology 2001;220(1):90–6.

55. Zidi SH, Prat F, Le Guen O, et al. Performance characteristics of magnetic resonance cholangiography in the staging of malignant hilar strictures. Gut 2000; 46(1):103–6.

56. Yeh TS, Jan YY, Tseng JH, et al. Malignant perihilar biliary obstruction: magnetic resonance cholangiopancreatographic findings. Am J Gastroenterol 2000; 95(2):432–40.

57. Manfredi R, Brizi MG, Masselli G, et al. Malignant biliary hilar stenosis: MR cholangiography compared with direct cholangiography. Radiol Med 2001; 102(1–2):48–54 [in Italian].

58. Altehoefer C, Ghanem N, Furtwängler A, et al. Breathhold unenhanced and gadolinium-enhanced magnetic resonance tomography and magnetic resonance cholangiography in hilar cholangiocarcinoma. Int J Colorectal Dis 2001; 16(3):188–92.

59. Lee HY, Kim SH, Lee JM, et al. Preoperative assessment of resectability of hepatic hilar cholangiocarcinoma: combined CT and cholangiography with revised criteria. Radiology 2006;239(1):113–21.

60. Aloia TA, Charnsangavej C, Faria S, et al. High-resolution computed tomography accurately predicts resectability in hilar cholangiocarcinoma. Am J Surg 2007;193(6):702–6.

61. Tillich M, Mischinger HJ, Preisegger KH, et al. Multiphasic helical CT in diagnosis and staging of hilar cholangiocarcinoma. AJR Am J Roentgenol 1998; 171(3):651–8.

62. Cha JH, Han JK, Kim TK, et al. Preoperative evaluation of Klatskin tumor: accuracy of spiral CT in determining vascular invasion as a sign of unresectability. Abdom Imaging 2000;25(5):500–7.

63. Petrowsky H, Wildbrett P, Husarik DB, et al. Impact of integrated positron emission tomography and computed tomography on staging and management of gallbladder cancer and cholangiocarcinoma. J Hepatol 2006;45(1): 43–50.

64. Anderson CD, Rice MH, Pinson CW, et al. Fluorodeoxyglucose PET imaging in the evaluation of gallbladder carcinoma and cholangiocarcinoma. J Gastrointest Surg 2004;8(1):90–7.

65. Kim JY, Kim MH, Lee TY, et al. Clinical role of 18F-FDG PET-CT in suspected and potentially operable cholangiocarcinoma: a prospective study compared with conventional imaging. Am J Gastroenterol 2008;103(5):1145–51.
66. Jarnagin WR, Weber S, Tickoo SK, et al. Combined hepatocellular and cholangiocarcinoma: demographic, clinical, and prognostic factors. Cancer 2002; 94(7):2040–6.
67. Rotellar F, Pardo F. Laparoscopic staging in hilar cholangiocarcinoma: is it still justified? World J Gastrointest Oncol 2013;5(7):127–31.
68. Bhattacharjya S, Bhattacharjya T, Baber S, et al. Prospective study of contrast-enhanced computed tomography, computed tomography during arterioportography, and magnetic resonance imaging for staging colorectal liver metastases for liver resection. Br J Surg 2004;91(10):1361–9.
69. Onishi H, Murakami T, Kim T, et al. Hepatic metastases: detection with multidetector row CT, SPIO-enhanced MR imaging, and both techniques combined. Radiology 2006;239(1):131–8.
70. Numminen K, Isoniemi H, Halavaara J, et al. Preoperative assessment of focal liver lesions: multidetector computed tomography challenges magnetic resonance imaging. Acta Radiol 2005;46(1):9–15.
71. Kulemann V, Schima W, Tamandl D, et al. Preoperative detection of colorectal liver metastases in fatty liver: MDCT or MRI? Eur J Radiol 2011; 79(2):e1–6.
72. van Kessel CS, van Leeuwen MS, van den Bosch MA, et al. Accuracy of multislice liver CT and MRI for preoperative assessment of colorectal liver metastases after neoadjuvant chemotherapy. Dig Surg 2011;28(1):36–43.
73. Koh DM, Collins DJ, Wallace T, et al. Combining diffusion-weighted MRI with Gd-EOB-DTPA-enhanced MRI improves the detection of colorectal liver metastases. Br J Radiol 2012;85(1015):980–9.
74. Macera A, Lario C, Petracchini M, et al. Staging of colorectal liver metastases after preoperative chemotherapy. Diffusion-weighted imaging in combination with Gd-EOB-DTPA MRI sequences increases sensitivity and diagnostic accuracy. Eur Radiol 2013;23(3):739–47.
75. Knowles B, Welsh FK, Chandrakumaran K, et al. Detailed liver-specific imaging prior to pre-operative chemotherapy for colorectal liver metastases reduces intra-hepatic recurrence and the need for a repeat hepatectomy. HPB (Oxford) 2012;14(5):298–309.
76. Hammerstingl R, Huppertz A, Breuer J, et al. Diagnostic efficacy of gadoxetic acid (Primovist)-enhanced MRI and spiral CT for a therapeutic strategy: comparison with intraoperative and histopathologic findings in focal liver lesions. Eur Radiol 2008;18(3):457–67.
77. Shindoh J, Loyer EM, Kopetz S, et al. Optimal morphologic response to preoperative chemotherapy: an alternate outcome end point before resection of hepatic colorectal metastases. J Clin Oncol 2012;30(36):4566–72.
78. Ramos E, Valls C, Martinez L, et al. Preoperative staging of patients with liver metastases of colorectal carcinoma. Does PET/CT really add something to multidetector CT? Ann Surg Oncol 2011;18(9):2654–61.
79. Briggs RH, Chowdhury FU, Lodge JP, et al. Clinical impact of FDG PET-CT in patients with potentially operable metastatic colorectal cancer. Clin Radiol 2011;66(12):1167–74.
80. Llamas-Elvira JM, Rodríguez-Fernández A, Gutiérrez-Sáinz J, et al. Fluorine-18 fluorodeoxyglucose PET in the preoperative staging of colorectal cancer. Eur J Nucl Med Mol Imaging 2007;34(6):859–67.

81. Tanaka K, Takakura H, Takeda K, et al. Importance of complete pathologic response to prehepatectomy chemotherapy in treating colorectal cancer metastases. Ann Surg 2009;250(6):935–42.

82. Auer RC, White RR, Kemeny NE, et al. Predictors of a true complete response among disappearing liver metastases from colorectal cancer after chemotherapy. Cancer 2010;116(6):1502–9.

83. Elias D, Youssef O, Sideris L, et al. Evolution of missing colorectal liver metastases following inductive chemotherapy and hepatectomy. J Surg Oncol 2004; 86(1):4–9.

84. Benoist S, Brouquet A, Penna C, et al. Complete response of colorectal liver metastases after chemotherapy: does it mean cure? J Clin Oncol 2006;24(24): 3939–45.

85. Tan MC, Linehan DC, Hawkins WG, et al. Chemotherapy-induced normalization of FDG uptake by colorectal liver metastases does not usually indicate complete pathologic response. J Gastrointest Surg 2007;11(9):1112–9.

86. van Kessel CS, Buckens CF, van den Bosch MA, et al. Preoperative imaging of colorectal liver metastases after neoadjuvant chemotherapy: a meta-analysis. Ann Surg Oncol 2012;19(9):2805–13.

87. Bischof DA, Clary BM, Maithel SK, et al. Surgical management of disappearing colorectal liver metastases. Br J Surg 2013;100(11):1414–20.

88. Mullen JT, Ribero D, Reddy SK, et al. Hepatic insufficiency and mortality in 1,059 noncirrhotic patients undergoing major hepatectomy. J Am Coll Surg 2007; 204(5):854–62 [discussion: 862–4].

89. Kishi Y, Abdalla EK, Chun YS, et al. Three hundred and one consecutive extended right hepatectomies: evaluation of outcome based on systematic liver volumetry. Ann Surg 2009;250(4):540–8.

90. Shindoh J, Truty MJ, Aloia TA, et al. Kinetic growth rate after portal vein embolization predicts posthepatectomy outcomes: toward zero liver-related mortality in patients with colorectal liver metastases and small future liver remnant. J Am Coll Surg 2013;216(2):201–9.

91. Truty MJ, Vauthey JN. Uses and limitations of portal vein embolization for improving perioperative outcomes in hepatocellular carcinoma. Semin Oncol 2010;37(2):102–9.

92. Abdalla EK, Barnett CC, Doherty D, et al. Extended hepatectomy in patients with hepatobiliary malignancies with and without preoperative portal vein embolization. Arch Surg 2002;137(6):675–80 [discussion: 680–1].

93. Lu DS, Yu NC, Raman SS, et al. Radiofrequency ablation of hepatocellular carcinoma: treatment success as defined by histologic examination of the explanted liver. Radiology 2005;234(3):954–60.

94. Brace CL. Radiofrequency and microwave ablation of the liver, lung, kidney, and bone: what are the differences? Curr Probl Diagn Radiol 2009;38(3):135–43.

Prognostication Systems as Applied to Primary and Metastatic Hepatic Malignancies

CrossMark

Clifford S. Cho, MD

KEYWORDS

- Prognostication • Hepatic • Malignancy • Primary • Metastatic

KEY POINTS

- The disease biology of primary and metastatic cancers of the liver does not always fit well into the conventional tumor-node-metastasis staging paradigm.
- The impact of surgical resection on long-term survival has led to the incorporation of anatomic and biological measures of resectability into prognostication systems for primary and metastatic cancers of the liver.
- Efforts to refine the prediction of individual oncologic outcomes have used nomograms to accommodate the reality that some prognostic factors are continuous variables, and that some prognostic factors are more important than others.

INTRODUCTION

The traditional tumor-node-metastasis (TNM) framework that underlies the staging of many epithelial malignancies is based on 2 fundamental observations regarding cancer biology. First, cancers seem to progress in a sequential manner, characterized by primary tumors progressing in size or anatomic depth of tissue involvement, lymphatic spread into regional lymph nodes, and distant hematogenous progression into discontiguous organ sites. Second, the presence of nodal metastases typically carries more prognostic weight than disease progression at the primary site, and the presence of distant metastases typically carries more prognostic impact than disease progression either at the primary site or in regional lymph nodes. The same TNM staging paradigm that has successfully enabled the development of prognostic staging systems for many cancers has never been useful for prognostic stratification of patients with hepatic malignancies. For one thing, many hepatic neoplasms are manifestations of metastatic disease; the uniform assignment of all patients into a single stage IV

The author has nothing to disclose.
Section of Surgical Oncology, Department of Surgery, University of Wisconsin School of Medicine and Public Health, J4/703 Clinical Sciences Center, 600 Highland Avenue, Madison, WI 53792, USA
E-mail address: cho@surgery.wisc.edu

Surg Oncol Clin N Am 24 (2015) 41–56
http://dx.doi.org/10.1016/j.soc.2014.09.010
1055-3207/15/$ – see front matter © 2015 Elsevier Inc. All rights reserved.
surgonc.theclinics.com

category does little to permit subtle distinctions of expected survival outcomes. In addition, nodal metastases (often a dominant factor in the estimation of prognosis for patients with epithelial malignancies) are often rare and occasionally of unclear prognostic significance in primary and metastatic hepatic tumors. Moreover, prognosis for patients with hepatic tumors is often determined by the technical feasibility of surgical resection; as a result, variables that describe the anatomic location (eg, involvement of critical vascular structures) or distribution of tumors (eg, the presence of bilateral disease) must be included in any meaningful prognostication scheme. In addition, many primary hepatic malignancies arise in a setting of compromised liver function, so the severity of that liver dysfunction often dictates prognosis as much as (if not more than) traditional oncologic parameters like tumor size or number. In order to accommodate this diversity and heterogeneity of prognostically informative variables, efforts to stratify expected survival for patients with hepatic malignancies have resulted in a multitude of nontraditional staging and scoring systems. This article provides an overview of the prognostication systems that have been proposed for patients with primary and metastatic hepatic malignancies.

PRIMARY HEPATIC MALIGNANCIES
Hepatocellular Carcinoma

Overview
Hepatocellular carcinoma (HCC) is a leading cause of mortality worldwide. Because conditions of chronic inflammation and chronic hepatocellular death and regeneration also favor hepatocarcinogenesis, the risk of HCC is significantly higher among patients with chronic viral hepatitis and long-standing cirrhosis. In addition, these conditions effectively cause the liver to become a carcinogenic substrate, promoting the development of multifocal tumors and recurrent tumors after successful treatment. The range of treatment options for HCC include systemic chemotherapy, transarterial delivery of bland embolization particles, chemoembolization, selective internal radiation therapy, tumoral injection with cytotoxic ethanol, thermal ablation using radiofrequency or microwave energy, resection, and total hepatectomy with orthotopic allotransplantation. To a large extent, the development of such a wide breadth of treatment options has been necessary because many patients with HCC are not candidates for aggressive interventions.[1]

Prognostic variables
Retrospective series have determined that traditional oncologic metrics like tumor size and number are reflective of disease progression and eventual prognosis. The United Network of Organ Sharing and University of California San Francisco criteria used to select patients with HCC who are most likely to benefit from liver transplantation are based on tumor size and number.[2,3] The relationship between tumor size and prognosis is unlikely to be linear, because several series have reported potentially favorable outcomes among patients undergoing resection of solitary, large HCC[4–8]; the ability of tumors in these highly selected patient cohorts to reach massive proportions without showing more ominous signs of progression such as metastatic disease is probably a reflection of indolent intrinsic disease biology. The prognostic significance of regional (hilar or perihepatic) lymph node metastases remains incompletely defined; although the presence of such nodal metastases seems to be an ominous sign, the prevalence of nodal metastases seems to be low.[9–12] Although the development of extrahepatic metastases portends a poor outcome, the preneoplastic nature of chronic liver diseases often makes the risk of intrahepatic recurrence higher than the risk of distant metastasis.[13,14]

One prognostic variable that has consistently been shown to indicate a higher likelihood of recurrent disease after resection or transplantation is vascular invasion by tumor.[13,15–23] Although cases of macrovascular invasion into the portal or hepatic veins can be diagnosed radiographically, the more common circumstance of microvascular invasion can be difficult to exclude before resection or transplantation. The heavy prognostic impact of microvascular invasion has led some investigators to recommend routine core biopsies of HCC tumors before transplantation.[24,25] Several investigations have pointed out the possibility that other negative prognostic markers such as advanced tumor grade, marked increase of serum levels of alpha fetoprotein (AFP), or large tumor size may be surrogates of microvascular invasion.[24,26–29]

Because of the causal relationship that exists between chronic viral hepatitis or cirrhosis and HCC, the presence of these carcinogenic conditions is a strong predictor of disease recurrence following therapy.[13,30–34] In addition, because advanced cirrhosis limits the feasibility of aggressive liver-directed therapies, metrics like the Child-Turcotte-Pugh score[35,36] or MELD (Model for End-stage Liver Disease) score[37] that quantify hepatic dysfunction can be as important as more traditional oncologic descriptors in determining long-term prognosis and treatment morbidity and mortality. For example, although a patient with preserved liver function and 2 left-sided HCC tumors measuring 3 cm each may be eligible for potentially curative resection, a patient with advanced liver insufficiency and a solitary 2-cm HCC may be ineligible to receive life-prolonging therapy.

Several series reporting outcomes after resection of HCC have indicated that perioperative outcomes such as estimated blood loss[22,38] and postoperative complications[39] may directly affect expected survival outcomes.

Prognostication systems

Early staging systems attempted to impose the traditional TNM scheme onto HCC prognostication (**Table 1**). In an effort to incorporate the important prognostic variables of tumor size, tumor number, and presence of vascular invasion, the 1997 American Joint Committee on Cancer (AJCC) staging system used complex combinations of these 3 variables in 10 distinct T classes.[40] This complexity was partially ameliorated by the International Hepato-Pancreato-Biliary Association (IHPBA) staging system, which relied on a scoring system based on the absence or presence of 3 criteria (>2 cm maximal tumor dimension, multiple tumors, and vascular invasion) to define 4 distinct T classes.[41] Both systems relied on a maximal tumor diameter cutoff of 2 cm to measure tumor size. The recognition that a cutoff of 5 cm permitted more accurate stratification of outcomes led to the Vauthey staging system,[42] and this improvement was incorporated into the next iteration, the 2002 AJCC staging system.[43]

One potential limitation of these systems was that they did not accommodate liver dysfunction as a prognostic or treatment selection variable. An early attempt to incorporate both tumor-specific and liver function–specific variables was the Okuda staging system, which was first described in 1985.[44] Using 4 criteria (tumor extension involving >50% of the liver parenchyma, presence of ascites, serum albumin ≤3 mg/dL, and serum bilirubin ≥3 mg/dL), this system categorizes patients into 3 stages (stage A, no criteria; B, 1–2 criteria; C, 3–4 criteria) that accurately stratify expected survival outcomes. The Cancer of the Liver Italian Program (CLIP) staging system used gradations of liver function as assessed by Child-Pugh class, tumor burden as characterized by morphologic assessments of tumor number and extent of hepatic parenchymal involvement, and the prognostic variables of AFP and portal vein thrombosis into a prognostically informative numerical scoring system that ranged from 0 to 6.[46] The Barcelona Clinic Liver Cancer (BCLC) system, first described

Table 1
Prognostic variables included in staging systems for hepatocellular carcinoma

Staging System	Adverse Prognostic Variables
AJCC system, 5th edition[40]	Tumor size >2 cm Multiple tumors Bilateral tumors Microvascular invasion Major vascular invasion Extrahepatic invasion
IHPBA system[41]	Tumor size >2 cm Multiple tumors Vascular invasion
Vauthey system[42]	Tumor size >5 cm Multiple tumors Microvascular invasion Major vascular invasion
AJCC system, 6th edition[43]	Tumor size >5 cm Multiple tumors Microvascular invasion Major vascular invasion
Okuda system[44]	Disease involving >50% liver parenchyma Ascites Albumin $\leq$ 3 mg/dL Bilirubin $\geq$ 3 mg/dL
BCLC system[45]	Tumor size >3 cm Tumor size >5 cm Multiple tumors Vascular invasion Extrahepatic invasion Symptoms Child-Pugh class
CLIP system[46]	Multiple tumors Disease involving >50% liver parenchyma AFP $\geq$ 400 ng/mL Portal vein thrombosis
JIS[47]	Tumor size >2 cm Multiple tumors Vascular invasion Child-Pugh score

Abbreviations: AJCC, American Joint Committee on Cancer; BCLC, Barcelona Clinic Liver Cancer; CLIP, Cancer of the Liver Italian Program; IHPBA, International Hepato-Pancreato-Biliary Association; JIS, Japanese Integrated System.

in 1999, also incorporated factors that described tumor burden and liver function but also introduced an overall assessment of performance status; as such, the BCLC system was developed as a means to streamline the triage of patients into appropriate treatment strategies.[45] Stage A patients were largely patients with limited disease burden, preserved hepatic function, and excellent performance status who would be best served with liver transplantation. Stage B patients were patients with preserved hepatic function and performance status whose tumor burden exceeded criteria for transplantation; as a result, these patients were generally treated with hepatic resection. Stage C patients were those whose performance status or disease burden rendered them ineligible for resection or transplantation and who were best treated with transarterial therapies, and stage D patients were patients whose combination of liver function, performance status, and tumor burden were best managed with supportive care only. In this way, the BCLC system was designed as a means of triaging patients into appropriate treatment strategies and not strictly as a means of prognostication The merit of incorporating both traditional tumor-specific and hepatic functional metrics into prognostication for HCC was shown by the Japanese Integrated System (JIS), which relied on a combination of the IHPBA staging system and the Child-Pugh classification into a simple scoring system that stratified expected survival outcomes after resection of HCC.[47]

In 2008, the Memorial Sloan-Kettering Cancer Center (MSKCC) experience with 184 patients with HCC treated with partial hepatectomy was examined in an effort to validate these prognostication systems.[22] As expected, most of these systems were able to stratify overall and recurrence-free survival outcomes into distinct prognostic categories. However, none of these systems permitted accurate stratification of individual survival outcomes. In this analysis, a concordance index (c-index) was calculated for each system's ability to properly predict the longer survivor between 2 randomly selected pairs of patients. When calculated based on every possible random pair of patients, a c-index of 1.0 indicates that a system is able to properly predict the longer survivor 100% of the time; a c-index of 0.5 indicates that a system is able to properly predict the longer survivor 50% of the time (indicating an individual predictive capacity no better than a coin toss). The c-indices for the various systems ranged between 0.54 and 0.59, and only the 2002 AJCC staging system had a 95% confidence interval that exceeded 0.5, indicating that all other staging systems were incapable of stratifying expected survival outcomes on an individual basis. In an effort to enhance individual risk prediction, the data set was used to generate a prognostic nomogram in which prognostic factors were assigned weighted scores based on the magnitude of their association with survival. In this way, a scoring system that incorporated the variables of patient age, estimated operative blood loss, margin status, presence of satellite lesions, presence of vascular invasion, tumor size, and AFP level was developed to determine the specific likelihood of overall or recurrence-free survival for individual patients. In addition to being able to allow for some variables being more prognostically informative than others, nomograms also enable the incorporation of continuous variables (eg, estimated blood loss) into risk calculation. The MSKCC HCC nomogram had a c-index of 0.74 (95% confidence interval, 0.68–0.80) in the prediction of overall survival, and a c-index of 0.67 (95% confidence interval, 0.61–0.73) in the prediction of recurrence-free survival, which indicates that the use of a prognostic nomogram can enhance the precision of individual prognostication.

Cholangiocarcinoma

Overview
Arising from the cholangiocytes populating the biliary tree, cholangiocarcinoma (CCA) can present as intrahepatic and hilar variants (with extrahepatic CCA being outside the present article's focus on hepatic malignancies). Associations exist between CCA and hepatitis C, chronic biliary parasitic infestations, and primary sclerosing cholangitis. However, CCA differs from HCC in that most cases arise outside the context of a known predisposing hepatocellular or biliary disorder. Like HCC, CCA is optimally treated with resection; consequently, anatomic factors associated with resectability serve as prognostic indicators as well. The insidious ability of CCA to grow longitudinally along the biliary tree has led to an aggressive approach to tumoral extirpation, which is particular evident with hilar CCA, for which optimal therapy involves resection not only of the biliary tumor but of the upstream hemiliver and the contiguous biliary

radicles within. In addition to longitudinal growth, CCA has the ability to grow in a radial manner, often invading from the biliary duct into the adjacent portal venous and hepatic arterial structures that make up the remainder of the portal triad. The anatomic confines of the hepatic hilus, with the close proximity of the portal veins and hepatic arteries to the hepatic ducts, means that significant bilateral involvement of critical hilar structures may render a small focus of CCA unresectable.[1]

Prognostic variables

Like other epithelial malignancies, CCA seems to follow a familiar pattern of local tumor progression that begins with intramucosal atypia and eventually progresses to transmural invasion. Also like other epithelial malignancies, CCA has a tendency to metastasize to local hilar lymph nodes.[1] As with HCC, tumor size and tumor number have been shown to be reliable prognostic indicators for patients undergoing surgical resection. The prevalence of hilar lymph node metastases is higher for CCA than for HCC, and the presence of nodal metastases has proved to be a powerfully negative prognostic factor. The presence of intratumoral lymphovascular invasion, which may be a surrogate marker of nodal metastases, has similarly been found to negatively affect survival outcomes.[48–50] Tumor differentiation has also been shown to be associated with differences in survival.[51,52] Marked increases in serum tumor markers like carbohydrate antigen 19-9 (CA19-9) and carcinoembryonic antigen (CEA) have also been associated with poorer outcomes.[53–55] To an extent greater than that seen with HCC, it is common for CCA to present with distant extrahepatic metastases, and their presence clearly portends a poor prognostic outlook. As stated, CCA has an ability to grow longitudinally along biliary structures with microscopic extension beyond areas of grossly visible tumor involvement. The ability to effect a microscopically negative resection margin has been associated with improved survival outcomes.[56–60]

Prognostic systems

Intrahepatic cholangiocarcinoma The typical pattern of primary tumoral progression, nodal metastasis, and hematogenous dissemination to distant organ sites has allowed a traditional TNM approach to CCA staging (**Table 2**). Early staging systems for intrahepatic CCA were based on parameters of tumor size and number that were similar to those used for hepatocellular carcinoma.[61] In 2001, Okabayashi and colleagues[62] from the National Cancer Center Hospital in Tokyo used their experience with 60 patients with resected intrahepatic CCA to identify hilar lymph node metastasis, multiple tumors, tumor-related symptoms, and microscopic or macroscopic invasion of any vascular structure as prognostic factors on multivariate analysis. Using these variables, they proposed a novel staging system in which stage I disease was defined as

Table 2	
Prognostic variables included in staging systems for intrahepatic CCA	
Staging System	**Adverse Prognostic Variables**
UICC system[61]	Tumor size >2 cm Multiple tumors Bilateral tumors Microvascular invasion Major vascular invasion
Okabayashi system[62]	Multiple tumors Vascular invasion

Abbreviation: UICC, Union for International Cancer Control.

the presence of solitary tumors without vascular invasion, stage II disease was defined by the presence of solitary tumors with vascular invasion, stage IIIA disease was defined by the presence of multiple tumors, stage IIIB disease was defined by the presence of nodal metastases, and stage IV disease was defined by the presence of distant metastases. The ability of this staging system to stratify recurrence-free and overall survival outcomes ultimately led to the inclusion of these criteria into the current AJCC staging system, which uses a T classification system based on tumor number and presence of vascular invasion, with T3 tumors defined by tumor extension into extrahepatic tissues and T4 tumors defined by diffusely infiltrative, periductal tumor infiltration.[63] Several investigators have since suggested that tumor number should be included as a prognostic factor.[64,65] In 2013, Wang and colleagues[55] developed a prognostic nomogram based on CEA level, CA19-9 level, vascular invasion, nodal metastases, direction of invasion into extrahepatic structures, tumor number, and maximal tumor diameter. Using methodology similar to that used by Cho and colleagues,[22] they used their data set of 367 patients treated with partial hepatectomy to show that this prognostic nomogram outperformed the seventh edition of the AJCC staging system (with concordance indices of 0.74 vs 0.65). A similar prognostic nomogram with a concordance index of 0.69 was recently proposed by Hyder and colleagues[66] using the prognostic variables of age, vascular invasion, nodal metastases, tumor number, maximal tumor diameter, and presence of cirrhosis using an international data set of 514 patients who underwent resection of intrahepatic CCA.

Hilar cholangiocarcinoma Early AJCC staging systems that relied on tumor size for T staging did not apply well to hilar CCA, in which small but unfortunately located tumors could be unresectable (**Table 3**). In 1975, Bismuth and Corlette[67] proposed an anatomic classification system for hilar CCA that could be used to determine operative approach and resectability. Subsequent work from MSKCC proposed an alternative T classification system that incorporated adjacent vascular involvement to stratify patients based on resectability.[58] The MSKCC system also stratified expected survival outcomes, because patients with technically unresectable disease experienced earlier demise than patients with technically resectable disease.[60] Acknowledging the particular anatomic ramifications of local tumor invasion within the hepatic hilus, the most

Table 3
Prognostic variables included in staging systems for hilar CCA

Staging System	Adverse Prognostic Variables
MSKCC system[58]	Unilateral hepatic duct involvement Ipsilateral hepatic hemiatrophy Ipsilateral portal vein involvement Bilateral hepatic duct involvement Main portal vein encasement
AJCC system, 7th edition[63]	Tumor extension into adipose tissue beyond duct wall Tumor extension into adjacent hepatic parenchyma Unilateral portal vein or hepatic artery involvement Main or bilateral portal vein involvement Common hepatic artery involvement Contralateral portal vein involvement Contralateral hepatic artery involvement Tumor extension into bilateral second-order biliary radicles Regional lymph node metastases Para-aortic, paracaval, celiac artery, or superior mesenteric artery lymph node metastases

recent AJCC staging system for hilar CCA adopts elements of the MSKCC staging system into the determination of T stage.[63] A distinction between the Bismuth-Corlette and MSKCC systems is that the former communicates more information (eg, right-sided vs left-sided involvement) for purposes of anatomic description and operative planning; in a similar but more comprehensive way, Deoliveira and colleagues[68] recently proposed a detailed anatomic classification system that communicates not only right versus left sidedness and presence of nodal and distant metastases but also tumor size, morphology, presence of underlying liver disease, anticipated postresection future liver remnant, and the anatomic extent of bile duct, portal vein, and hepatic artery involvement by tumor.

HEPATIC COLORECTAL ADENOCARCINOMA METASTASES
Overview

Unlike other manifestations of systemically disseminated cancer, hepatic metastases from colorectal adenocarcinoma offer unique opportunities for surgical intervention. The liver is often the solitary site of metastasis in colorectal cancer. Long-term follow-up of patients following hepatic metastasectomy suggests that approximately one-fifth of patients undergoing resection of their hepatic metastases are cured of their disease.[69,70] Moreover, the management and outcomes of metastatic colorectal adenocarcinoma have undergone dramatic improvements over the past several decades. These improvements have come about in small part from advancements in operative and perioperative techniques, and in large part from advancements in systemic chemotherapy. These improvements have enabled surgeons to offer therapeutic interventions to patients who were once considered ineligible for operative therapy, and have allowed patients with metastatic colorectal cancer to live far longer than was possible in the past. A byproduct of these evolutionary changes in therapy is that the prognostic variables associated with long-term survival outcomes may also have changed.[71-74]

Prognostic Variables

The prognostic variables that have historically been found to influence survival outcomes after hepatic colorectal adenocarcinoma metastasectomy can be divided into 4 categories. The first of these relates to features of the primary tumor that reflect individual cancer biology. Several analyses have found that primary tumor variables such as transserosal (>T3) invasion of the initial colorectal tumor or the presence of nodal metastases (N1) seems to affect outcomes after resection of metastatic disease, suggesting that intrinsic features of disease biology manifested by the primary tumor may also influence outcomes after metastasectomy.[75-79] The second category of prognostic factors describes the pace of disease progression. Multiple analyses have found that synchronous presentation of hepatic metastases portends a worse prognosis than metachronous presentation, and that the disease-free interval of time between primary and metastatic diagnosis is inversely related to survival duration after metastasectomy.[75-77,79,80] The third category of factors describes the disease burden and/or technical resectability of the hepatic metastases, and includes variables like tumor size, tumor number, bilateral involvement, or serum levels of CEA.[75-79,81] The fourth category of factors describes responsiveness to systemic chemotherapy. Earlier studies suggested that radiographic response of hepatic metastases to neoadjuvant chemotherapy was associated with favorable outcomes after resection.[82-84] As systemic chemotherapy has become more effective (and as the likelihood of disease progression on chemotherapy has decreased), the prognostic impact of this variable has become less clear.[85] More recent studies have shown that biological predictors of responsiveness to specific therapeutic agents (eg, K-ras mutational status as a predictor of responsiveness to cetuximab) may be highly informative prognostic variables.[86–88]

Prognostic Systems

As surgical intervention for hepatic metastases from colorectal adenocarcinoma became more common, it became evident that a specific staging system was needed to further stratify survival expectations for patients who, by definition, would be uniformly categorized as having stage D or stage IV disease in the standard Duke, Astler-Collins, and AJCC staging systems of the day. Beginning in the late 1990s, several prognostic scoring systems were proposed around the variables that seemed to carry prognostic weight for patients undergoing hepatic metastasectomy: the presence of nodal metastases in the primary tumor; the time interval between primary tumor and metastatic tumor development; the number, size, and anatomic distribution of hepatic tumors; and CEA levels. A brief overview of proposed scoring systems shows a remarkable level of uniformity (**Table 4**), suggesting the likelihood that these

Table 4	
Prognostic variables included in risk scoring systems for hepatic colorectal metastases	
Study	**Adverse Prognostic Variables**
Nordlinger et al,[89] 1996	Age $\geq$ 60 y Serosal involvement of primary tumor Node-positive primary Disease-free interval <2 y Hepatic metastasis size $\geq$5 cm Hepatic metastasis number $\geq$4 Hepatic resection margin $\leq$1 cm
Iwatsuki et al,[90] 1999	Disease-free interval $\leq$30 mo Hepatic metastasis size $\geq$8 cm Hepatic metastasis number $\geq$2 Bilateral hepatic metastases Positive hepatic resection margin Extrahepatic metastases
Fong et al,[77] 1999	Node-positive primary Disease-free interval <1 y Hepatic metastasis size $\geq$5 cm Hepatic metastasis number >1 CEA>200 ng/mL
Nagashima et al,[91] 2004	Serosal involvement of primary tumor Node-positive primary tumor Hepatic metastasis size $\geq$5 cm Hepatic metastasis number >1 Resectable extrahepatic metastases
Rees et al,[92] 2008	Node-positive primary tumor Moderately differentiated primary tumor Poorly differentiated primary tumor CEA 6–60 ng/mL CEA>60 ng/mL Hepatic metastasis number >3 Hepatic metastasis size 5–10 cm Hepatic metastasis size >10 cm Positive hepatic resection margin Extrahepatic metastases

investigators were separately characterizing the same biological reality. The system that had the highest degree of adoption was the Clinical Risk Score (CRS) or Fong score, named after the author who first proposed the system based on his analysis of the MSKCC experience.[77] Fong and colleagues[77] identified 7 prognostically informative variables: positive resection margin, presence of extrahepatic disease, node-positive primary tumor, disease-free interval between primary and metastatic diagnosis less than 12 months, multifocal (>1) tumor, maximal tumor diameter greater than 5 cm, and CEA level greater than 200 ng/mL. Of these, they excluded margin status (on the argument that this could not be reliably assessed preoperatively) and extrahepatic disease (on the argument that this should be a contraindication to hepatic metastasectomy), and used the remaining 5 criteria to create a simple 0 to 5 scoring system that clearly stratified patients into 6 distinct prognostic categories. This scoring system has been validated by several other institutions, and remains in use as a means of stratifying expected outcomes.[93,94]

In 2008, Kattan and colleagues[95] revisited the MSKCC experience to develop a nomogram to predict individual disease-specific survival following hepatic metastasectomy. Although the CRS is a simple scoring system that gives equal weight to each of the prognostic variables and treats each of them as categorical variables, use of a nomogram with 5 additional prognostic variables again allowed differential weighting and the incorporation of continuous variables. The investigators determined that the MSKCC nomogram, which incorporated the variables of patient age, gender, site of primary tumor (colon vs rectum), disease-free interval, CEA level, number of tumors, maximal diameter of largest tumor, need for bilateral resection, tumoral involvement of more than 1 hemiliver, and nodal status of primary tumor, outperformed the original CRS in discriminating survival outcomes of patients who were treated after the development of the CRS in 1998 (c-index of 0.688 vs 0.648; $P = .03$).

As noted earlier, outcomes for patients with hepatic colorectal metastases have been transformed by the development of newer and more effective forms of chemotherapy. Note that these scoring systems, including the MSKCC nomogram, were largely developed using data collected from patients treated before the use of contemporary systemic chemotherapy. More recent analyses have suggested that, in the current era of oxaliplatin, irinotecan, and biological agents like bevacizumab and cetuximab, factors that once held prognostic weight may no longer be relevant in the determination of prognosis. For example, a recent study determined that overall survival after hepatic metastasectomy was influenced by the nodal status of the primary tumor in the era before the adoption of perioperative oxaliplatin and irinotecan, but that this influence disappeared thereafter.[96] An analysis of 305 patients treated at MD Anderson Cancer Center with neoadjuvant oxaliplatin or irinotecan before hepatic metastasectomy found that the only variables that remained independently associated with differences in survival were surgical resection margin status and radiographic response to chemotherapy, which raises the possibility that, in the setting of effective systemic chemotherapy, prognostication for hepatic colorectal metastasectomy may be reduced to a technical question of whether liver metastases can be completely resected.[97]

SUMMARY

Staging systems are means of (1) acknowledging the great variability of outcomes that can be seen with cancer and (2) predicting outcomes for individuals who have cancer. The staging and prognostication of hepatic malignancies has been particularly challenging, because primary and metastatic liver cancers differ greatly in the array of manifestations that reflect prognosis and in their responsiveness to therapeutic intervention. As understanding of these diseases has evolved and matured, so have the prognostication systems for these cancers. This evolution has included the use of traditional TNM staging configurations extensively modified to fit the unique manifestations of hepatic cancer biology, and novel scoring systems designed to accommodate prognostically informative variables that do not fit naturally into the TNM schema. Although these systems enable the stratification of patients into prognostically distinct categories, the recent use of nomograms to reflect the differential importance of various prognostic factors permits a shift in focus from group stratification toward prediction of individual oncologic outcomes. The trajectory of incremental refinements in prognostication discussed in this article will undoubtedly continue into the future.

REFERENCES

1. Cho C, Fong Y. Benign and malignant primary liver neoplasms. In: Zinner MJ, Ashley SW, editors. Maingot's abdominal operations. New York: McGraw-Hill; 2013. p. 927–54.
2. Mazzaferro V, Regalia E, Doci R, et al. Liver transplantation for the treatment of small hepatocellular carcinomas in patients with cirrhosis. N Engl J Med 1996; 334(11):693–9.
3. Yao FY, Ferrell L, Bass NM, et al. Liver transplantation for hepatocellular carcinoma: expansion of the tumor size limits does not adversely impact survival. Hepatology 2001;33(6):1394–403.
4. Lee NH, Chau GY, Lui WY, et al. Surgical treatment and outcome in patients with a hepatocellular carcinoma greater than 10 cm in diameter. Br J Surg 1998;85(12): 1654–7.
5. Regimbeau JM, Farges O, Shen BY, et al. Is surgery for large hepatocellular carcinoma justified? J Hepatol 1999;31(6):1062–8.
6. Poon RT, Fan ST, Wong J. Selection criteria for hepatic resection in patients with large hepatocellular carcinoma larger than 10 cm in diameter. J Am Coll Surg 2002;194(5):592–602.
7. Pawlik TM, Poon RT, Abdalla EK, et al. Critical appraisal of the clinical and pathologic predictors of survival after resection of large hepatocellular carcinoma. Arch Surg 2005;140(5):450–7.
8. Liau KH, Ruo L, Shia J, et al. Outcome of partial hepatectomy for large (>10 cm) hepatocellular carcinoma. Cancer 2005;104(9):1948–55.
9. Uenishi T, Hirohashi K, Shuto T, et al. The clinical significance of lymph node metastases in patients undergoing surgery for hepatocellular carcinoma. Surg Today 2000;30(10):892–905.
10. Jaeck D. The significance of hepatic pedicle lymph node metastases in surgical management of colorectal liver metastases and of other liver malignancies. Ann Surg Oncol 2003;10(9):1007–11.
11. Grobmyer SR, Wang L, Gonen M, et al. Perihepatic lymph node assessment in patients undergoing partial hepatectomy for malignancy. Ann Surg 2006; 244(2):260–4.
12. Xiaohong S, Huikai L, Feng Q, et al. Clinical significance of lymph node metastasis in patients undergoing partial hepatectomy for hepatocellular carcinoma. World J Surg 2010;34(5):1028–33.
13. Cha C, Fong Y, Jarnagin WR, et al. Predictors and patterns of recurrence after resection of hepatocellular carcinoma. J Am Coll Surg 2003;197(5):753–8.

14. Yang Y, Nagano H, Ota H, et al. Patterns and clinicopathologic features of extra-hepatic recurrence of hepatocellular carcinoma after curative resection. Surgery 2007;141(2):196–202.
15. Ringe B, Pichlmayr R, Wittekind C, et al. Surgical treatment of hepatocellular carcinoma: experience with liver resection and transplantation in 198 patients. World J Surg 1991;15(2):270–85.
16. Chen MF, Hwang TL, Jeng LB, et al. Hepatic resection in 120 patients with hepatocellular carcinoma. Arch Surg 1989;124(9):1025–8.
17. Vauthey JN, Klimstra D, Francheschi D, et al. Factors affecting long-term outcome after hepatic resection for hepatocellular carcinoma. Am J Surg 1995;169(1):28–34.
18. Lau H, Fan ST, Ng IO, et al. Long term prognosis after hepatectomy for hepatocellular carcinoma: a survival analysis of 204 consecutive patients. Cancer 1998;83(11):2303–11.
19. Tsai TJ, Chau GY, Lui WY, et al. Clinical significance of microscopic tumor venous invasion in patients with resectable hepatocellular carcinoma. Surgery 2000;127(6):603–8.
20. Cho CS, Knechtle SJ, Heisey DM, et al. Analysis of tumor characteristics and survival in liver transplant recipients with incidentally diagnosed hepatocellular carcinoma. J Gastrointest Surg 2001;5(6):594–601.
21. Shah SA, Cleary SP, Wei AC, et al. Recurrence after liver resection for hepatocellular carcinoma: risk factors, treatment, and outcomes. Surgery 2007;141(3):330–9.
22. Cho CS, Gonen M, Shia J, et al. A novel prognostic nomogram is more accurate than conventional staging systems for predicting survival after resection of hepatocellular carcinoma. J Am Coll Surg 2008;206(2):281–91.
23. Sumie S, Kuromatsu R, Okuda K, et al. Microvascular invasion in patients with hepatocellular carcinoma and its predictable clinicopathological factors. Ann Surg Oncol 2008;15(5):1375–82.
24. Esnaola NF, Lauwers GY, Mirza NQ, et al. Predictors of microvascular invasion in patients with hepatocellular carcinoma who are candidates for orthotopic liver transplantation. J Gastrointest Surg 2002;6(2):224–32.
25. Tamura S, Kato T, Berho M, et al. Impact of histological grade of hepatocellular carcinoma on the outcome of liver transplantation. Arch Surg 2001;136(1):25–30.
26. Shijo H, Okazaki M. Prediction of portal vein invasion by hepatocellular carcinoma: a correlation between portal vein tumor thrombus and biochemical test. Jpn J Clin Oncol 1991;21(2):94–9.
27. Pawlik TM, Delman KA, Vauthey JN, et al. Tumor size predicts vascular invasion and histologic grade: Implications for selection of surgical treatment for hepatocellular carcinoma. Liver Transpl 2005;11(9):1086–92.
28. Cillo U, Vitale A, Navaglia F, et al. Role of blood AFP mRNA and tumor grade in the preoperative prognostic evaluation of patients with hepatocellular carcinoma. World J Gastroenterol 2005;11(44):6920–5.
29. Cucchetti A, Piscaglia F, Grigioni AD, et al. Preoperative prediction of hepatocellular carcinoma tumour grade and micro-vascular invasion by means of artificial neural network: a pilot study. J Hepatol 2010;52(6):880–8.
30. Kubo S, Hirohashi K, Tanaka H, et al. Effect of viral status on recurrence after liver resection for patients with hepatitis B virus-related hepatocellular carcinoma. Cancer 2000;88(5):1016–24.
31. Ahmad SA, Bilimoria MM, Wang X, et al. Hepatitis B or C virus serology as a prognostic factor in patients with hepatocellular carcinoma. J Gastrointest Surg 2001;5(5):468–76.

32. Sasai Y, Yamada T, Tanaka H, et al. Risk of recurrence in a long-term follow-up after surgery in 217 patients with hepatitis B- or hepatitis C-related hepatocellular carcinoma. Ann Surg 2006;244(5):771–80.

33. Bozorgzadeh A, Orloff M, Abt P, et al. Survival outcomes in liver transplantation for hepatocellular carcinoma, comparing impact of hepatitis C versus other etiology of cirrhosis. Liver Transpl 2007;13(6):807–13.

34. Cescon M, Cucchetti A, Grazi GL, et al. Role of hepatitis B virus infection in the prognosis after hepatectomy for hepatocellular carcinoma in patients with cirrhosis: a Western dual-center experience. Arch Surg 2009;144(10): 906–13.

35. Child CG, Turcotte JG. Surgery and portal hypertension. In: Child CG, editor. The liver and portal hypertension. Philadelphia: WB Saunders; 1964. p. 50–62.

36. Pugh RN, Murray-Lyon IM, Dawson JL, et al. Transection of the oesophagus for bleeding oesophageal varices. Br J Surg 1973;60(8):646–9.

37. Kamath PS, Wiesner RH, Malinchoc M, et al. A model to predict survival in patients with end-stage liver disease. Hepatology 2001;33(2):464–70.

38. Katz SC, Shia J, Liau KH, et al. Operative blood loss independently predicts recurrence and survival after resection of hepatocellular carcinoma. Ann Surg 2009;249(4):617–23.

39. Kusano T, Sasaki A, Kai S, et al. Predictors and prognostic significance of operative complications in patients with hepatocellular carcinoma who underwent hepatic resection. Eur J Surg Oncol 2009;35(11):1179–85.

40. American Joint Committee on Cancer. Liver (including intrahepatic bile ducts). In: Fleming ID, et al, editors. AJCC cancer staging manual. Philadelphia: Lippincott-Raven; 1998. p. 98–126.

41. Makuuchi M, Belghiti J, Belli G, et al. IHPBA concordant classification of primary liver cancer: working group report. J Hepatobiliary Pancreat Surg 2003;10(1): 26–30.

42. Vauthey JN, Lauwers GY, Esnaola NF, et al. Simplified staging for hepatocellular carcinoma. J Clin Oncol 2002;20(6):1527–36.

43. American Joint Committee on Cancer. Liver (including intrahepatic bile ducts). In: Greene FL, et al, editors. AJCC cancer staging manual. New York: Springer; 2002. p. 131–8.

44. Okuda K, Ohtsuki T, Obata H. Natural history of hepatocellular carcinoma and prognosis in relation to treatment: study of 850 patients. Cancer 1985;56(4): 918–28.

45. Llovet JM, Bru C, Bruix J. Prognosis of hepatocellular carcinoma: the BCLC staging classification. Semin Liver Dis 1999;19(3):329–38.

46. Prospective validation of the CLIP score: a new prognostic system for patients with cirrhosis and hepatocellular carcinoma. The Cancer of the Liver Italian Program (CLIP) Investigators. Hepatology 2000;31(4):840–5.

47. Kudo M, Chung H, Osaki Y, et al. Prognostic staging system for hepatocellular carcinoma (CLIP score): its value and limitations, and a proposal for a new staging system, the Japan Integrated Staging Score (JIS score). J Gastroenterol 2003;38(3):207–15.

48. Weber SM, Jarnagin WR, Klimstra D, et al. Intrahepatic cholangiocarcinoma: resectability, recurrence pattern, and outcomes. J Am Coll Surg 2001;193(4): 384–91.

49. Uenishi T, Hirohashi K, Kubo S, et al. Clinicopathological factors predicting outcome after resection of mass-forming cholangiocarcinoma. Br J Surg 2001; 88(7):969–74.

50. Suzuki S, Sakaguchi T, Yokoi Y, et al. Clinicopathological prognostic factors and impact of surgical treatment of mass-forming intrahepatic cholangiocarcinoma. World J Surg 2002;26(6):687–93.

51. Shirabe K, Mano Y, Taketomi A, et al. Clinicopathological prognostic factors after hepatectomy for patients with mass-forming intrahepatic cholangiocarcinoma: relevance of the lymphatic invasion index. Ann Surg Oncol 2010;17(7):1816–22.

52. Saxena A, Chua TC, Sarkar A, et al. Clinicopathologic and treatment-related factors influencing recurrence and survival after hepatic resection intrahepatic cholangiocarcinoma: a 19-year experience from an established Australian hepatobiliary unit. J Gastrointest Surg 2010;14(7):1128–38.

53. Ohtsuka A, Ito H, Kimura F, et al. Results of surgical treatment for intrahepatic cholangiocarcinoma and clinicopathological factors influencing survival. Br J Surg 2002;89(12):1525–31.

54. Cho SY, Park SJ, Kim SH, et al. Survival analysis of intrahepatic cholangiocarcinoma after resection. Ann Surg Oncol 2010;17(7):1823–30.

55. Wang Y, Li J, Xia Y, et al. Prognostic nomogram for intrahepatic cholangiocarcinoma after partial hepatectomy. J Clin Oncol 2013;31(9):1188–95.

56. Cherqui D, Tantawi B, Alon R, et al. Intrahepatic cholangiocarcinoma. Results of aggressive surgical management. Arch Surg 1995;130(10):1073–8.

57. Su H, Tsay SH, Wu CC, et al. Factors influencing postoperative morbidity, mortality, and survival after resection for hilar cholangiocarcinoma. Ann Surg 1996;223(4):384–94.

58. Burke EX, Jarnagin WR, Hochwald SN, et al. Hilar cholangiocarcinoma: patterns of spread, the importance of hepatic resection for curative operation, and a presurgical clinical staging system. Ann Surg 1998;228(3):385–94.

59. Tsao JI, Nimura Y, Kamiya J, et al. Management of hilar cholangiocarcinoma: comparison of an American and a Japanese experience. Ann Surg 2000;232(2):166–74.

60. Jarnagin WR, Fong Y, DeMatteo RP, et al. Staging, resectability, and outcome in 225 patients with hilar cholangiocarcinoma. Ann Surg 2001;234(4):507–17.

61. International Union Against Cancer. TNM classification of malignant tumours. New York: Wiley-Liss; 1997.

62. Okabayashi T, Yamamoto K, Kosuge T, et al. A new staging system for mass-forming intrahepatic cholangiocarcinoma: analysis of preoperative and postoperative variables. Cancer 2001;92(9):2374–83.

63. American Joint Committee on Cancer. Liver. In: Edge SB, et al, editors. AJCC Cancer Staging Manual. New York: Springer; 2010. p. 191–210.

64. Nathan H, Aloia TA, Vauthey JN, et al. A proposed staging system for intrahepatic cholangiocarcinoma. Ann Surg Oncol 2009;16(10):14–22.

65. Jiang W, Zeng ZC, Tang ZY, et al. A prognostic scoring system based on clinical features of intrahepatic cholangiocarcinoma: the Fudan score. Ann Oncol 2011;22(7):1644–52.

66. Hyder O, Marques H, Pulitano C, et al. A nomogram to predict long-term survival after resection for intrahepatic cholangiocarcinoma: an Eastern and Western experience. JAMA Surg 2014;149(5):432–8.

67. Bismuth H, Corlette MB. Intrahepatic cholangioenteric anastomosis in carcinoma of the hilus of the liver. Surg Gynecol Obstet 1975;140(2):170–8.

68. Deoliveira ML, Schulick RD, Nimua Y, et al. New staging system and a registry for perihilar cholangiocarcinoma. Hepatology 2011;53(4):1363–71.

69. Tomlinson JS, Jarnagin WR, DeMatteo RP, et al. Actual 10-year survival after resection of colorectal liver metastases defines cure. J Clin Oncol 2007;25(29):4575–80.

70. Pulitano C, Castillo F, Aldrighette L, et al. What defined 'cure' after liver resection for colorectal metastases? Results after 10 years of follow-up. HPB (Oxford) 2010; 12(4):244–9.

71. Choti MA, Sitzmann JV, Tiburi MF, et al. Trends in long-term survival following liver resection for hepatic colorectal metastases. Ann Surg 2002;235(6):759–66.

72. Andres A, Majno PE, Morel P, et al. Improved long-term outcome of surgery for advanced colorectal liver metastases: reasons and implications for management on the basis of a severity score. Ann Surg Oncol 2008;15(1):134–43.

73. House MG, Ito H, Gonen M, et al. Survival after hepatic resection for metastatic colorectal cancer: trends in outcomes for 1,600 patients during two decades at a single institution. J Am Coll Surg 2010;210(5):752–5.

74. Vigano L, Russolillo N, Ferrero A, et al. Evolution of long-term outcome of liver resection for colorectal metastases: analysis of actual 5-year survival rates over two decades. Ann Surg Oncol 2012;19(6):2035–44.

75. Schlag P, Hohenberger P, Herfarth C. Resection of liver metastases in colorectal cancer – competitive analysis of treatment results in synchronous versus metachronous metastases. Eur J Surg Oncol 1990;16(4):360–5.

76. Scheele J, Stang R, Altendort-Hofmann A, et al. Resection of colorectal liver metastases. World J Surg 1995;19(1):59–71.

77. Fong Y, Fortner J, Sun RL, et al. Clinical score for predicting recurrence after hepatic resection for metastatic colorectal cancer: analysis of 1001 consecutive cases. Ann Surg 1999;230(3):309–21.

78. Ambiru S, Miyazaki M, Isono T, et al. Hepatic resection for colorectal metastases: analysis of prognostic factors. Dis Colon Rectum 1999;42(5):632–9.

79. Yamada H, Kondo S, Okushiba S, et al. Analysis of predictive factors for recurrence after hepatectomy for colorectal liver metastases. World J Surg 2001; 25(9):1121–33.

80. Tsai MS, Su YH, Ho MC, et al. Clinicopathological features and prognosis in resectable synchronous and metachronous colorectal liver metastasis. Ann Surg Oncol 2007;14(2):786–94.

81. Cady B, Stone MD, McDermott WV Jr, et al. Technical and biological factors in disease-free survival after hepatic resection for colorectal cancer metastases. Arch Surg 1992;127(5):561–8.

82. Allen PJ, Kemeny N, Jarnagin W, et al. Importance of response to neoadjuvant chemotherapy in patients undergoing resection of synchronous colorectal liver metastases. J Gastrointest Surg 2003;7(1):109–15.

83. Small RM, Lubezky N, Schmueli E, et al. Response to chemotherapy predicts survival following resection of hepatic colo-rectal metastases in patients treated with neoadjuvant therapy. J Surg Oncol 2009;99(2):93–8.

84. Broquet A, Abdalla EK, Kopetz S, et al. High survival rate after two-stage resection of advanced colorectal liver metastases: response-based selection and complete resection define outcome. J Clin Oncol 2011;29(8):1083–90.

85. Gallagher DJ, Zheng J, Capanu M, et al. Response to neoadjuvant chemotherapy does not predict overall survival for patients with synchronous colorectal hepatic metastases. Ann Surg Oncol 2009;16(7):1844–51.

86. Khambata-Ford S, Garrett CR, Meropol NJ, et al. Expression of epiregulin and amphiregulin and K-ras mutation status predict disease control in metastatic colorectal cancer patients treated with cetuximab. J Clin Oncol 2007;25(2):3230–7.

87. Karapetis CS, Khambata-Ford S, Jonker DJ, et al. K-ras mutations and benefit from cetuximab in advanced colorectal cancer. N Engl J Med 2008;359(17): 1757–65.

88. Levi F, Karaboue A, Gorden L, et al. Cetuximab and circadian chronomodulated chemotherapy as salvage treatment for metastatic colorectal cancer (mCRC): safety, efficacy and improved secondary surgical resectability. Cancer Chemother Pharmacol 2011;67(2):339–48.

89. Nordlinger B, Guiguet M, Vaillant JC, et al. Surgical resection of colorectal carcinoma metastases to the liver. A prognostic scoring system to improve case selection, based on 1568 patients. Association Francaise de Chirurgie Cancer 1996; 77(7):1254–62.

90. Iwatsuki S, Dvorchik I, Madariaga JR, et al. Hepatic resection for metastatic colorectal adenocarcinoma: a proposal of a prognostic scoring system. J Am Coll Surg 1999;189(3):291–9.

91. Nagashima I, Takada T, Matsuda K, et al. A new scoring system to classify patients with colorectal liver metastases: proposal of criteria to select candidates for hepatic resection. J Hepatobiliary Pancreat Surg 2004;11(2):79–83.

92. Rees M, Tekkis PP, Welsh FK, et al. Evaluation of long-term survival after hepatic resection for metastatic colorectal cancer: a multifactorial model of 929 patients. Ann Surg 2008;247(1):125–35.

93. Merkel S, Bialecki D, Meyer T, et al. Comparison of clinical risk scores predicting prognosis after resection of colorectal liver metastases. J Surg Oncol 2009; 100(5):349–57.

94. Rahbari NN, Reissfelder C, Schulze-Bergkamen H, et al. Adjuvant therapy after resection of colorectal liver metastases: the predictive value of the MSKCC clinical risk score in the era of modern chemotherapy. BMC Cancer 2014;14:174.

95. Kattan MW, Gonen M, Jarnagin WR, et al. A nomogram for predicting disease-specific survival after hepatic resection for metastatic colorectal cancer. Ann Surg 2008;247(2):282–7.

96. Thomay AA, Nagorney DM, Cohen SJ, et al. Modern chemotherapy mitigates adverse prognostic effect of regional nodal metastases in stage IV colorectal cancer. J Gastrointest Surg 2014;18(1):69–74.

97. Blazer DG 3rd, Kishi Y, Maru DM, et al. Pathologic response to preoperative chemotherapy: a new outcome end point after resection of hepatic colorectal metastases. J Clin Oncol 2008;26(33):5344–51.

Modern Technical Approaches in Resectional Hepatic Surgery

Christoph W. Michalski, MD[a], Kevin G. Billingsley, MD[b],*

KEYWORDS

- Liver surgery • Primary liver tumors • Liver metastasis • Surgical techniques

KEY POINTS

- Major liver surgery can be performed safely.
- Precise preoperative treatment planning is required.
- Intraoperative ultrasound facilitates management of inflow and outflow to and from the liver.
- Low central venous pressure and meticulous transection are important for minimizing blood loss.

INTRODUCTION

Techniques and indications for resection of liver tumors have considerably evolved during the last 2 decades. Liver surgery can be performed more safely than ever and the number of liver resections has increased in the past years.[1–3] Multimodal treatment for colorectal liver metastases has expanded the group of patients who are potentially eligible for liver resection. Surgical approaches to complex resection have been further augmented by a variety of electrosurgical devices and the increasing use of preoperative portal vein embolization to augment the size and function of the planned liver remnant.

The critical elements for safety in resectional hepatic surgery include meticulous preoperative evaluation, including assessment of liver function and delineation of hepatic anatomy. Intraoperative management involves the use of a low central venous pressure anesthetic technique and seamless communication between the anesthesiologist and the surgeon. Resection involves techniques to control the inflow into the liver, techniques to control the vascular outflow (hepatic veins), and techniques to

The authors have nothing to disclose.

[a] Division of Surgical Oncology, Oregon Health and Science University, 3181 Southwest Sam Jackson Park Road, Portland, OR 97239, USA; [b] Division of Surgical Oncology, Department of Surgery, Oregon Health and Science University, 3181 Southwest Sam Jackson Park Road, Portland, OR 97239, USA

* Corresponding author.

E-mail address: billingk@ohsu.edu

Surg Oncol Clin N Am 24 (2015) 57–72
http://dx.doi.org/10.1016/j.soc.2014.09.007
surgonc.theclinics.com

divide the liver parenchyma and navigate within the liver. This article reviews these elements in detail.

INDICATIONS FOR LIVER RESECTION

Although most resectional surgery is performed for primary or metastatic liver cancer, in selected cases liver resection is also performed for benign disease.

Benign Neoplasms

The most common benign neoplasm requiring resection is hepatic adenoma. These lesions may grow to be large and symptomatic. They are associated with a small risk of malignant transformation,[4] and a risk of rupture. Both focal nodular hyperplasia (FNH) and hemangioma are benign lesions, and resection is only indicated if patients are clearly symptomatic from the tumor. Because FNH is an entirely benign neoplasm, resection is restricted only to situations in which the neoplasm is associated with life-limiting symptomatology. These symptoms often involve persistent abdominal pain, fullness, and early satiety. Hepatic adenomas are associated with a risk of hemorrhage and a small risk of malignant transformation.[5] Resection is generally recommended for lesions that are more than 5 cm in diameter, particularly if all hormonal therapy has been terminated and no additional regression in the size of the lesion has occurred. Unlike with malignant neoplasia, surgical margins are not critical in determining outcome and surgeons should not risk critical inflow or outflow structures in an effort to obtain wide surgical margins.

Metastatic Colorectal Cancer

Resectable metastatic colorectal cancer is the most common indication for liver resection. The prognosis after complete resection of colorectal liver metastases is variable and is associated with factors such as number of lesions, size of lesions, synchronicity of disease, extent of lymph node involvement.[6–8] Patients that are treated with complete resection may be afforded long term survival. The 5 year survival rate varies between 30% and 45%.[6,8]

From an oncologic standpoint, the most important aim is to clear all liver disease and to achieve negative margins. Because most liver resections are performed for colorectal cancer liver metastasis (CRLM), they frequently involve multimodal treatment, mainly preoperative chemotherapy with regimens including either oxaliplatin or irinotecan as the principle chemotherapeutic agent. A randomized trial conducted by the European Organisation for Research and Treatment of Cancer (EORTC) demonstrated that perioperative oxaliplatin-based chemotherapy improves progression-free but not overall survival.[9,10] In addition to disease control, preoperative chemotherapy has the ability to render unresectable disease resectable in a small subset of patients, by virtue of substantial disease response. The optimal extent of surgical margin remains controversial; however, evidence suggests that microscopically positive surgical margins are associated with increased disease recurrence. Therefore, microscopically negative margins remain a focus for all hepatic resections. Numerous articles have shed light on this issue, and although it has been controversially discussed for some time, agreement now exists that a negative margin is a clear prognostic factor and that at least 1 mm is required for the definition of a negative margin.

Neuroendocrine Liver Metastases

Neuroendocrine tumors, particularly carcinoid, although often multifocal within the liver, tend to be indolent in progression, and patients will derive survival benefit from resection of liver disease.[11] These operations often involve multiple resections of small lesions. These patients are also treated with nonresection liver-directed therapy.[12]

Noncolorectal Nonneuroendocrine Metastases

Few definitive data exist to support resection of other metastatic tumors from the liver. However, long-term disease control may be provided after liver resection in a variety of histologies, including renal cell cancer, breast cancer, anal cancer, melanoma, and rare cases lung cancer. Liver resection should not be considered standard for most individuals with these tumors, and decision making should be performed on an individual basis by a multidisciplinary team.

Hepatocellular Cancer

Resection is a potentially curative treatment for patients with hepatocellular carcinoma (HCC). However, most patients in North America with the disease are not surgical candidates because of the presence of cirrhosis or extensive disease. Generally, if no liver disease is present and the lesion is technically amenable to resection, surgery should be the first option, unless transplantation, according to current criteria, is an option. If liver disease is present, treatment is dictated by the extent of the disease. To this end, the Barcelona Clinic Liver Cancer classification is used.[13] Patients with disease stages 0 and A may be suitable for resection, whereas patients with advanced disease stages B to D have a worse prognosis and should probably not undergo resection. However, recent data show that some patients with BCLC stage B disease may actually be able to undergo resection and may benefit from surgery.[14]

Cholangiocellular Cancer

Of the 3 types of cholangiocellular carcinoma (CCC)—intrahepatic, perihilar, and distal—intrahepatic and perihilar CCC can be approached surgically, if the extent of disease technically allows resection and no extrahepatic disease is present. Although technical considerations for intrahepatic CCC are comparable to those of CRLM and HCC, perihilar CCCs (Klatskin tumors) almost always require hepatic resection combined with resection of a part of the biliary tree.[15] Orthotopic liver transplantation is highly controversial and is performed in only a few centers worldwide.[16] Distal CCC generally involves the intrapancreatic component of the bile duct, and surgical therapy requires pancreaticoduodenectomy.

This article provides an overview of the patient selection process, perioperative management, and technical details of modern liver surgery. Treatment of CRLM is emphasized because this condition is now the most common indication for liver surgery, and its management integrates many subspecialties into complex treatment schemes.

PREOPERATIVE FUNCTIONAL EVALUATION

Preoperative prediction of size and function of the liver remnant is important mainly for resections in patients with underlying liver disease (eg, fibrosis/cirrhosis, chemotherapy-induced liver damage) and for extended resections with presumably small future liver remnants (FLRs). Of these, right trisectionectomy (or extended right hepatectomy, including resection of segments 4a and 4b) is the most common extended variation. FLR prediction can be performed using different approaches, including imaging-based volume calculations and/or functional assessment analyses such as the indocyanine green clearance rate.[17,18] In healthy livers, FLR volumes of approximately 30% are sufficient for postoperative liver function. Although the imaging calculations provide an exact prediction of the FLR volume, extensive clinical experience is required to determine which patients may actually do well with an extended resection, particularly if the FLR volume is less than 30%. In surgery for metastatic colorectal cancer, extended preoperative treatment with chemotherapy may be associated with chemotherapy-associated steatohepatitis.[19] This chemotherapy-associated process will compromise liver regeneration and must be considered when contemplating extensive resection. To increase the number of patients eligible for extended resection, portal vein embolization and staged hepatectomies have been introduced.[20–22] Portal vein embolization increases the FLR volume in many cases, and this allows for resection of disease deemed unresectable initially.[22–24]

ANATOMY AND TERMINOLOGY OF LIVER RESECTION

Couinaud[25] outlined the anatomic framework for modern liver surgery by defining the segments of the liver according to the portal vein inflow. However, the recent increase in liver resection, its wide implementation in clinical practice, and the development of extended liver resections necessitated a more practical classification for daily clinical use. The scientific committee of the International Hepato-Pancreato-Biliary Association defined a joint classification in 2000 (the Brisbane classification).[26] This classification defines 3 orders of liver resection: (1) right or left hepatectomy or hemihepatectomy; (2) right or left, anterior or posterior sectionectomy, and right or left hepatectomy plus left medial or right anterior section, respectively; and (3) segmentectomies. This comprehensive classification provides increased precision in describing resectional liver operations. It has been widely adopted in reporting outcomes of liver surgery; however, major confusion still stems from mistakenly using the term *trisegmentectomy* for *trisectionectomy* (extended right or left hepatectomy). This article uniformly uses the Brisbane terminology (**Table 1**).

TECHNICAL CONSIDERATIONS AND OUTCOMES AFTER LIVER SURGERY

Compared with other major abdominal operations, surgery of the liver still carries a higher risk of perioperative or even intraoperative mortality. Hemorrhage and postoperative liver failure are the major factors associated with postoperative mortality. Technical advances have thus been mainly achieved through better resolution and use of intraoperative ultrasound, and the development of techniques allowing for meticulous inflow and outflow control. In addition, recent years have brought increasing focus on blood-sparing transection and more exact preoperative prediction of size and function of the liver remnant.

Intraoperative ultrasound of the liver should be used in all cases to determine the exact anatomy of the portal pedicles (inflow and indirect visualization of the biliary tree) and the hepatic veins (outflow), and the localization and extension of the tumors. To achieve this, high-resolution ultrasound is required, which incorporates duplex function and vascular Doppler capability. Ultrasound also helps determine whether additional lesions are present in the liver, particularly in the future liver remnant, and helps assess the relationship of the tumors to the intrahepatic vascular and biliary structures.

Once the exact anatomy has been determined, extensive mobilization of the right or left liver lobe (or both) is advisable. Although potentially time-consuming, this allows for inflow and outflow control, which limits blood loss in situations wherein intrahepatic control is difficult. Blood-sparing transection can be performed using a wide variety of techniques and devices, of which none has been shown to be clearly superior.[27]

Table 1
Brisbane classification and terminology of liver anatomy and resection

Anatomic Term	Liver Segments	Term for Surgical Resection
First-order division		
Right hemiliver OR Right liver	5–8 (+/− 1)	Right hepatectomy OR Right hemihepatectomy (+/− segment 1)
Left hemiliver OR Left liver	2–4 (+/− 1)	Left hepatectomy OR Left hemihepatectomy (+/− segment 1)
Second-order division		
Right anterior section	5,8	Add "-ectomy" to any of the anatomic terms, as in *right anterior sectionectomy*
Right posterior section	6,7	Right posterior sectionectomy
Left medial section	4	Left medial sectionectomy OR Resection segment 4 OR Segmentectomy 4
Left lateral section	2,3	Left lateral sectionectomy OR Bisegmentectomy 2,3
Right hemiliver plus left medial section	4–8 (+/− 1)	Right trisectionectomy OR Extended right hepatectomy OR Extended right hemihepatectomy
Left hemiliver plus right anterior section	2–4 plus 5,8 (+/− 1)	Left trisectionectomy OR Extended left hepatectomy OR Extended left hemihepatectomy
Third-order division		
Segments 1–9	Any one of segment1 to segment9	Segmentectomy
2 contiguous segments	Any one of Sg1 to Sg9 in continuity	Bisegmentectomy

Adapted from The Terminology Committee of the IHPBA. The Brisbane 2000 terminology of hepatic anatomy and resections. HPB 2000;2:333–9; with permission.

Acceptable techniques[28] include clamp fracture,[29] staple transection,[30] water jet dissection,[31] and ultrasonic dissection.[32] Although perhaps more time-consuming than other methods, many surgeons favor ultrasonic dissection for its ability to allow precise identification and control of intrahepatic pedicles and veins.[32]

POSITIONING AND SETUP

Patients should be positioned supine with both arms extended. This positioning provides access to both arms for intravenous therapy and provides the opportunity to extend a right subcostal incision laterally. The exception to this is if the surgeon anticipates using a right thoracoabdominal incision, which is sometimes used for very large tumors of the right liver. In this case, the ideal setup involves suspending the right arm over the patient's head with an airplane splint and elevating the right chest slightly to facilitate chest exposure.

The operating lights should be positioned exactly before the patient is prepared. Because intraoperative ultrasound is required for precise definition of liver anatomy, placing the ultrasound device in the surgeon's field of vision before starting the procedure is advisable. Once positioning and setup of the instrumentation is completed, a team time-out is performed. This procedure emphasizes the interaction of the surgeons with the anesthesiologists and nurses, and is the time to reiterate the potential risks of liver surgery, such as blood loss and hemodynamic instability. The need for a low central venous pressure, particularly during the transection phase, and for blood products in the operating room should also be discussed at this point.

INCISIONS AND RETRACTION

A multitude of potential incisions can be performed in open liver surgery, depending on the extent of resection and the preference of the surgeon. For (extended) right hepatectomy, the authors usually use a right subcostal incision with midline extension. The subcostal incision is performed at approximately a 3-fingers width below the costal margin, with a maximal extension to the iliac crest line on the right side. The midline incision is extended up to the xiphoid, sometimes along the sides of the xiphoid up to the sternum, to allow for better exposure of the suprahepatic vena cava and the hepatic veins. If mobilization of the liver is difficult, the incision may be extended to the left subcostally. In cases of large right-sided liver tumors, a thoracoabdominal incision is sometimes required. This procedure involves a midline incision with an extension across the right hemiabdomen, with additional extension to the right chest. The costal margin is divided and the chest is opened in the eighth or ninth intercostal space. The peripheral diaphragm is divided and later repaired. The left liver can also usually be accessed with the right subcostal incision with midline extension. If the left lateral segments are large and extensive mobilization of the left side is required, a bilateral subcostal incision (with or without midline extension) may be helpful.

Before the retractors are placed, the ligamentum of teres and the falciform ligament should be divided. This technique prevents unwanted tearing of the liver capsule and the parenchyma. A large number of self-retaining retractor systems are available, which allow for forced retraction of the upper and lower parts of the incision, using bilateral crossbars on top and 2 angled arms below. Several body wall retractors are used to expose as much of the liver as possible, whereas the porta hepatis is exposed with malleables.

INTRAOPERATIVE ULTRASONOGRAPHY

The authors use intraoperative ultrasonography and duplex ultrasound in all liver resections. After mobilization of the liver, the portal pedicle and hepatic vein anatomy are analyzed. Portal venous and hepatic arterial flow to the right and left side of the liver is determined; this is the baseline analysis, which is used for comparison after test-clamping the pedicles to the side of resection.

Hepatic venous anatomy is analyzed, with a particular emphasis on the route of the middle hepatic vein, which in many cases is precisely within the line of transection. Larger branches of the middle hepatic vein can be marked with electrocautery on the surface of the liver; this allows for early recognition of those during parenchymal transection.

The liver is then scanned for the tumor or metastasis. The findings are compared with the preoperative imaging, and additional lesions may be identified. The relation of the tumors to the portal pedicles and the hepatic veins is determined. The plane of resection is defined accordingly.

HEPATIC MOBILIZATION

Except for superficial wedge resections, mobilization of the involved side of the liver is generally mandated. For right hepatectomy, mobilization of the right liver is usually sufficient and advisable to prevent kinking of the remnant. For left hepatectomy, complete mobilization of the liver is most of the time required to allow for control of the inferior vena cava (IVC).

Mobilization of the right liver is started with a dissection toward the hepatic veins, taking particular care not to injure these vessels. The right coronary and triangular ligaments are divided, allowing for retraction of the liver to the left side. The vena cava is then carefully exposed and the adrenal gland is dissected off of the IVC. Small veins from the adrenal gland to the IVC are tied off. If the IVC feels filled and firm, communication with the anesthesiologist is paramount to start reducing the central venous pressure. Proceeding with mobilization of the liver off the vena cava at a central venous pressure of greater than 5 may lead to considerable blood loss if there is injury to a retrohepatic vein. The liver is retracted further to the left side and stepwise exposure of the short hepatic veins is achieved. At this point, it is important to control as many small veins toward the left side as possible to facilitate IVC control during the transection phase. The caudate lobe sometimes extends on the IVC to the right side of the liver, necessitating its division with a stapler device. Depending on the planned extent of resection and the individual anatomy, the right hepatic vein (and potentially the middle hepatic vein) is dissected and controlled with vessel loops. At the cephalad aspect of the liver, a circumferential band of tissue that encircles the IVC is inevitably present below the hepatic veins. This so-called caval ligament may be divided with a stapling device or electrosurgical device. Once this band is divided, access to the right hepatic vein is optimized.

Mobilization of the left side of the liver is started similarly with dissection of the triangular ligament and the ventral border of the left hepatic vein. The left lateral segments are mobilized by dividing the gastrohepatic and left coronary ligaments. The left (and possibly the middle) hepatic veins are dissected and controlled with vessel loops. If the caudate lobe must be resected, complete mobilization is best achieved through controlling the small vein branches to the IVC from both the right and the left sides in a step-by-step fashion.

APPROACH TO INFLOW CONTROL

Among the different ways to gain inflow control to the liver, the authors use the 2 general methods depending on the underlying disease and the planned extent of resection. They use intrahepatic control during transection of the liver most of the time for resections of liver metastases and intrahepatic cholangiocarcinomas, and mainly perform extrahepatic portal dissection and division of the respective vessels for hilar cholangiocarcinoma or in clinical situations in which the disease is particularly close to the hilus. However, a combination of both techniques is particularly useful for fibrotic/cirrhotic liver resections, wherein the time of intermittent Pringle maneuvers must be kept as short as possible.[33–35]

Intrahepatic/Intraparenchymal Inflow Control

Because dissection of the porta hepatis presents a risk of inadvertent injury to the biliary tree, particularly also devascularization of parts of the bile ducts of the liver remnant, intrahepatic control of the portal pedicles is a reasonable approach to liver metastasis and intrahepatic cholangiocarcinoma resections. If intraoperative ultrasonography demonstrates regular anatomy and patent inflow to both liver lobes, the plane of transection is scored on the liver surface and the parenchyma is divided toward the main right or left portal pedicle. It is not necessary to control the pedicles within the liver before transection. Intermittent inflow control using the Pringle maneuver controls bleeding, and the pedicles may be approached by simply dividing the liver parenchyma along the line of planned transection until the pedicles are encountered and are dissected circumferentially. In the authors' practice, the ultrasonic dissector is preferred, which is ideal for precise skeletonization of the pedicles.

When the pedicles are reached, they are carefully dissected without injuring the biliary system, and then are encircled and test-clamped. Repeat ultrasound after test-clamping is used to ensure that the inflow to the future liver remnant is patent. Division of the respective portal pedicle is performed using vascular staplers or clamps and suturing techniques. If possible, from an oncologic standpoint, dissecting the subpedicles is advisable in case a right hepatectomy is planned (eg, the right anterior and posterior portal pedicles). This approach allows for safe identification of the right versus the left portal structures and, in the case of a right hepatectomy, for avoiding injury to the left main portal pedicle. For left hepatectomy, the left main portal pedicle may be dissected at the base of the umbilical fissure (after ensuring that the disease does not encroach on this area). Control of the left pedicle at this point assures complete inflow control to the anatomic left liver while also providing a margin of safety to avoid damage to the right portal pedicle. This approach decreases the risk of compromising the portal inflow to the (left) liver remnant. Often little room is available for the division of the anterior and posterior pedicles because of a close margin to the tumor. In these cases, the authors use an DST Series TA 45 stapler (Coviden, Mansfield, Massachusetts, USA) on the remnant side and cut the specimen side open, and then generously oversew the vessels/bile ducts on the specimen side. During intraparenchymal dissection of the main portal pedicles, large branches of the middle hepatic vein may be encountered; pretransection ultrasonography can help determining this risk. Careful dissection of these branches close to the portal pedicles allows for a blood-sparing approach to intraparenchymal portal pedicle division.

During parenchymal transection, the authors perform intermittent Pringle maneuvers for 5 to 10 minutes, and then open the inflow to the liver for 3 to 5 minutes. In their experience, this has not hampered the outcome of resection on noncirrhotic livers but has allowed for low blood loss surgeries.[36]

However, in cases of large tumors approaching the main right or left portal pedicles, or in patients with fibrotic/cirrhotic livers and a low reserve, extrahepatic dissection and early ligation of the hepatic artery and portal vein to the involved hemiliver may be required.

Extrahepatic/Porta Hepatis Inflow Control

When the liver disease is close to the hilus, it is appropriate to perform hilar dissection and extrahepatic control of hilar structures. To gain access to the extrahepatic main portal structures, the cystic and hilar plates are lowered and the right or left hepatic artery is encountered. The respective artery is controlled with vessel loops at this point and the portal vein is dissected and controlled extrahepatically with vessel loops. The artery is divided after adequate dissection has been performed to assure understanding of the hepatic arterial anatomy. Doppler ultrasound is performed to confirm the extrahepatic portal anatomy. Because access to the portal vein bifurcation is usually only possible after dividing the right (or left) hepatic artery, the respective artery is transected at this point. Once the portal vein bifurcation is safely identified, the respective branches to the right or left side of the liver are divided, either using a vascular stapler device or vascular clamps and suturing techniques. For cases in which this is difficult, test-clamping of the respective main portal vein branch is performed, followed by Duplex ultrasound of the future liver remnant.

APPROACH TO OUTFLOW CONTROL

As depicted in "Hepatic Mobilization," outflow control is achieved using several distinct approaches. First, control of the right and/or middle and/or left hepatic veins is achieved through careful dissection around the respective vessels during mobilization of the liver. The small hepatic veins into the IVC are controlled during mobilization of the liver off the IVC. Control of as many of these small veins as possible is advisable to prevent tearing during liver parenchymal transection, particularly because congestion of the caudate lobe is rare and usually does not lead to overt postoperative complications. Thus, the small veins draining the caudate lobe can be transected safely.

The respective hepatic veins are divided after dividing the inflow to the respective side of the liver during the transection phase. Division of the hepatic veins is performed using a vascular stapler. It is important to carefully check the systemic blood pressure after closing but before firing the stapler. In rare cases, division of one of the major hepatic veins compromises the blood flow through the IVC and back to the heart. If the blood pressure decreases, the clamp should be removed and repositioned so no obstruction to caval flow is present. Duplex ultrasound should also be used to document flow in the other hepatic veins. If no venous outflow is present from the planned remnant, the vein should not be divided. This situation is rare but necessitates termination of the operation.

TECHNIQUES OF PARENCHYMAL TRANSECTION

A wide variety of parenchymal transection techniques exists, of which none has been proven to be superior.[29,30,37,38] However, meticulous transection techniques have recently gained increasing attention, whereas finger fracture and clamp crushing are less frequently used. For anatomic liver resections, the authors use the harmonic scalpel to divide the first 1 to 2 cm of liver parenchyma, followed by ultrasonic dissection. Depending on the tissue density, ultrasonic dissection allows the extent of fragmentation capability to be defined. Small vessels are controlled with either electrocautery or any bipolar energy vessel-sealing instrument.

Larger pedicles are divided using clips, ties, or vascular staplers. In nonanatomic resections, such as wedge resections, ultrasonic shears and/or bipolar vessel-sealing instruments together with clamp crushing can be used efficiently without increasing the rate of complications. **Table 2** summarizes the advantages of the available instruments for hepatic transection.

SPECIFIC PROCEDURES
Right Hemihepatectomy

The crucial initial step in right hemihepatectomy is complete mobilization of the right liver. Intraoperative ultrasound is used to define the anatomy of the main right portal pedicle and its relation to the middle hepatic vein. The line of transection is scored through the gallbladder fossa and on top of the liver toward the plane between the right and the middle hepatic vein. It is taken down just to the right of the gallbladder fossa, toward the caudate lobe and the IVC. The authors always open the anterior plane first

Table 2
Liver tissue transection devices

Authors	Technique	Resection Major	Resection Minor	Transfusion (n)	EBL (mL)	Pringle Maneuver (n)
Arnoletti & Brodsky,[41] 1999	Finger fracture with vascular occlusion	49	0	N/A	500	49
Arru et al,[42] 2007	Ultrasonic dissector and harmonic scalpel	69	31	N/A	500	58
Ayav et al,[43] 2008	Habib 4X	11	51	1	267	0
Lupo et al,[44] 2007 (randomized)	Crush clamp	10	19	13	N/A	N/A
	Linear RFA	11	19	8	N/A	N/A
Cho et al,[45] 2009	Harmonic scalpel and water dissection	19	28	N/A	620	0
Wagman et al,[46] 2009	Habib 4X	31	45	11	427	20
Schmidbauer et al,[47] 2002	Ultracision	8	50	11	820	58
Takayama et al,[48] 2001 (randomized)	Ultrasonic dissector	24	42	N/A	515	48
	Crush clamp	24	42	N/A	452	52

Abbreviations: EBL, estimated blood loss; N/A, not available; RFA, radiofrequency ablation.
Data from Wagman LD, Lee B, Castillo E, et al. Liver resection using a four-prong radiofrequency transection device. Am Surg 2009;75(10):991–4.

and transect down to the main right portal pedicle. This pedicle is carefully dissected out and, if possible and oncologically reasonable, the right anterior and posterior pedicles are exposed selectively. At this point, it is important not to deviate too far to the left side, particularly to avoid injury to the left-sided bile ducts. Test-clamping is crucial before dividing the pedicles to determine inflow to the left liver remnant. The pedicles are divided using a vascular stapler if possible. Alternatively, a TA stapler can be used or the pedicles can be clamped, divided, and oversewn. The right hepatic vein can then be divided with a vascular stapler to allow for even more mobilization of the liver.

During further transection toward the liver dome, the likelihood of encountering the middle hepatic vein increases significantly. To avoid bleeding from this vessel, the transection must be advanced forward carefully and small branches must be dissected and controlled selectively. Depending on the position of the lesion, the transection can be advanced on the right or left side of the middle hepatic vein. However, a left-sided transection may result in (some) congestion of segments 4a/b, and good drainage through the left hepatic vein is required.

Once the decision has been made regarding whether the middle hepatic vein should be preserved, this vessel may need to be dissected out and divided with a vascular stapler. Particular care must be taken at the final step of transection near the IVC to avoid overt bleeding from one of the vein remnants.

Extended Right Hepatectomy

With the increased use and efficacy of portal vein embolization of the right liver and the portal pedicles to segment 4, extended right hepatectomies have become significantly safer, and thus more common, resections. Again, the liver should be mobilized as much as possible, including the left lateral segments. All hepatic veins must be controlled. The line of transection will be right next to the falciform ligament; depending on the anatomy of the middle hepatic vein and the location of the lesion, the vein may be preserved. In addition, and with intraparenchymal inflow control, the transection plan will need to be taken parallel to the porta hepatis right above the hilar plate toward the gallbladder fossa and down to the caudate lobe. When an in-continuity caudate lobe resection is required, full mobilization of segment 1 must precede transection; in addition, a hepatotomy will need to be made on top of the caudate lobe, just below the left lateral segments and along the line of the ligamentum venosum. The anterior plane is opened first but, unlike with right hemihepatectomy, several larger pedicles into segment 4 will be encountered that need to be controlled with either ties or staplers. When advancing the transection down toward the main portal pedicle, particular care will need to be taken not to injure the left-sided portal structures. The transection will then be advanced along the portal bifurcation toward the right side, and can be completed as described in the section for right hemihepatectomies. Before dividing the pedicle, precise duplex ultrasound is recommended. In cases of Klatskin tumors extending to the left side, a partial resection of the left bile duct system may be required. This procedure frequently results in the division of several smaller bile ducts that will need to be reconstructed using a Roux en Y hepaticojejunostomy. Completion of transection at the dome of the liver again requires meticulous dissection of the middle hepatic vein to avoid bleeding. Because the liver remnant will be rather mobile, the authors advocate reattaching the triangular ligaments with several interrupted sutures.

Left Hemihepatectomy

Similar to right hemihepatectomy, the principal plane of resection is between segments 5/8 and 4a/b. Although it is a less frequently performed procedure, it is not particularly technically difficult. Mobilization of the right hemiliver is usually not required, except when the caudate lobe must also be resected. The central venous pressure should be kept as low as possible. The line of transection is scored along the segment 5/8 and 4a/b border and is taken down to the gallbladder fossa toward the left side of the liver, along the ligamentum venosum into the caudate lobe and on the ventral side of the IVC. For in-continuity caudate lobe resections, the transection is taken from the left main portal pedicle straight down toward the IVC. As in right hemihepatectomy, intraoperative ultrasound is mandated to guarantee preserved inflow to the right liver. The left main portal pedicle is divided at the base of the umbilical fissure, distal to the takeoff of the caudate lobe inflow, unless the caudate is being resected. The left hepatic vein is divided, usually in an intraparenchymal location, when advancing the transection toward the dome of the liver.

Central Hepatectomy

For larger tumors of the liver that involve segments IV, V, and VIII, a central hepatectomy may be an ideal approach. This resection will allow adequate tumor clearance and preserve functional liver on the right and left sides of the liver. **Fig. 1** depicts the surgical approach and shows the major structures that need to be transected.

The operation proceeds through generous mobilization of the right liver to facilitate exposure and dissection. The gallbladder is disengaged from the porta hepatis and the cystic artery and cystic duct are divided. The liver parenchyma is then opened to the right side of the umbilical fissure and the inflow pedicles to segment IV are transected with stapler or suture ligature (**Fig. 2**). Then, from a suprahilar position within the liver, the dissection is advanced laterally above the right main portal pedicle until the right anterior sectoral pedicle (V, VIII) is identified (**Fig. 3**). This pedicle is encircled and

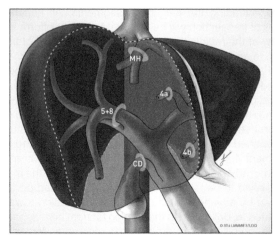

Fig. 1. Overview. CD, cystic duct; MH, middle hepatic vein.

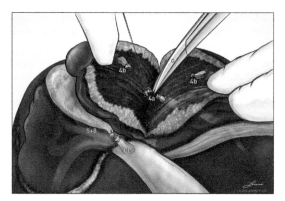

Fig. 2. Take down of portal pedicles 4a and 4b.

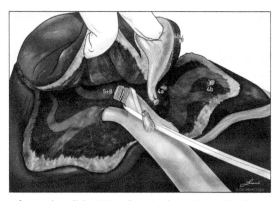

Fig. 3. Take down of portal pedicle 5/7 and cystic duct. CD, cystic duct.

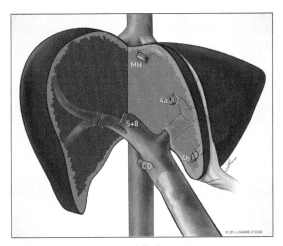

Fig. 4. Completion. CD, cystic duct; MH, middle hepatic vein.

test clamped. Preservation of flow to the right posterior sector should be demonstrated via duplex ultrasonography before this pedicle is transected. Demarcation of the right anterior sectoral pedicle should be evident (see **Fig. 3**). The pedicle should be divided, and the transection then completed by dividing the plane between segments 5/8 and 6/7. While transecting toward the base of segment 8, care should be taken to preserve the right hepatic vein. The middle hepatic vein will be divided close to the IVC, which completes the resection and allows for passing the specimen off of the table (**Fig. 4**).

Segmental Resections

Segmental and wedge resections are useful for selected indications, such as for treating multiple bilobar metastases and desired clearance of one lobe within a staged resection; for treating disease recurrence in the liver remnant; potential small for size liver remnant; when there is a need for short operative time because of patient comorbidities; and in debulking of a multitude of carcinoid/neuroendocrine tumor liver metastases. Although segmental resections have an advantage in terms of tissue preservation, this must be weighed against increased blood loss and a considerable risk of biliary complications.[39,40] Furthermore, these resections are more frequently associated with positive margins and, depending on their location, may lead to inadvertent injury to important portal structures. In the case of a planned staged resection, such an injury may render the second operation impossible. On the other hand, segmental resections can often be performed laparoscopically, reducing the inpatient time considerably.

REFERENCES

1. Dimick JB, Wainess RM, Cowan JA, et al. National trends in the use and outcomes of hepatic resection. J Am Coll Surg 2004;199(1):31–8.
2. Dokmak S, Fteriche FS, Borscheid R, et al. 2012 Liver resections in the 21st century: we are far from zero mortality. HPB 2013;15(2):908–15.
3. Jarnagin WR, Gonen M, Fong Y, et al. Improvement in perioperative outcome after hepatic resection: analysis of 1,803 consecutive cases over the past decade. Ann Surg 2002;236(4):397–406 [discussion: 406–7].

4. Karkar AM, Tang LH, Kashikar ND, et al. Management of hepatocellular adenoma: comparison of resection, embolization and observation. HPB (Oxford) 2013;15(3):235–43.
5. Bieze M, Busch OR, Tanis PJ, et al. Outcomes of liver resection in hepatocellular adenoma and focal nodular hyperplasia. HPB (Oxford) 2014;16(2):140–9.
6. de Jong MC, Pulitano C, Ribero D, et al. Rates and patterns of recurrence following curative intent surgery for colorectal liver metastasis: an international multi-institutional analysis of 1669 patients. Ann Surg 2009;250(3):440–8.
7. Scheele J, Stangl R, Altendorf-Hofmann A. Hepatic metastases from colorectal carcinoma: impact of surgical resection on the natural history. Br J Surg 1990; 77(11):1241–6.
8. Tomlinson JS, Jarnagin WR, DeMatteo RP, et al. Actual 10-year survival after resection of colorectal liver metastases defines cure. J Clin Oncol 2007;25(29): 4575–80.
9. Nordlinger B, Sorbye H, Glimelius B, et al. Perioperative chemotherapy with FOLFOX4 and surgery versus surgery alone for resectable liver metastases from colorectal cancer (EORTC Intergroup trial 40983): a randomised controlled trial. Lancet 2008;371(9617):1007–16.
10. Nordlinger B, Sorbye H, Glimelius B, et al. Perioperative FOLFOX4 chemotherapy and surgery versus surgery alone for resectable liver metastases from colorectal cancer (EORTC 40983): long-term results of a randomised, controlled, phase 3 trial. Lancet Oncol 2013;14(12):1208–15.
11. Frilling A, Modlin IM, Kidd M, et al. Recommendations for management of patients with neuroendocrine liver metastases. Lancet Oncol 2014;15(1):e8–21.
12. Mayo SC, Herman JM, Cosgrove D, et al. Emerging approaches in the management of patients with neuroendocrine liver metastasis: role of liver-directed and systemic therapies. J Am Coll Surg 2013;216(1):123–34.
13. Llovet JM, Fuster J, Bruix J, et al. The Barcelona approach: diagnosis, staging, and treatment of hepatocellular carcinoma. Liver Transpl 2004;10(2 Suppl 1): S115–20.
14. Zhong JH, Ke Y, Gong WF, et al. Hepatic resection associated with good survival for selected patients with intermediate and advanced-stage hepatocellular carcinoma. Ann Surg 2014;260(2):329–40.
15. Zaydfudim VM, Rosen CB, Nagorney DM. Hilar cholangiocarcinoma. Surg Oncol Clin N Am 2014;23(2):247–63.
16. Darwish Murad S, Kim WR, Harnois DM, et al. Efficacy of neoadjuvant chemoradiation, followed by liver transplantation, for perihilar cholangiocarcinoma at 12 US centers. Gastroenterology 2012;143(1):88–98.e3 [quiz: e14].
17. Hoekstra LT, de Graaf W, Nibourg GA, et al. Physiological and biochemical basis of clinical liver function tests: a review. Ann Surg 2013;257(1):27–36.
18. Ribero D, Amisano M, Bertuzzo F, et al. Measured versus estimated total liver volume to preoperatively assess the adequacy of the future liver remnant: which method should we use? Ann Surg 2013;258(5):801–6 [discussion: 806–7].
19. Chun YS, Laurent A, Maru D, et al. Management of chemotherapy-associated hepatotoxicity in colorectal liver metastases. Lancet Oncol 2009;10(3):278–86.
20. Huang SY, Aloia TA, Shindoh J, et al. Efficacy and safety of portal vein embolization for two-stage hepatectomy in patients with colorectal liver metastasis. J Vasc Interv Radiol 2014;25(4):608–17.
21. Shindoh J, Tzeng CW, Aloia TA, et al. Safety and efficacy of portal vein embolization before planned major or extended hepatectomy: an institutional experience of 358 patients. J Gastrointest Surg 2014;18(1):45–51.

22. Shindoh J, Vauthey JN, Zimmitti G, et al. Analysis of the efficacy of portal vein embolization for patients with extensive liver malignancy and very low future liver remnant volume, including a comparison with the associating liver partition with portal vein ligation for staged hepatectomy approach. J Am Coll Surg 2013; 217(1):126–33 [discussion: 133–4].

23. Correa D, Schwartz L, Jarnagin WR, et al. Kinetics of liver volume changes in the first year after portal vein embolization. Arch Surg 2010;145(4):351–4 [discussion: 354–5].

24. Shindoh J, Truty MJ, Aloia TA, et al. Kinetic growth rate after portal vein embolization predicts posthepatectomy outcomes: toward zero liver-related mortality in patients with colorectal liver metastases and small future liver remnant. J Am Coll Surg 2013;216(2):201–9.

25. Couinaud C. The liver: anatomical and surgical studies (in French). Paris: Masson; 1957.

26. The Terminology Committee of the IHPBA. The Brisbane 2000 terminology of hepatic anatomy and resections. HPB 2000;2:333–9.

27. Simillis C, Li T, Vaughan J, et al. Methods to decrease blood loss during liver resection: a network meta-analysis. Cochrane Database Syst Rev 2014;(4): CD010683.

28. Pamecha V, Gurusamy KS, Sharma D, et al. Techniques for liver parenchymal transection: a meta-analysis of randomized controlled trials. HPB (Oxford) 2009;11(4):275–81.

29. Rahbari NN, Elbers H, Koch M, et al. Randomized clinical trial of stapler versus clamp-crushing transection in elective liver resection. Br J Surg 2014;101(3):200–7.

30. Raoof M, Aloia TA, Vauthey JN, et al. Morbidity and mortality in 1,174 patients undergoing hepatic parenchymal transection using a stapler device. Ann Surg Oncol 2014;21(3):995–1001.

31. Rau HG, Duessel AP, Wurzbacher S. The use of water-jet dissection in open and laparoscopic liver resection. HPB (Oxford) 2008;10(4):275–80.

32. Lochan R, Ansari I, Coates R, et al. Methods of haemostasis during liver resection–a UK national survey. Dig Surg 2013;30(4–6):375–82.

33. Figueras J, Llado L, Ruiz D, et al. Complete versus selective portal triad clamping for minor liver resections: a prospective randomized trial. Ann Surg 2005;241(4): 582–90.

34. Hoekstra LT, van Trigt JD, Reiniers MJ, et al. Vascular occlusion or not during liver resection: the continuing story. Dig Surg 2012;29(1):35–42.

35. Sugiyama Y, Ishizaki Y, Imamura H, et al. Effects of intermittent Pringle's manoeuvre on cirrhotic compared with normal liver. Br J Surg 2010;97(7):1062–9.

36. Gur I, Diggs BS, Wagner JA, et al. Safety and outcomes following resection of colorectal liver metastases in the era of current perioperative chemotherapy. J Gastrointest Surg 2013;17(12):2133–42.

37. Muratore A, Mellano A, Tarantino G, et al. Radiofrequency vessel-sealing system versus the clamp-crushing technique in liver transection: results of a prospective randomized study on 100 consecutive patients. HPB (Oxford) 2014;16:707–12.

38. Savlid M, Strand AH, Jansson A, et al. Transection of the liver parenchyma with an ultrasound dissector or a stapler device: results of a randomized clinical study. World J Surg 2013;37(4):799–805.

39. Lee SY. Central hepatectomy for centrally located malignant liver tumors: a systematic review. World J Hepatol 2014;6(5):347–57.

40. Dokmak S, Agostini J, Jacquin A, et al. High risk of biliary fistula after isolated segment VIII liver resection. World J Surg 2012;36(11):2692–8.

41. Arnoletti JP, Brodsky J. Reduction of transfusion requirements during major hepatic resection for metastatic disease. Surgery 1999;125(2):166–71.
42. Arru M, Pulitano C, Aldrighetti L, et al. A prospective evaluation of ultrasonic dissector plus harmonic scalpel in liver resection. The American surgeon 2007; 73(3):256–60.
43. Ayav A, Jiao L, Dickinson R, et al. Liver resection with a new multiprobe bipolar radiofrequency device. Archives of surgery 2008;143(4):396–401; discussion 401.
44. Lupo L, Gallerani A, Panzera P, et al. Randomized clinical trial of radiofrequency-assisted versus clamp-crushing liver resection. The British journal of surgery 2007;94(3):287–91.
45. Cho JY, Han HS, Yoon YS, et al. Outcomes of laparoscopic liver resection for lesions located in the right side of the liver. Archives of surgery 2009;144(1):25–9.
46. Wagman LD, Lee B, Castillo E, et al. Liver resection using a four-prong radiofrequency transection device. The American surgeon 2009;75(10):991–4.
47. Schmidbauer S, Hallfeldt KK, Sitzmann G, et al. Experience with ultrasound scissors and blades (UltraCision) in open and laparoscopic liver resection. Annals of surgery 2002;235(1):27–30.
48. Takayama T, Makuuchi M, Kubota K, et al. Randomized comparison of ultrasonic vs clamp transection of the liver. Archives of surgery 2001;136(8):922–8.

Complications Following Hepatectomy

Maria C. Russell, MD

KEYWORDS

- Hepatectomy • Venous thromboembolism • Bile leak
- Post hepatectomy liver failure

KEY POINTS

- As the number of liver resections in the United States has increased, operations are more commonly performed on older patients with multiple comorbidities.
- The advent of effective chemotherapy, as well as techniques such as portal vein embolization, have compounded the number of increasingly complex resections taking up to 75% of healthy livers. As a result, although the operations have become safer from a mortality standpoint, the morbidity from liver resections has not decreased.
- Four potentially devastating complications of liver resection include postoperative hemorrhage, venous thromboembolism, bile leak, and post-hepatectomy liver failure.

Liver resection remains the most effective curative treatment of primary liver malignancies, including cholangiocarcinoma and hepatocellular carcinoma (HCC), as well metastatic disease, such as colorectal liver metastases. The number of liver resections performed in the United States nearly doubled between 1988 and 2000, with more than 7000 liver resections performed between 1996 and 2000.[1] As the incidence of these primary and metastatic cancers to the liver increase, the number of liver resections will grow.

Recent advances in patient selection and operative technique have substantially reduced the risk of mortality, from a historical high of 20% to current risk of 1% to 5%.[2–6] Despite this, morbidity rates still range from 20% to 56%, depending on the patient, the extent of resection, the disease process, and the hospital and surgeon.[2–8]

Most studies on complications after hepatectomy have been from single institutions. Jarnagin and colleagues[5] refuted the 13% to 20% operative mortality published in 1977 by Foster and Berman[3] when they published a retrospective review from more than 1800 patients undergoing hepatic resection at Memorial Sloan Kettering between 1991 and 2001. Operative mortality decreased from 4.0% to 1.3% over the course of the review, with a 45% overall complication rate. Benzoni and colleagues[9] evaluated 134 patients undergoing liver resection for HCC and 153 patients undergoing

The author has nothing to disclose.
Division of Surgical Oncology, Department of Surgery, Emory University Hospital, 550 Peachtree Street Northeast, 9th Floor MOT, Atlanta, GA 30308, USA
E-mail address: maria.c.russell@emory.edu

Surg Oncol Clin N Am 24 (2015) 73–96
http://dx.doi.org/10.1016/j.soc.2014.09.008
1055-3207/15/$ – see front matter © 2015 Elsevier Inc. All rights reserved.

liver metastasectomies in a single institution and found a 4.5% mortality rate and 47.7% morbidity rate. Significant increases in complications were found in major hepatectomies, extended hepatectomy, Pringle longer than 20 minutes, and blood transfusions greater than 600 mL. Additionally, Childs B and C classification and histopathologic grading were associated with increased complications in patients with HCC. Sadamori and colleagues[10] evaluated major morbidity following liver resection for HCC and found significantly higher rates of bile leakage (12.8% overall) and organ/space surgical-site infections (8.6% overall) in patients undergoing repeat hepatectomy and prolonged surgery. In 2007, however, Virani and colleagues[11] used the National Surgical Quality Improvement Program–Patient Safety in Surgery (NSQIP-PSS) initiative to look at 30-day morbidity and mortality after liver resection among 14 hospitals in the United States. Overall complications occurred in 22.6% of patients, with 5.2% requiring return to the operating room for complications. Of these, sepsis, wound infection, urinary tract infection, and organ space infection were the most common. Patients who had any complications remained at significantly higher risk of death. In light of this information, identifying patients who are more likely to experience post-hepatectomy complications is the first step toward preventing them.

The steady to increasing rates of complications following liver resections are multifactorial. In general, operations are being offered to patients at increasing age with significant comorbidities. The operations are becoming increasingly complex with more extended resections and more repeat hepatectomies. Additionally, with increasingly effective chemotherapy regimens for colorectal liver metastases, previously unresectable patients are converted to resectable, but with livers that are more subject to steatosis, steatohepatitis, and sinusoidal compromise after months of chemotherapy. As these patients are increasingly offered surgical resection, the rates of morbidity remain high.

When discussing outcomes following hepatectomy, it is imperative to define the extent of resection. Liver resections range from a small, nonanatomic wedges to trisegmentectomies in which more than 75% of the liver parenchyma is removed. In general, "major hepatectomy" is defined as resection of 3 or more liver segments as defined by Couinaud. Some studies demonstrate similar morbidity across the board, whereas others show significant differences according to the extent of resection. Zimmitti and colleagues[12] analyzed postoperative complications based on increasingly complex liver resections. They found that, with the exception of biliary leak, the rates of complications did not increase as complexity of the operation increased. Li and colleagues[13] also looked at patients undergoing minor or major hepatectomy versus ablation for HCC. Rates of major complication between minor and major hepatectomy and ablation were 21.3%, 35.1%, and 9.3% ($P<.01$), respectively. Overall complications were 26.9%, 41.0%, and 11.5% ($P<.01$), respectively. As compared with minor hepatectomy, major hepatectomy was associated with higher rates of infectious (organ/space, superficial skin infections, pneumonia, sepsis, septic shock), pulmonary (unplanned reintubation, prolonged ventilator support), renal (progressive renal insufficiency, acute renal failure), and hematologic (bleeding within 72 hours requiring transfusions, deep venous thrombosis [DVT]) complications.

The importance of the pathology of the underlying liver is also paramount when discussing complications. In HCC, at least 80% of patients have hepatic fibrosis or frank cirrhosis.[14] As such, the remnant liver is already damaged and perhaps more susceptible to additional insult. Whether to resect or transplant these livers remains controversial.[15–19] In fact, some studies show a significantly improved overall survival rate (65.7% vs 43.8%, $P = .005$) and recurrence-free survival (85.3% vs 22.7%, $P<.001$) for patients who undergo resection within Milan Criteria, especially for patients with underlying chronic hepatitis C infection.[19] Other studies maintain that surgical resection of solitary HCC in patients with preserved liver function remains the preferable approach.[20–22] Nevertheless, when discussing complications after liver resection, it is important to note that some livers, including those with cirrhosis, fibrosis, and/or steatosis, may be more susceptible to baseline injury than an otherwise healthy liver.

Patients who undergo hepatic resection are subject to the "routine" complications, such as wound infections, sepsis, pneumonia, and other morbidity commensurate with any operation. For purposes of this article, we focus on complications particular to hepatic resection, including post-hepatectomy bleeding, venous thromboembolism (VTE), bile leak, and liver failure.

POST-HEPATECTOMY HEMORRHAGE

In 1977, Foster and Berman[3] reported operative mortality for major liver resection to be 20%, with 20% of these deaths resulting from hemorrhage. Over time, however, with improved imaging, meticulous operative technique, and advances in perioperative management, the need for transfusions has decreased. Given the possible association of postoperative transfusions with adverse outcomes, this is an important focus to decrease morbidity.[23] Recent studies document the incidence of postoperative hemorrhage from 0.6% to 8.0%.[5,24–27]

A challenge remains to define precisely what postoperative bleeding means. Definitions range from requiring a certain number of packed red blood cells (PRBCs) to bleeding requiring reexploration to "hemorrhage from the operative site" to bleeding via a drain.[11,28–33] In 2011, the International Study Group of Liver Surgery (ISGLS) set forth guidelines for the definition of post-hepatectomy hemorrhage.[24] The consensus definition was a drop in hemoglobin greater than 3 g/dL postoperatively compared with postoperative baseline (immediately after surgery) and/or any postoperative transfusion of PRBCs for a falling hemoglobin and/or the need for invasive reintervention (embolization or relaparotomy) to stop the bleeding. They further categorize the definition by grade based on requirements for less than 2 units of PRBCs (grade A), more than 2 units of PRBCs (grade B), or the need for interventional radiologic intervention or reoperation (grade C) (**Box 1**). This definition was validated in an 835-patient sample that correlated well with in-hospital mortality for grades A, B, and C of 0%, 17%, and 50%, respectively. Although it is important to have this definition now, previous studies did not have a uniform definition.

Risk Factors

Although it is difficult to identify definitive risk factors for postoperative hemorrhage, Lim and colleagues[27] suggest that cirrhotic livers bleed more; they also report that the outflow system may be affected by central venous pressure, which changes after extubation. Yang and colleagues[34] recently analyzed risk factors for postoperative mortality after relaparotomy for hemorrhage. Patients who underwent late relaparotomy (>6 hours) had a 25% mortality, which was significantly higher than those undergoing early relaparotomy (8.6% mortality; $P = .001$).[34] Independent risk factors contributing to increased hospital mortality included early time period (1997–2004), cirrhosis, ineffective hemostasis secondary to coagulopathy, late relaparotomy, postoperative liver failure, and postoperative renal failure requiring dialysis (all $P<.05$).

Management

Most cases of postoperative hemorrhage occur within the first 48 hours after an operation from the liver surface or the diaphragm.[35] Unfortunately, preexisting drains or

> **Box 1**
> **Postoperative hemorrhage**
>
> ISGLS definition of post-hepatectomy hemorrhage:
>
> 1. Drop in hemoglobin >3 g/dL after establishing a postoperative baseline
> 2. Any postoperative transfusion for a falling hemoglobin and/or the need for any reintervention (embolization or relaparotomy) to stop bleeding
> 3. Evidence of bleeding, such as blood loss via drains or active hemorrhage by imaging.
>
> Grade A: Bleeding requiring transfusion of up to 2 units PRBCs
>
> Grade B: Bleeding requiring transfusion of >2 units PRBCs but without invasive intervention
>
> Grade C: Bleeding requiring interventional treatment or relaparotomy
>
> Excluded: Patients requiring immediate postoperative transfusion secondary to intraoperative blood loss
>
> *Abbreviations:* ISGLS, International Study Group of Liver Surgery; PRBCs, packed red blood cells.
> *From* Rahbari NN, Garden OJ, Padbury R, et al. Post-hepatectomy haemorrhage: a definition and grading by the International Study Group of Liver Surgery (ISGLS). HPB (Oxford) 2011;13:531; with permission.

interventional radiology–placed drains are seldom useful, owing to the propensity for a clot to form within them. Close hemodynamic monitoring for hypotension and tachycardia, correction of coagulopathy, and blood transfusions are recommended. The indications for relaparotomy are often based on multiple factors. Reasonable considerations for relaparotomy include blood loss exceeding 1 L or the ongoing need for transfusion, hemoglobin decreases by 3 to 4 points, necessitating transfusion, or hemodynamic instability requiring transfusion.[27,35]

Of patients who experience post-hepatectomy hemorrhage, 1% to 8% of these will require repeat laparotomy, which carries a mortality of 17% to 83%.[24,36–38] The potential for morbidity and subsequent mortality associated with postoperative hemorrhage is high.

POST-HEPATECTOMY VENOUS THROMBOSIS/THROMBOEMBOLISM

Studies have shown the patients at greatest risk of VTE are those undergoing abdominal or pelvic surgery for cancer.[39–41] The consequences of VTE cannot be overstated. Mortality from VTE has been estimated at 8 years to be between 12% and 50%.[42,43] A recent population-based study demonstrated a 30-day mortality for DVT of 3% and 31% for pulmonary embolism (PE) versus 0.4% for the comparison group without VTE. Although the most dramatic increase in mortality was in the first year, the overall 30-year mortality rate ratios also were significant, with a rate of 1.55 (95% confidence interval [CI] 1.53–1.57) for DVT and 2.77 (95% CI 2.74–2.81) for PE.[44]

Despite this potentially deadly complication, many surgeons have been reluctant to use pharmacologic prophylaxis in the setting of liver resection, citing risk of postoperative bleeding, impaired postoperative liver function, and "auto-anticoagulation."[45–47] Recent publications, however, have demonstrated that the rate of pulmonary embolus after liver resection is 6% and the rate of VTE approaches that of other abdominal operations for malignancy.[45,48] For this reason, the paradigm of pharmacologic prophylaxis may be shifting.

One major challenge in comparing across studies is the lack of standard postoperative prophylaxis. Although some studies mention the exact pharmacologic regimens used, most of them have left this up to surgeon discretion, making the precise contribution of prophylaxis unclear. Additionally, early ambulation and sequential compression devices are difficult to track in the postoperative patient, contributing to additional possible inconsistencies across studies.

Risk Factors

There are no prospective, randomized, controlled trials evaluating VTE risk in patients undergoing hepatectomy. Multiple retrospective studies and 1 prospective study have been performed to establish the incidence and risk factors of VTE (**Table 1**).[45,46,49–52] Factors such as higher body mass index, longer operative times, and major liver resection are cited in multiple studies to put patients at risk for VTE.[45,49,50,52] Other potential risk factors, including previous DVT, postoperative complications, and longer length of stay also could contribute to the VTE.[45,49,52]

Interestingly, the rationale of "auto-anticoagulation" with elevated international normalized ratio (INR) was shown by Nathan and colleagues[49] to actually put patients at increased risk for VTE. In their discussion, it is emphasized that INR gives an "incomplete view of a patient's coagulation profile," as previously reported by

Table 1
Incidence and risk factors for post-hepatectomy VTE

Study	Rate	Risk Factors
Ejaz et al[52] (variable pharmacologic prophylaxis)	4.7% VTE 1.8% PE 3.3% DVT	History of VTE Prolonged operative time Increased length of stay
Nathan et al[49] (variable pharmacologic prophylaxis)	2.6% VTE 1.7% PE 1.1% DVT	Advanced age Higher BMI Longer procedure time Major complication Higher postoperative INR
Tzeng et al[45] (no data on prophylaxis)	2.9% VTE 1.3% PE 1.9% DVT	Major hepatectomy Male gender Preoperative AST >27 IU/L ASA class ≥3 OR time >222 min Postoperative organ space infection Length of stay ≥7 d
Reddy et al[46] (variable pharmacologic prophylaxis)	3.6% VTE 2.9% PE 0.7% DVT	Pharmacologic thromboprophylaxis
Melloul et al[50] (pharmacologic and mechanical prophylaxis)	6% PE	BMI >25 kg/m² Major liver resection Normal or minimally fibrotic liver parenchyma
Morris-Stiff et al[51] (prophylaxis not clear)	2.1% VTE 1.3% PE 0.7% DVT	History of DVT or PE

Abbreviations: ASA, American Society of Anesthesiologists; AST, aspartate aminotransferase; BMI, body mass index; DVT, deep vein thrombosis; INR, international normalized ratio; OR, operating room; PE, pulmonary embolism; VTE, venous thromboembolism.

Chitlur.[53] It is further cautioned that an elevated INR is more indicative of the amount of liver resected than as a protective factor against VTE, which was also confirmed by Tzeng and colleagues[45] from M.D. Anderson.

Management

In the case of VTE, prevention may be the best management, although the evidence-based literature behind this is mostly extrapolated from general surgery literature. Reddy and colleagues[46] left the administration, timing, and type of pharmacologic prophylaxis to the discretion of the surgeon, whereas mechanical prophylaxis and early ambulation were standard across patients. The only significant variable associated with VTE was that patients treated with pharmacologic prophylaxis had lower rates of VTE when compared with those not receiving prophylaxis (6.3% vs 2.2%, $P = .03$).[49] Nathan and colleagues[49] examined the timing of prophylaxis and found no difference (immediate, early, late/never) between low molecular weight heparin and unfractionated heparin as a predictor for VTE. Similarly, Ejaz and colleagues[52] demonstrated that even the "current best practice prophylaxis for VTE" does not necessarily prevent VTE, with 70.4% of patients who developed VTE having received postoperative VTE prophylaxis within 24 hours. Although chemoprophylaxis decreases the incidence of VTE by approximately 75% in general surgery patients, it is an accepted fact that, even with adherence to chemoprophylaxis, there will still be patients who will have VTEs.[54,55]

Although a major concern for administration of prophylaxis is postoperative bleeding, this had not been collaborated in current studies. Tzeng and colleagues[45] examined NSQIP data and found that the incidence of VTE far exceeds the risk of major bleeding events, thereby supporting the recommendation for chemoprophylaxis in patients without bleeding disorders or overt postoperative bleeding. Likewise, Reddy and colleagues[46] found lower rates of postoperative red blood cell transfusion (16.7% vs 26.4%, $P = .02$) and similar rates of overall transfusions (35.0% vs 30.6%, $P = .36$) in patients receiving VTE prophylaxis. These 2 studies support the use of VTE prophylaxis with data refuting increased bleeding complications.

Although the role for VTE prophylaxis in liver surgery has not undergone rigorous testing with randomized studies, the most recent studies indicate that this is not an uncommon, but potentially deadly, event. These studies have, likewise, refuted the long-held belief that prophylaxis will increase bleeding complication. It therefore seems prudent to at least consider routine chemoprophylaxis in patients undergoing major hepatectomy, at least until a more effective method of prevention is discovered.

POST-HEPATECTOMY PORTAL VEIN AND HEPATIC ARTERY THROMBOSIS

Vascular complications, such as thrombosis of the portal vein or hepatic artery, are rarely reported complications after hepatectomy. The vast majority of these events are best described in the transplantation literature. As more aggressive liver resections are undertaken, such as those with hepatic artery and portal vein reconstructions, however, the risk factors and frequency of these complications may become more relevant.

Hepatic artery thrombosis (HAT) is a rare complication and generally reported in the literature only when associated with arterial reconstruction in liver resection or in transplantation. Even with hepatic artery resection, Azoulay and colleagues[56] recently reported a patency of 100% in the 5 patients in their series undergoing hepatic artery reconstruction for cholangiocarcinoma. The transplantation literature, on the other hand, reports a 3% to 9% risk of HAT that results in acute graft loss.[57] This complication may present acutely with graft failure, sepsis, or abscess. In a delayed fashion, it may present as cholangitis, bile leak, or altered liver function tests.[57,58]

Again, most of the literature regarding postoperative portal vein thrombosis (PVT) is taken from the transplantation literature, where there is a 2% to 6% risk of thrombosis.[59,60] PVT after hepatectomy may go unrecognized because of the lack of specific symptoms. Patients may present with abdominal pain if it involves the superior mesenteric vessels and produces bowel congestion or ischemia. Alternatively, patients can present with nausea, vomiting, anorexia, weight loss, diarrhea, or increased abdominal distention secondary to ascites.[61,62] If acute thrombosis is unrecognized, collateral vessels will develop and the patient will progress to cavernous transformation of the portal vein and portal hypertension, which may manifest as varices, splenomegaly, and hemorrhage.[63]

Risk Factors

A recent review and meta-analysis of vascular resection in the treatment of hilar cholangiocarcinoma not surprisingly found that vascular complications, including PVT or HAT, stenosis, or pseudoaneurysms were more common in patients undergoing vascular resections (odds ratio [OR] 8.8, 95% CI 3.5–22; $P<.0001$).[64] Additionally, there was a significantly higher mortality in patients undergoing vascular resection (OR 2.07, 95% CI 1.21–3.57; $P = .008$), but an even higher mortality rate in patients undergoing hepatic artery resection (4.48, 95% CI 1.97–10.16; $P = .0003$). Extrapolating from the transplantation literature, relevant risk factors for hepatic artery complications include small artery diameter, older donor age (>60), prolonged ischemia time, blood transfusions, prolonged operative time, bile leak, and cholangitis.[57,65,66] Other studies have demonstrated that extra-anatomic anastomosis was the only multivariate factor independently associated with hepatic artery complications in the living donor transplant recipient.[67]

HAT in the transplantation literature usually is discovered on serial Doppler ultrasounds, which are an integral component of postoperative care for the patient after transplantation; however, computed tomography (CT) scans also may provide information on HAT. As there are no large series of hepatic artery resection in liver resection, it is difficult to definitively identify relevant risk factors in this population of patients.

Like HAT, PVT can be identified by Doppler ultrasound, CT, or MRI. Color Doppler is especially helpful to confirm the diagnosis of PVT and cavernous transformation of the portal vein and is superior to CT for diagnostic purposes, but this modality is extremely user dependent.[61,68] Magnetic resonance angiography can provide dynamic images to look at flow and anatomy, but is time-consuming and expensive. Finally, portal venography is not only diagnostic, but can also be therapeutic; obviously, however, this is an invasive procedure with the potential for complications.

Management

The severity of HAT can dictate the management. In patients with a weak signal, but normal liver function, initial management can be conservative, including heparin and volume administration. Interventional radiology–based procedures, such as angioplasty, can be considered; however, urgent surgical thrombectomy may be required to reestablish flow.[67]

PVT can be managed in various ways, as reviewed by Thomas and Ahmad[68] in 2010. Anticoagulation with intravenous heparin followed by long-term warfarin has reduced the risk of thrombotic events and promoted the recanalization of the vein.[63,69] There are some data that this should be instituted as quickly as possible for the highest likelihood of recanalization.[70,71] Again, looking toward the transplantation literature for guidance, there are reports of successful treatment with thrombolysis, angioplasty, and stent repair.[72,73] Thrombolytic therapy yields excellent results, especially with early intervention, and may provide superior results to systemic anticoagulation.[68] Finally, open surgical thrombectomy has been used to reestablish flow in the portal system.[61] This intervention is usually reserved for patients suffering from ischemic bowel secondary to porto-mesenteric vein thrombosis. The advantages of this approach are that it allows for immediate resolution of thrombosis, as well as operative revision of any previous vascular anastomosis that may have contributed to the thrombosis. It obviously carries with it, however, the associated risks of a major operation.

BILE LEAK

Bile leak remains a considerable complication after liver resection. The incidence is a substantial cause of associated morbidity, ranging from 2.6% to 33.0%.[74–77] Zimmitti and colleagues[12] recently examined liver resections at M.D. Anderson Cancer Center and found a 9.8% rate of liver-related complications, including 4.8% rate of bile leak. Although intraoperative blood loss and rates of transfusion fell over time, there was a rising incidence of bile leak from 3.7% in the early period of the study to 5.9% in the later time period. Despite decreasing mortality and improvements in other complication rates, biliary complications remain a significant concern.

The term "bile leak" has many definitions, from drainage of bile from the abdominal wound or drain, intra-abdominal collection identified at drainage or reoperation, and cholangiographic evidence of biliary leakage or stricture.[76] A definition for bile leak was standardized by the ISGLS as a bilirubin level in a drain 3 times the serum concentration on or after pod 3 or the need for radiologic or operative intervention from a biliary collection or bile peritonitis.[78]

Bile leaks may result in prolonged hospitalization, need for additional imaging, and increased interventions. Major bile leaks are associated with intra-abdominal sepsis, with a morality as high as 40% to 50%.[79–81] Additionally, bile leak can increase hospitalization of 8 days versus 12 days ($P<.001$).

Risk Factors

Several studies have explored risk factors for bile leak (**Table 2**). Lo and colleagues[76] found advanced age, preoperative leukocytosis, left-sided hepatectomy, and prolonged operating times as significant risk factors. Nagano and colleagues[82] demonstrated advanced age, a large incisional surface area, and high-risk operations to be risk factors for leak.[83] Benzoni and colleagues[9] found additional factors of Pringle greater than 20 minutes, transfusion greater than 600 mL, pleural effusion, and extended hepatectomy to be associated with postoperative bile leak. Advanced age may or may not be associated with increased risk depending on the study.[76,84]

Even when looking at risk factors for bile leak in patients with HCC, there are many of the same risk factors, including cirrhosis, major resection, and operative time, and leak rate does not appear to significantly differ from non-HCC cases (**Table 3**).[85] Sadamori and colleagues[10] evaluated an HCC resection population and found univariate factors of repeat hepatectomy, operating room time of at least 300 minutes, blood loss greater than 2 L, blood transfusion, and duration of liver transection as significant factors in postoperative bile leak; repeat hepatectomy and duration of operation greater than 300 minutes persisted on multivariate analysis. Although there are numerous studies examining risk factors for bile leak, the lack of standard definition and the variation in study design make comparison difficult.

Table 2 Factors in bile leak		
Study Author	**% Leak**	**Significant Factors**
Lo et al[76]	8.1	Age ⸱ Childs B and C

Study Author	**% Leak**	**Significant Factors**	
Lo et al[76]	8.1	Age	Childs B and C
		Non-HCC	Major hepatectomy
		Mean hemoglobin	Caudate resection
		Estimated blood loss	T-tube drainage
		Platelets	Concomitant bilioenteric
		Noncirrhotic livers	or bowel anastomosis
			Mean operative time
		Logistic Regression:	Left hepatectomy
		Advanced age	Prolonged operative time
		Preoperative leukocytosis	
Sadamori et al[10] (all HCC)	12.9	Trisegmentectomy	OR time >300 min
		Repeat hepatectomy	Blood transfusion
		MVA	
		OR time >300 min	
Zimmitti et al[12]	4.8	Preoperative jaundice	Bile duct resection/reconstruction
		Portal vein embolization	Liver-associated procedures
		Biliary tumors	OR time >180 min
		Repeat hepatectomy	EBL >1000 mL
		Two-stage resection	Tumor diameter >30 mm
		Extended resection	Portal node dissection
		Caudate resection	Intraoperative transfusion
		En bloc diaphragm resection	
		MVA	En bloc diaphragm resection
		Repeat hepatectomy	Extended hepatectomy
		Bile duct resection	
		Intraoperative transfusion	
Benzoni et al[9]	6	Major hepatectomy	Segmentectomy/wedge
		Left hepatectomy	Pringle >20 min
		Trisegmentectomy	Transfusion >600 mL
		Bisegmentectomy/left	Abscess
		lobectomy	Liver dysfunction
			Pleural effusion
Sadamori et al[83]	12.8	Repeat hepatectomy	Blood transfusion
		OR time >300 min	Duration of parenchymal
		EBL >2000 mL	transection
		MVA	
		Repeat hepatectomy	
		OR time >300 min	
Nagano et al[82]	5.4	Age	
		Cut surface area	
		High-risk operation	
Okumura et al[85]	6.5	Fibrosis or cirrhosis	Hepatectomy including Couinaud
		OR time >5 h	segment 4 or segment 5
		Major hepatic resection	
		MVA	
		OR time	
		Resection of segment 4	

Abbreviations: EBL, estimated blood loss; HCC, hepatocellular carcinoma; MVA, multivariate analysis; OR, operating room.

Table 3
Bile leak across various pathologies

Study Author	Pathology (number)	Leak Rate Number (%)
Tanaka et al,[103] 2002	HCC (316)	23 (7.3%)
	CCC (9)	3 (33.3%)
	Metastatic (33)	0 (0%)
	Other (5)	0 (0%)
Nagano et al,[82] 2003	HCC (126)	9 (7.1%)
	Metastatic (187)	17 (5.4%)
Sadamori et al,[10] 2013	HCC (359)	46 (12.8%)

Abbreviations: CCC, cholangiocarcinoma; HCC, hepatocellular carcinoma.

Management

The best management of any complication is to prevent it. There have been many publications on strategies to prevent bile leak or to detect and repair it intraoperatively.[86–92] Unfortunately, there are no techniques of liver resection that are immune to bile leak; clamp-crushing technique, stapling, Cavitron Ultrasonic Surgical Aspirator (CUSA), radiofrequency dissecting sealer, harmonic scalpel, and the vessel sealing system all have an associated risk of bile leak. A recent meta-analysis demonstrated a decreased risk of bile leak using the vessel-sealing system when compared with the crush clamping, CUSA, and radiofrequency dissecting sealer, but randomized controlled trials are needed to fully appreciate the impact of these transection techniques on outcomes such as bile leak.[93] Likewise, there are multiple publications on the use of fibrin glues and omental wrapping, but no large randomized or multi-institutional studies exist, and there is no clear consensus on the usefulness of these maneuvers.[94–97]

The next best strategy to prevent bile leak would be intraoperative detection and repair of the injury. There have been many studies for intraoperative detection of bile leak, each with strengths and weaknesses. Zimmitti and colleagues[98] recently published data from M.D. Anderson describing the "air leak test" for intraoperative bile duct leaks. There were significantly fewer postoperative bile leaks after the air leak test (1.9%) than the non–air leak test (10.8%; $P = .008$). Similarly, indocyanine green and methylene blue have been recommended for detection of bile leaks, but these dyes tend to stain surrounding parenchyma, making it difficult to pinpoint the areas of leak after the first injection.[74,99] The saline link test can also detect bile duct injuries, but the clear nature of the saline can allow for missed injuries and a randomized controlled trial by Ijichi and colleagues[100] did not find a significant difference in postoperative bile leak (6% vs 4%, $P = .99$). Li and colleagues[101] recently reported that intraductal injection of 5% fat emulsion, "the white test," to detect bile duct injury resulted in a 5.3% bile leak in the experimental group compared with 22.9% leak rate in the control group ($P<.01$), but this was in a small group of patients (137) at a single institution. Finally, Kaibori and colleagues[102] recently described an intraoperative indocyanine green (ICG) fluorescent cholangiography for intraoperative detection of bile leak with a 10% incidence of bile leakage in the control group and a 0% incidence in the ICG fluorescence group ($P = .019$). Although some promising studies exist, most of these studies have been performed on small groups of patients in single institutions and larger multi-institutional studies are needed to address this very important complication.

In many patients, the bile leaks will resolve spontaneously. In 2002, Tanaka and colleagues[103] published their results of 363 patients undergoing hepatic resection, including 42% of 316 patients with hepatocellular carcinoma who had liver cirrhosis. With a 7.2% (26/338) postoperative bile leak rate, 69% of these (18/26) healed on their own without additional treatments. Nagano and colleagues[82] in 2003 published similar results with most bile leaks healing at an average of 37.8 days with drainage alone when a fistulogram was negative. Vigano and colleagues[104] looked at their series of 593 patients who had a bile leak and found a 5.7% risk of the complication. Similarly, 76.5% of these patients had spontaneous healing. Multivariate analysis found the only factor for failure of conservative management was a drain output of greater than 100 mL per day.

In patients without preexisting and well-functioning drains, interventional radiology is frequently used to place drain(s) to treat intraperitoneal collections and to treat or prevent sepsis. In patients with a persistent leak, endoscopic retrograde pancreatico-cholangiograms (ERPCs) versus percutaneous transhepatic cholangiograms (PTCs) are often performed to improve biliary-enteric drainage, with the aim of reducing bile flow out of the injured bile duct. The ability to place a PTC is often limited by the lack of ductal dilation early in the postoperative course. ERPC has recently been associated with a high rate of success in providing biliary decompression and permitting the closure of leaks, but is usually not an option after operative biliary diversion.[105,106]

Small leaks also can be managed with fibrin glue in some cases. There are limited data on the volume of leak that is amenable to fibrin glue treatment, but some investigators suggest that leakage of less than 50 mL per day could be addressed by this procedure.[74,103] This method of treatment is somewhat controversial.

Reoperation for bile leak is associated with a high mortality rate. The liver has already suffered significant injury and may not have the reserve to tolerate another major operation. Additionally, these leaks often occur when the postoperative inflammatory response is greatest, marking the highest risk for adhesions. One study demonstrated a 37.5% mortality associated with reoperation.[76,107] Lo and colleagues[76] found that of the 5 patients who required reoperation, only 1 patient survived.

POST-HEPATECTOMY LIVER FAILURE

Liver failure is perhaps the most devastating complication after liver resection. Although temporary support systems are under development, there is little treatment for this potentially lethal complication other than vigilant supportive care. The incidence of post-hepatectomy liver failure (PHLF) ranges from 4% to 19%, secondary to the variable patient population and extent of resection.[108–112] In recent literature, the incidence is less than 10%, owing to improved preoperative assessment and intraoperative and postoperative management.[78,113] Liver failure still remains a major factor in post-hepatectomy mortality, accounting for 18% to 75% of deaths in some series,[114–116] and up to 60% to 100% of deaths in other series.[117–119]

There have been in excess of 50 studies that have defined PHLF. Many investigators incorporate laboratory values, such as bilirubin and INR, whereas others make the definition based on clinical variables like hepatic encephalopathy and presence of ascites; still others use some combination of laboratory and clinical variables.[6,78,120–122] The time period in which liver failure is defined is also contentious. For example, the "50-50 criteria" uses both bilirubin level and INR on postoperative day 5 to predict post-hepatectomy mortality.[123] Hyder and colleagues,[4] on the other hand, derived a comprehensive algorithm for predicting PHLF. Additionally, Mullen and colleagues[6] proposed a peak total serum bilirubin of greater than 7 mg/dL to define liver failure in the postoperative setting. In 2011, the ISGLS defined PHLF as the "impaired ability of the liver to maintain its synthetic, excretory and detoxifying functions, which are characterized by and increased international normalized ratio and concomitant hyper-bilirubinemia (according to the normal limits of the local laboratory) on or after postop-erative day 5."[78] This group further differentiated severity by classification A, B, or C. Finally, Etra and colleagues[124] recently published that a postoperative day 3 bilirubin greater than 3 mg/dL was a sensitive and specific early predictor of postoperative liver insufficiency. These hosts of definitions over the past decade make comparisons across studies difficult.

Risk Factors

It is essential to define risk factors for PHLF to identify these patients before submitting them to a potentially deadly surgery. One way to look at risk factors is to delineate those related to patients and the disease from those related to intraoperative and postoperative management of patients (**Table 4**).

Patient and disease factors

Although sex and age have been examined as potential factors in PHLF, the results from studies are contradictory. Many studies demonstrate no difference in outcomes in well-selected elderly patients undergoing hepatectomy, whereas other data report increasing risk of postoperative liver insufficiency after age 65, especially in an extended resection.[123,125–131] At least from a regenerative standpoint, a recent study by Fernandes and colleagues[132] found no difference in liver regeneration between those younger than 65 and those older than 65. Additionally, male sex is also debat-ably one of the nonmodifiable risk factors for increasing postoperative hepatic insuf-ficiency, with some studies demonstrating a doubling of the risk.[6,133]

As neoadjuvant and conversion chemotherapeutic strategies improve, the per-centage of patients undergoing liver resections after exposure to chemotherapy is increasing.[134] Common regimens for the treatment of colorectal cancer include 5-fluorouracil combined with oxaliplatin, irinotecan, and the targeted agents bevaci-zumab and cetuximab. Although these regimens have helped to make previously unresectable metastases sometimes resectable, their prolonged use can result in steatosis, steatohepatitis, and sinusoidal congestion.[135–141]

In 2006, Karoui[142] published their findings of the impact of preoperative chemo-therapy in major hepatectomy. Postoperative morbidity was correlated with the

Table 4 Risk factors for post-hepatectomy liver failure	
Category	Risk Factor
Patient related	Age Male Comorbidities Preexisting liver disease Steatosis Fibrosis Cirrhosis Chemotherapy-induced liver damage
Surgery/Postoperative	Prolonged operating room time Excessive blood loss Small future liver remnant/extent of resection Ischemia/reperfusion Infection

number of preoperative chemotherapy cycles. Although there was no postoperative liver failure in the control group, the chemotherapy group had an 11% rate of transient liver failure (P = .046). In these patients, 90% had steatosis involving more than 50% of hepatocytes after a median number of 15 cycles of chemotherapy. In a similar study, Shindoh and colleagues[143] reviewed 194 patients undergoing no chemotherapy, short-course (≤12 weeks) chemotherapy, or long-duration (>12 weeks) chemotherapy. Postoperative hepatic insufficiency was 0%, 5.1%, and 16.3% (P = .04) in patients receiving no, short-duration, and long-duration chemotherapy, respectively. Recommendations from this article were to increase the mandatory future liver remnant (FLR) from 20% to 30% in patients having received more than 12 weeks of chemotherapy to potentially decrease the rates of postoperative hepatic insufficiency. Although there are not many modifiable risk factors in patients having hepatectomy, this is at least something to consider.

In addition to chemotherapy-induced toxicity, cirrhosis is a major consideration when operating on patients, especially in the HCC population. These patients often have reduced functional reserves, as well as diminished regenerative capacity, making the operation itself higher risk and often requiring a larger FLR to avoid PHLF. In patients with cirrhosis, PHLF rates range between 2% and 19%.[144–151] Unfortunately, although Child-Pugh score and Model for End-Stage Liver Disease can give some information about the degree of cirrhosis, they may underestimate the ability of a patient to withstand resection. In these patients, at least in Asia, preoperative tests for functional liver reserve, such as ICG clearance, are considered essential.[139,152] In patients with cirrhosis, the recommended FLR is greater than 40%.[153–155] In patients who have further reduction in functional reserve as demonstrated by ICG-R15 of 10% to 20%, some investigators recommend FLR greater than 50% before liver resection to decrease the risk of postoperative hepatic failure.[153,156]

Intraoperative and Postoperative Risk Factors

There are actual operative and postoperative factors that can affect rates of postoperative hepatic insufficiency. Among these, FLR, hepatic inflow occlusion time, overall operative time, and blood loss are all associated with the development of postoperative hepatic insufficiency.

In a normal liver, an FLR of 20% to 25% is generally considered adequate to avoid liver insufficiency; however, in heavily pretreated chemotherapy livers and/or in those with cirrhosis, steatosis, or fibrosis, the FLR necessary should be at least 40% to limit postoperative complications.[154,157] Techniques such as portal vein embolization are now used to help ensure there is adequate FLR. It is critical that the surgeon consider FLR before embarking on liver resection.[133,158]

The ability of the liver to tolerate the ischemia/reperfusion cycle of the Pringle maneuver (hepatic pedicle inflow occlusion) may be limited and may result in reduced postoperative liver function. There have been several studies on the best technique, whether it be intermittent or continuous clamping. Additionally, Clavien and colleagues[159] demonstrated that ischemic preconditioning (10 minutes of ischemia followed by 10 minutes of reperfusion) is a useful strategy in patients with a planned 30-minute inflow occlusion and found increased benefit in younger patients, patients with longer inflow occlusion, and in cases of lower resected liver volume, as well as those with steatosis. Some studies have shown improvement in function with intermittent clamping, whereas others maintain that continuous clamping is associated with less blood loss and shorter transection time.[159–161] One important point is that in cirrhotic livers, the method of occluding blood flow must be carefully weighed. There is some suggestion that a selective inflow occlusion, if absolutely necessary, may be used to permit the future liver to maintain blood supply via the hepatic artery for the duration of the portal occlusion.[162]

Blood loss and the need for blood transfusions have a direct correlation with increased hepatic insufficiency.[5,23,75] Although studies point to different values, a blood loss greater than 1000 to 1250 mL is associated with increasing complications. Increasing blood loss is associated with volume shifts, including hypotension, possibly tachycardia, and the need for blood products.[163] Additionally, it is associated with coagulopathy, which perpetuates the need for more blood products, as well as predisposes to infection.[23] Immunomodulatory effects from blood also have been shown to affect recurrence.[23,164] Each of these factors affects the liver during the critical regenerative post period.

Rates of postoperative infection after major resection may be as high as 50%, with bacterial infection developing in up to 80% of patients in postoperative liver failure.[119] These infections can cause or exacerbate liver failure secondary to the inhibitory effect of sepsis on liver regeneration.[116] Additionally, the liver failure actually increases the likelihood of infection secondary to alterations in immunologic defense and sepsis.[165] Kupffer cells, which have a responsibility in both the innate immune system to regeneration of the liver, are affected doubly by both the liver resection itself and the bacterial endotoxins, which may increase as a result of translocation from the liver and portal blood flow. This complex series of events puts additional strain on the liver and can worsen liver insufficiency.

Treatment

The best treatment of postoperative liver failure is prevention. This involves optimizing a patient's comorbid conditions, careful consideration of duration of preoperative chemotherapy, adequate assessment of FLR with portal vein embolization if necessary, limiting operative time with meticulous operative technique with control of blood loss, and careful monitoring of the postoperative liver enzymes, coagulation, and mental status. Once the patient sets on the course of liver failure, there are limited options for treatment.

Patients exhibiting signs of liver failure should be transferred to a monitored setting. Goal-directed therapy aimed at maintaining pulmonary, renal, and circulatory function should be initiated.[166] Fresh-frozen plasma, vitamin K, albumin, and diuretics should be used to support the liver. Intubation and dialysis should be considered in patients.

There are 2 main liver support systems that are available for temporary support of patients. The molecular absorbent recirculating system is an albumin dialysis machine that has been used in several studies, but whose actual efficacy is yet to be determined.[167,168] The Prometheus system uses a similar dialysis principle but may have a better detoxifying capacity.[166] Future studies are needed in both of these systems to prove efficacy. Finally, liver transplantation can be considered, but, given that most liver resections are for malignancy, most patients are not candidates for this modality.

SUMMARY

The number of liver resections performed in the United States is increasing. With the increasing numbers are more complicated patients undergoing extensive operations. Although the mortality from liver resections has improved dramatically, the morbidity from these cases is staying steady, or even increasing, as some studies have shown. Despite the number of studies evaluating these complications, there are conflicting data on what preoperative and intraoperative factors can improve outcomes.

The implications of these complications cannot be overstated. The United States spent $2.3 trillion on health care expenditures in 2008, up 4.4% from 2007.[169] Postoperative complications are seen as a marker of quality in the health care forum.[170–172] A recent study from Switzerland looked at the economic consequences of complications from hepatobiliary, colorectal, and bariatric procedures.[173] Thirty-day mortality for liver surgery was 3.1%, with an overall morbidity of 56%; however, 29% of patients had more than 1 complication. The cost of surgery without complications was a mean of $13,625, but skyrocketed to $69,369 when complications were considered. Obviously, the more complications that a patient had, the more the cost increased. In another study, patients with complications averaged 15.0 ± 12.2 days in the hospital compared with 7.3 ± 4.5 days for those without complications ($P<.001$). Additionally, those with complications were more likely to return to the operating room within 30 days (OR = 9.7; 95% CI 4.9–19.5).

A recent publication by Lucas and colleagues[174] used the American College of Surgeons NSQIP to look at the timing of these complications and readmission rates after hepatopancreatobiliary surgery. The overall complication rate was 20.9%, but they found that there were significant differences in the timing of the complications. They observed that urinary tract infections, respiratory complications, reoperative bleeding, and cardiac complications were more likely to occur in the initial inpatient setting while the patient was under medical supervision. In contrast, wound complications, deep and organ space infections, and dehiscence more commonly presented in outpatients. Those patients with inpatient complications did not have a significant risk for readmission, whereas outpatient complications, whether minor or major, frequently resulted in readmission with adjusted risk ratio of 3.13 and 8.45, respectively. As hospitals are increasingly penalized for readmissions, improving outpatient management of these conditions will become progressively important.

Surgeons are increasingly performing complex operations on an aging population with multiple comorbidities and heavily pretreated or hepatitis-damaged livers, and although mortality rates have decreased, these patients are having more complications. There are multiple problems comparing different types of liver resections with different baseline liver functions for different disease processes and no standard definitions for complications. The ISGLS has attempted to put in definable terms several high-morbidity complications, which should make it easier to define the actual incidence of these complications. The next vital step, however, is to identify preoperative factors that contribute to postoperative morbidity and mortality to select appropriate patients for these high-risk operations.

REFERENCES

1. Dimick JB, Wainess RM, Cowan JA, et al. National trends in the use and outcomes of hepatic resection. J Am Coll Surg 2004;199:31–8.
2. Asiyanbola B, Chang D, Gleisner AL, et al. Operative mortality after hepatic resection: are literature-based rates broadly applicable? J Gastrointest Surg 2008;12:842–51.
3. Foster JH, Berman MM. Solid liver tumors. Major Probl Clin Surg 1977;22:1–342.
4. Hyder O, Pulitano C, Firoozmand A, et al. A risk model to predict 90-day mortality among patients undergoing hepatic resection. J Am Coll Surg 2013;216: 1049–56.
5. Jarnagin WR, Gonen M, Fong Y, et al. Improvement in perioperative outcome after hepatic resection: analysis of 1,803 consecutive cases over the past decade. Ann Surg 2002;236:397–406 [discussion: 406–7].

6. Mullen JT, Ribero D, Reddy SK, et al. Hepatic insufficiency and mortality in 1,059 noncirrhotic patients undergoing major hepatectomy. J Am Coll Surg 2007;204: 854–62 [discussion: 862–4].
7. McKay A, Sutherland FR, Bathe OF, et al. Morbidity and mortality following multivisceral resections in complex hepatic and pancreatic surgery. J Gastrointest Surg 2008;12:86–90.
8. Mathur AK, Ghaferi AA, Osborne NH, et al. Body mass index and adverse perioperative outcomes following hepatic resection. J Gastrointest Surg 2010;14: 1285–91.
9. Benzoni E, Cojutti A, Lorenzin D, et al. Liver resective surgery: a multivariate analysis of postoperative outcome and complication. Langenbecks Arch Surg 2007;392:45–54.
10. Sadamori H, Yagi T, Shinoura S, et al. Risk factors for major morbidity after liver resection for hepatocellular carcinoma. Br J Surg 2013;100:122–9.
11. Virani S, Michaelson JS, Hutter MM, et al. Morbidity and mortality after liver resection: results of the patient safety in surgery study. J Am Coll Surg 2007; 204:1284–92.
12. Zimmitti G, Roses RE, Andreou A, et al. Greater complexity of liver surgery is not associated with an increased incidence of liver-related complications except for bile leak: an experience with 2,628 consecutive resections. J Gastrointest Surg 2013;17:57–64 [discussion: 64–5].
13. Li GZ, Speicher PJ, Lidsky ME, et al. Hepatic resection for hepatocellular carcinoma: do contemporary morbidity and mortality rates demand a transition to ablation as first-line treatment? J Am Coll Surg 2014;218:827–34.
14. Okuda K. Hepatocellular carcinoma. J Hepatol 2000;32:225–37.
15. Adam R, Azoulay D, Castaing D, et al. Liver resection as a bridge to transplantation for hepatocellular carcinoma on cirrhosis: a reasonable strategy? Ann Surg 2003;238:508–18 [discussion: 518–9].
16. Bigourdan JM, Jaeck D, Meyer N, et al. Small hepatocellular carcinoma in Child A cirrhotic patients: hepatic resection versus transplantation. Liver Transpl 2003; 9:513–20.
17. Cha CH, Ruo L, Fong Y, et al. Resection of hepatocellular carcinoma in patients otherwise eligible for transplantation. Ann Surg 2003;238:315–21 [discussion: 321–3].
18. Margarit C, Escartin A, Castells L, et al. Resection for hepatocellular carcinoma is a good option in Child-Turcotte-Pugh class A patients with cirrhosis who are eligible for liver transplantation. Liver Transpl 2005;11:1242–51.
19. Squires MH 3rd, Hanish SI, Fisher SB, et al. Transplant versus resection for the management of hepatocellular carcinoma meeting Milan Criteria in the MELD exception era at a single institution in a UNOS region with short wait times. J Surg Oncol 2014;109:533–41.
20. Bismuth H, Majno PE. Hepatobiliary surgery. J Hepatol 2000;32:208–24.
21. Arii S, Yamaoka Y, Futagawa S, et al. Results of surgical and nonsurgical treatment for small-sized hepatocellular carcinomas: a retrospective and nationwide survey in Japan. The Liver Cancer Study Group of Japan. Hepatology 2000;32:1224–9.
22. Bruix J, Sherman M, Llovet JM, et al. Clinical management of hepatocellular carcinoma. Conclusions of the Barcelona-2000 EASL conference. European Association for the Study of the Liver. J Hepatol 2001;35:421–30.
23. Kooby DA, Stockman J, Ben-Porat L, et al. Influence of transfusions on perioperative and long-term outcome in patients following hepatic resection for colorectal metastases. Ann Surg 2003;237:860–9 [discussion: 869–70].

24. Rahbari NN, Garden OJ, Padbury R, et al. Post-hepatectomy haemorrhage: a definition and grading by the International Study Group of Liver Surgery (ISGLS). HPB (Oxford) 2011;13:528–35.
25. Belghiti J, Hiramatsu K, Benoist S, et al. Seven hundred forty-seven hepatectomies in the 1990s: an update to evaluate the actual risk of liver resection. J Am Coll Surg 2000;191:38–46.
26. Schroeder RA, Marroquin CE, Bute BP, et al. Predictive indices of morbidity and mortality after liver resection. Ann Surg 2006;243:373–9.
27. Lim C, Dokmak S, Farges O, et al. Reoperation for post-hepatectomy hemorrhage: increased risk of mortality. Langenbecks Arch Surg 2014;399:735–40.
28. Fujii M, Shimada M, Satoru I, et al. A standardized safe hepatectomy; selective Glissonean transection using endolinear stapling devices. Hepatogastroenterology 2007;54:906–9.
29. Fujii Y, Shimada H, Endo I, et al. Management of massive arterial hemorrhage after pancreatobiliary surgery: does embolotherapy contribute to successful outcome? J Gastrointest Surg 2007;11:432–8.
30. Ogata S, Belghiti J, Farges O, et al. Sequential arterial and portal vein embolizations before right hepatectomy in patients with cirrhosis and hepatocellular carcinoma. Br J Surg 2006;93:1091–8.
31. Cho JY, Suh KS, Kwon CH, et al. Mild hepatic steatosis is not a major risk factor for hepatectomy and regenerative power is not impaired. Surgery 2006;139: 508–15.
32. Azoulay D, Lucidi V, Andreani P, et al. Ischemic preconditioning for major liver resection under vascular exclusion of the liver preserving the caval flow: a randomized prospective study. J Am Coll Surg 2006;202:203–11.
33. Vauthey JN, Pawlik TM, Abdalla EK, et al. Is extended hepatectomy for hepatobiliary malignancy justified? Ann Surg 2004;239:722–30 [discussion: 730–2].
34. Yang T, Li LL, Zhong Q, et al. Risk factors of hospital mortality after re-laparotomy for post-hepatectomy hemorrhage. World J Surg 2013;37:2394–401.
35. Jin S, Fu Q, Wuyun G, et al. Management of post-hepatectomy complications. World J Gastroenterol 2013;19:7983–91.
36. Tsao JI, Loftus JP, Nagorney DM, et al. Trends in morbidity and mortality of hepatic resection for malignancy. A matched comparative analysis. Ann Surg 1994;220:199–205.
37. Finch MD, Crosbie JL, Currie E, et al. An 8-year experience of hepatic resection: indications and outcome. Br J Surg 1998;85:315–9.
38. Sitzmann JV, Greene PS. Perioperative predictors of morbidity following hepatic resection for neoplasm. A multivariate analysis of a single surgeon experience with 105 patients. Ann Surg 1994;219:13–7.
39. Catheline JM, Capelluto E, Gaillard JL, et al. Thromboembolism prophylaxis and incidence of thromboembolic complications after laparoscopic surgery. Int J Surg Investig 2000;2:41–7.
40. Agnelli G, Bolis G, Capussotti L, et al. A clinical outcome-based prospective study on venous thromboembolism after cancer surgery: the @RISTOS project. Ann Surg 2006;243:89–95.
41. Alcalay A, Wun T, Khatri V, et al. Venous thromboembolism in patients with colorectal cancer: incidence and effect on survival. J Clin Oncol 2006;24: 1112–8.
42. Flinterman LE, van Hylckama Vlieg A, Cannegieter SC, et al. Long-term survival in a large cohort of patients with venous thrombosis: incidence and predictors. PLoS Med 2012;9:e1001155.

43. Ng AC, Chung T, Yong AS, et al. Long-term cardiovascular and noncardiovascular mortality of 1023 patients with confirmed acute pulmonary embolism. Circ Cardiovasc Qual Outcomes 2011;4:122–8.
44. Sogaard KK, Schmidt M, Pedersen L, et al. 30-year mortality following venous thromboembolism: a population-based cohort study. Circulation 2014;130:829–36.
45. Tzeng CW, Katz MH, Fleming JB, et al. Risk of venous thromboembolism outweighs post-hepatectomy bleeding complications: analysis of 5651 National Surgical Quality Improvement Program patients. HPB (Oxford) 2012;14:506–13.
46. Reddy SK, Turley RS, Barbas AS, et al. Post-operative pharmacologic thromboprophylaxis after major hepatectomy: does peripheral venous thromboembolism prevention outweigh bleeding risks? J Gastrointest Surg 2011;15:1602–10.
47. Kakkar AK, Levine M, Pinedo HM, et al. Venous thrombosis in cancer patients: insights from the FRONTLINE survey. Oncologist 2003;8:381–8.
48. De Martino RR, Goodney PP, Spangler EL, et al. Variation in thromboembolic complications among patients undergoing commonly performed cancer operations. J Vasc Surg 2012;55:1035–40.e4.
49. Nathan H, Weiss MJ, Soff GA, et al. Pharmacologic prophylaxis, postoperative INR, and risk of venous thromboembolism after hepatectomy. J Gastrointest Surg 2014;18:295–302 [discussion: 302–3].
50. Melloul E, Dondero F, Vilgrain V, et al. Pulmonary embolism after elective liver resection: a prospective analysis of risk factors. J Hepatol 2012;57:1268–75.
51. Morris-Stiff G, White A, Gomez D, et al. Thrombotic complications following liver resection for colorectal metastases are preventable. HPB (Oxford) 2008;10:311–4.
52. Ejaz A, Spolverato G, Kim Y, et al. Defining incidence and risk factors of venous thromboembolism after hepatectomy. J Gastrointest Surg 2014;18:1116–24.
53. Chitlur M. Challenges in the laboratory analyses of bleeding disorders. Thromb Res 2012;130:1–6.
54. Collins R, Scrimgeour A, Yusuf S, et al. Reduction in fatal pulmonary embolism and venous thrombosis by perioperative administration of subcutaneous heparin. Overview of results of randomized trials in general, orthopedic, and urologic surgery. N Engl J Med 1988;318:1162–73.
55. Mismetti P, Laporte S, Darmon JY, et al. Meta-analysis of low molecular weight heparin in the prevention of venous thromboembolism in general surgery. Br J Surg 2001;88:913–30.
56. Azoulay D, Pascal G, Salloum C, et al. Vascular reconstruction combined with liver resection for malignant tumours. Br J Surg 2013;100:1764–75.
57. Silva MA, Jambulingam PS, Gunson BK, et al. Hepatic artery thrombosis following orthotopic liver transplantation: a 10-year experience from a single centre in the United Kingdom. Liver Transpl 2006;12:146–51.
58. Bhattacharjya S, Gunson BK, Mirza DF, et al. Delayed hepatic artery thrombosis in adult orthotopic liver transplantation—a 12-year experience. Transplantation 2001;71:1592–6.
59. Woo DH, Laberge JM, Gordon RL, et al. Management of portal venous complications after liver transplantation. Tech Vasc Interv Radiol 2007;10:233–9.
60. Wozney P, Zajko AB, Bron KM, et al. Vascular complications after liver transplantation: a 5-year experience. AJR Am J Roentgenol 1986;147:657–63.
61. Cohen J, Edelman RR, Chopra S. Portal vein thrombosis: a review. Am J Med 1992;92:173–82.
62. Witte CL, Brewer ML, Witte MH, et al. Protean manifestations of pylethrombosis. A review of thirty-four patients. Ann Surg 1985;202:191–202.

63. Sheen CL, Lamparelli H, Milne A, et al. Clinical features, diagnosis and outcome of acute portal vein thrombosis. QJM 2000;93:531–4.
64. Abbas S, Sandroussi C. Systematic review and meta-analysis of the role of vascular resection in the treatment of hilar cholangiocarcinoma. HPB (Oxford) 2013;15:492–503.
65. Varotti G, Grazi GL, Vetrone G, et al. Causes of early acute graft failure after liver transplantation: analysis of a 17-year single-centre experience. Clin Transplant 2005;19:492–500.
66. Langnas AN, Marujo W, Stratta RJ, et al. Vascular complications after orthotopic liver transplantation. Am J Surg 1991;161:76–82 [discussion: 82–3].
67. Iida T, Kaido T, Yagi S, et al. Hepatic arterial complications in adult living donor liver transplant recipients: a single-center experience of 673 cases. Clin Transplant 2014;28:1025–30.
68. Thomas RM, Ahmad SA. Management of acute post-operative portal venous thrombosis. J Gastrointest Surg 2010;14:570–7.
69. Condat B, Pessione F, Hillaire S, et al. Current outcome of portal vein thrombosis in adults: risk and benefit of anticoagulant therapy. Gastroenterology 2001;120:490–7.
70. Turnes J, Garcia-Pagan JC, Gonzalez M, et al. Portal hypertension-related complications after acute portal vein thrombosis: impact of early anticoagulation. Clin Gastroenterol Hepatol 2008;6:1412–7.
71. Plessier A, Darwish-Murad S, Hernandez-Guerra M, et al. Acute portal vein thrombosis unrelated to cirrhosis: a prospective multicenter follow-up study. Hepatology 2010;51:210–8.
72. Sobhonslidsuk A, Reddy KR. Portal vein thrombosis: a concise review. Am J Gastroenterol 2002;97:535–41.
73. Bhattacharjya T, Olliff SP, Bhattacharjya S, et al. Percutaneous portal vein thrombolysis and endovascular stent for management of posttransplant portal venous conduit thrombosis. Transplantation 2000;69:2195–8.
74. Yamashita Y, Hamatsu T, Rikimaru T, et al. Bile leakage after hepatic resection. Ann Surg 2001;233:45–50.
75. Imamura H, Seyama Y, Kokudo N, et al. One thousand fifty-six hepatectomies without mortality in 8 years. Arch Surg 2003;138:1198–206 [discussion: 1206].
76. Lo CM, Fan ST, Liu CL, et al. Biliary complications after hepatic resection: risk factors, management, and outcome. Arch Surg 1998;133:156–61.
77. Capussotti L, Ferrero A, Vigano L, et al. Bile leakage and liver resection: Where is the risk? Arch Surg 2006;141:690–4 [discussion: 695].
78. Rahbari NN, Garden OJ, Padbury R, et al. Posthepatectomy liver failure: a definition and grading by the International Study Group of Liver Surgery (ISGLS). Surgery 2011;149:713–24.
79. Kohno H, Nagasue N, Chang YC, et al. Comparison of topical hemostatic agents in elective hepatic resection: a clinical prospective randomized trial. World J Surg 1992;16:966–9 [discussion: 970].
80. Bismuth H, Chiche L, Castaing D. Surgical treatment of hepatocellular carcinomas in noncirrhotic liver: experience with 68 liver resections. World J Surg 1995;19:35–41.
81. Lai EC, Fan ST, Lo CM, et al. Hepatic resection for hepatocellular carcinoma. An audit of 343 patients. Ann Surg 1995;221:291–8.
82. Nagano Y, Togo S, Tanaka K, et al. Risk factors and management of bile leakage after hepatic resection. World J Surg 2003;27:695–8.

83. Sadamori H, Yagi T, Matsuda H, et al. Risk factors for major morbidity after hepatectomy for hepatocellular carcinoma in 293 recent cases. J Hepatobiliary Pancreat Sci 2010;17:709–18.

84. Yamanaka N, Okamoto E, Kuwata K, et al. A multiple regression equation for prediction of posthepatectomy liver failure. Ann Surg 1984;200:658–63.

85. Okumura K, Sugimachi K, Kinjo N, et al. Risk factors of bile leakage after hepatectomy for hepatocellular carcinoma. Hepatogastroenterology 2013;60:1717–9.

86. Kim J, Ahmad SA, Lowy AM, et al. Increased biliary fistulas after liver resection with the harmonic scalpel. Am Surg 2003;69:815–9.

87. Weber JC, Navarra G, Jiao LR, et al. New technique for liver resection using heat coagulative necrosis. Ann Surg 2002;236:560–3.

88. Poon RT, Fan ST, Wong J. Liver resection using a saline-linked radiofrequency dissecting sealer for transection of the liver. J Am Coll Surg 2005;200:308–13.

89. Delis SG, Bakoyiannis A, Karakaxas D, et al. Hepatic parenchyma resection using stapling devices: peri-operative and long-term outcome. HPB (Oxford) 2009;11:38–44.

90. Castaldo ET, Earl TM, Chari RS, et al. A clinical comparative analysis of crush/clamp, stapler, and dissecting sealer hepatic transection methods. HPB (Oxford) 2008;10:321–6.

91. Romano F, Garancini M, Caprotti R, et al. Hepatic resection using a bipolar vessel sealing device: technical and histological analysis. HPB (Oxford) 2007;9:339–44.

92. Geller DA, Tsung A, Maheshwari V, et al. Hepatic resection in 170 patients using saline-cooled radiofrequency coagulation. HPB (Oxford) 2005;7:208–13.

93. Alexiou VG, Tsitsias T, Mavros MN, et al. Technology-assisted versus clamp-crush liver resection: a systematic review and meta-analysis. Surg Innov 2013;20:414–28.

94. Kobayashi S, Nagano H, Marubashi S, et al. Fibrin sealant with PGA felt for prevention of bile leakage after liver resection. Hepatogastroenterology 2012;59:2564–8.

95. Sanjay P, Watt DG, Wigmore SJ. Systematic review and meta-analysis of haemostatic and biliostatic efficacy of fibrin sealants in elective liver surgery. J Gastrointest Surg 2013;17:829–36.

96. Nanashima A, Tobinaga S, Abo T, et al. Usefulness of omental wrapping to prevent biliary leakage and delayed gastric emptying in left hepatectomy. Hepatogastroenterology 2012;59:847–50.

97. de Boer MT, Boonstra EA, Lisman T, et al. Role of fibrin sealants in liver surgery. Dig Surg 2012;29:54–61.

98. Zimmitti G, Vauthey JN, Shindoh J, et al. Systematic use of an intraoperative air leak test at the time of major liver resection reduces the rate of postoperative biliary complications. J Am Coll Surg 2013;217:1028–37.

99. Lam CM, Lo CM, Liu CL, et al. Biliary complications during liver resection. World J Surg 2001;25:1273–6.

100. Ijichi M, Takayama T, Toyoda H, et al. Randomized trial of the usefulness of a bile leakage test during hepatic resection. Arch Surg 2000;135:1395–400.

101. Li J, Malago M, Sotiropoulos GC, et al. Intraoperative application of "white test" to reduce postoperative bile leak after major liver resection: results of a prospective cohort study in 137 patients. Langenbecks Arch Surg 2009;394:1019–24.

102. Kaibori M, Ishizaki M, Matsui K, et al. Intraoperative indocyanine green fluorescent imaging for prevention of bile leakage after hepatic resection. Surgery 2011;150:91–8.

103. Tanaka S, Hirohashi K, Tanaka H, et al. Incidence and management of bile leakage after hepatic resection for malignant hepatic tumors. J Am Coll Surg 2002;195:484–9.
104. Vigano L, Ferrero A, Sgotto E, et al. Bile leak after hepatectomy: predictive factors of spontaneous healing. Am J Surg 2008;196:195–200.
105. Sherman S, Shaked A, Cryer HM, et al. Endoscopic management of biliary fistulas complicating liver transplantation and other hepatobiliary operations. Ann Surg 1993;218:167–75.
106. Cheung KL, Lai EC. Endoscopic stenting for malignant biliary obstruction. Arch Surg 1995;130:204–7.
107. Pace RF, Blenkharn JI, Edwards WJ, et al. Intra-abdominal sepsis after hepatic resection. Ann Surg 1989;209:302–6.
108. Capussotti L, Muratore A, Amisano M, et al. Liver resection for hepatocellular carcinoma on cirrhosis: analysis of mortality, morbidity and survival–a European single center experience. Eur J Surg Oncol 2005;31:986–93.
109. Chok KS, Ng KK, Poon RT, et al. Impact of postoperative complications on long-term outcome of curative resection for hepatocellular carcinoma. Br J Surg 2009;96:81–7.
110. Kawano Y, Sasaki A, Kai S, et al. Short- and long-term outcomes after hepatic resection for hepatocellular carcinoma with concomitant esophageal varices in patients with cirrhosis. Ann Surg Oncol 2008;15:1670–6.
111. Mizuguchi T, Nagayama M, Meguro M, et al. Prognostic impact of surgical complications and preoperative serum hepatocyte growth factor in hepatocellular carcinoma patients after initial hepatectomy. J Gastrointest Surg 2009;13:325–33.
112. Okamura Y, Takeda S, Fujii T, et al. Prognostic significance of postoperative complications after hepatectomy for hepatocellular carcinoma. J Surg Oncol 2011;104:814–21.
113. Paugam-Burtz C, Janny S, Delefosse D, et al. Prospective validation of the "fifty-fifty" criteria as an early and accurate predictor of death after liver resection in intensive care unit patients. Ann Surg 2009;249:124–8.
114. Detroz B, Sugarbaker PH, Knol JA, et al. Causes of death in patients undergoing liver surgery. Cancer Treat Res 1994;69:241–57.
115. Simmonds PC, Primrose JN, Colquitt JL, et al. Surgical resection of hepatic metastases from colorectal cancer: a systematic review of published studies. Br J Cancer 2006;94:982–99.
116. Garcea G, Maddern GJ. Liver failure after major hepatic resection. J Hepatobiliary Pancreat Surg 2009;16:145–55.
117. McCall J, Koea J, Gunn K, et al. Liver resections in Auckland 1998-2001: mortality, morbidity and blood product use. N Z Med J 2001;114:516–9.
118. Sun HC, Qin LX, Wang L, et al. Risk factors for postoperative complications after liver resection. Hepatobiliary Pancreat Dis Int 2005;4:370–4.
119. Schindl MJ, Redhead DN, Fearon KC, et al. The value of residual liver volume as a predictor of hepatic dysfunction and infection after major liver resection. Gut 2005;54:289–96.
120. Pawlik TM, Olino K, Gleisner AL, et al. Preoperative chemotherapy for colorectal liver metastases: impact on hepatic histology and postoperative outcome. J Gastrointest Surg 2007;11:860–8.
121. Zorzi D, Chun YS, Madoff DC, et al. Chemotherapy with bevacizumab does not affect liver regeneration after portal vein embolization in the treatment of colorectal liver metastases. Ann Surg Oncol 2008;15:2765–72.

122. Adam R, Aloia T, Levi F, et al. Hepatic resection after rescue cetuximab treatment for colorectal liver metastases previously refractory to conventional systemic therapy. J Clin Oncol 2007;25:4593–602.
123. Balzan S, Belghiti J, Farges O, et al. The "50-50 criteria" on postoperative day 5: an accurate predictor of liver failure and death after hepatectomy. Ann Surg 2005;242:824–8 [discussion: 828–9].
124. Etra JW, Squires MH 3rd, Fisher SB, et al. Early identification of patients at increased risk for hepatic insufficiency, complications and mortality after major hepatectomy. HPB (Oxford) 2014;16:875–83.
125. Menon KV, Al-Mukhtar A, Aldouri A, et al. Outcomes after major hepatectomy in elderly patients. J Am Coll Surg 2006;203:677–83.
126. Aldrighetti L, Arru M, Caterini R, et al. Impact of advanced age on the outcome of liver resection. World J Surg 2003;27:1149–54.
127. Ferrero A, Vigano L, Polastri R, et al. Hepatectomy as treatment of choice for hepatocellular carcinoma in elderly cirrhotic patients. World J Surg 2005;29:1101–5.
128. Hanazaki K, Kajikawa S, Shimozawa N, et al. Hepatic resection for hepatocellular carcinoma in the elderly. J Am Coll Surg 2001;192:38–46.
129. Mastoraki A, Tsakali A, Papanikolaou IS, et al. Outcome following major hepatic resection in the elderly patients. Clin Res Hepatol Gastroenterol 2014;38:462–6.
130. Alfieri S, Carriero C, Caprino P, et al. Avoiding early postoperative complications in liver surgery. A multivariate analysis of 254 patients consecutively observed. Dig Liver Dis 2001;33:341–6.
131. Koperna T, Kisser M, Schulz F. Hepatic resection in the elderly. World J Surg 1998;22:406–12.
132. Fernandes AI, Tralhao JG, Abrantes A, et al. Functional hepatocellular regeneration in elderly patients undergoing hepatectomy. Liver Int 2013. [Epub ahead of print].
133. Shoup M, Gonen M, D'Angelica M, et al. Volumetric analysis predicts hepatic dysfunction in patients undergoing major liver resection. J Gastrointest Surg 2003;7:325–30.
134. Brouquet A, Nordlinger B. Neoadjuvant therapy of colorectal liver metastases: lessons learned from clinical trials. J Surg Oncol 2010;102:932–6.
135. Fowler WC, Eisenberg BL, Hoffman JP. Hepatic resection following systemic chemotherapy for metastatic colorectal carcinoma. J Surg Oncol 1992;51:122–5.
136. Bismuth H, Adam R, Levi F, et al. Resection of nonresectable liver metastases from colorectal cancer after neoadjuvant chemotherapy. Ann Surg 1996;224:509–20 [discussion: 520–2].
137. Shankar A, Leonard P, Renaut AJ, et al. Neo-adjuvant therapy improves resectability rates for colorectal liver metastases. Ann R Coll Surg Engl 2001;83:85–8.
138. King PD, Perry MC. Hepatotoxicity of chemotherapy. Oncologist 2001;6:162–76.
139. Makuuchi M, Kokudo N, Arii S, et al. Development of evidence-based clinical guidelines for the diagnosis and treatment of hepatocellular carcinoma in Japan. Hepatol Res 2008;38:37–51.
140. Rubbia-Brandt L, Lauwers GY, Wang H, et al. Sinusoidal obstruction syndrome and nodular regenerative hyperplasia are frequent oxaliplatin-associated liver lesions and partially prevented by bevacizumab in patients with hepatic colorectal metastasis. Histopathology 2010;56:430–9.
141. Soubrane O, Brouquet A, Zalinski S, et al. Predicting high grade lesions of sinusoidal obstruction syndrome related to oxaliplatin-based chemotherapy for

colorectal liver metastases: correlation with post-hepatectomy outcome. Ann Surg 2010;251:454–60.

142. Karoui M, Penna C, Amin-Hashem M, et al. Influence of preoperative chemotherapy on the risk of major hepatectomy for colorectal liver metastatses. Ann Surg 2006;243(1):1–7.

143. Shindoh J, Tzeng CW, Aloia TA, et al. Optimal future liver remnant in patients treated with extensive preoperative chemotherapy for colorectal liver metastases. Ann Surg Oncol 2013;20(8):2493–500.

144. Fong Y, Sun RL, Jarnagin W, et al. An analysis of 412 cases of hepatocellular carcinoma at a Western center. Ann Surg 1999;229:790–9 [discussion: 799–800].

145. Midorikawa Y, Kubota K, Takayama T, et al. A comparative study of postoperative complications after hepatectomy in patients with and without chronic liver disease. Surgery 1999;126:484–91.

146. Poon RT, Fan ST, Lo CM, et al. Extended hepatic resection for hepatocellular carcinoma in patients with cirrhosis: is it justified? Ann Surg 2002;236:602–11.

147. Hsu KY, Chau GY, Lui WY, et al. Predicting morbidity and mortality after hepatic resection in patients with hepatocellular carcinoma: the role of Model for End-Stage Liver Disease score. World J Surg 2009;33:2412–9.

148. Choi GH, Park JY, Hwang HK, et al. Predictive factors for long-term survival in patients with clinically significant portal hypertension following resection of hepatocellular carcinoma. Liver Int 2011;31:485–93.

149. Ruzzenente A, Valdegamberi A, Campagnaro T, et al. Hepatocellular carcinoma in cirrhotic patients with portal hypertension: is liver resection always contraindicated? World J Gastroenterol 2011;17:5083–8.

150. Cucchetti A, Ercolani G, Vivarelli M, et al. Is portal hypertension a contraindication to hepatic resection? Ann Surg 2009;250:922–8.

151. Capussotti L, Ferrero A, Vigano L, et al. Portal hypertension: contraindication to liver surgery? World J Surg 2006;30:992–9.

152. Scheingraber S, Richter S, Igna D, et al. Indocyanine green disappearance rate is the most useful marker for liver resection. Hepatogastroenterology 2008;55:1394–9.

153. Kubota K, Makuuchi M, Kusaka K, et al. Measurement of liver volume and hepatic functional reserve as a guide to decision-making in resectional surgery for hepatic tumors. Hepatology 1997;26:1176–81.

154. Shirabe K, Shimada M, Gion T, et al. Postoperative liver failure after major hepatic resection for hepatocellular carcinoma in the modern era with special reference to remnant liver volume. J Am Coll Surg 1999;188:304–9.

155. Zorzi D, Laurent A, Pawlik TM, et al. Chemotherapy-associated hepatotoxicity and surgery for colorectal liver metastases. Br J Surg 2007;94:274–86.

156. Makuuchi M, Kosuge T, Takayama T, et al. Surgery for small liver cancers. Semin Surg Oncol 1993;9:298–304.

157. de Santibanes E, Alvarez FA, Ardiles V. How to avoid postoperative liver failure: a novel method. World J Surg 2012;36:125–8.

158. Vauthey JN, Chaoui A, Do KA, et al. Standardized measurement of the future liver remnant prior to extended liver resection: methodology and clinical associations. Surgery 2000;127:512–9.

159. Clavien PA, Selzner M, Rudiger HA, et al. A prospective randomized study in 100 consecutive patients undergoing major liver resection with versus without ischemic preconditioning. Ann Surg 2003;238:843–50 [discussion: 851–2].

160. Serafin A, Rosello-Catafau J, Prats N, et al. Ischemic preconditioning increases the tolerance of fatty liver to hepatic ischemia-reperfusion injury in the rat. Am J Pathol 2002;161:587–601.

161. Petrowsky H, McCormack L, Trujillo M, et al. A prospective, randomized, controlled trial comparing intermittent portal triad clamping versus ischemic preconditioning with continuous clamping for major liver resection. Ann Surg 2006;244:921–8 [discussion: 928–30].

162. Jin S, Dai CL. Hepatic blood inflow occlusion without hemihepatic artery control in treatment of hepatocellular carcinoma. World J Gastroenterol 2010;16: 5895–900.

163. van den Broek MA, Olde Damink SW, Dejong CH, et al. Liver failure after partial hepatic resection: definition, pathophysiology, risk factors and treatment. Liver Int 2008;28:767–80.

164. Jensen LS, Andersen AJ, Christiansen PM, et al. Postoperative infection and natural killer cell function following blood transfusion in patients undergoing elective colorectal surgery. Br J Surg 1992;79:513–6.

165. Lipka JM, Zibari GB, Dies DF, et al. Spontaneous bacterial peritonitis in liver failure. Am Surg 1998;64:1155–7.

166. Schreckenbach T, Liese J, Bechstein WO, et al. Posthepatectomy liver failure. Dig Surg 2012;29:79–85.

167. van de Kerkhove MP, de Jong KP, Rijken AM, et al. MARS treatment in posthepatectomy liver failure. Liver Int 2003;23(Suppl 3):44–51.

168. Chiu A, Chan LM, Fan ST. Molecular adsorbent recirculating system treatment for patients with liver failure: the Hong Kong experience. Liver Int 2006;26: 695–702.

169. Sisko A, Truffer C, Smith S, et al. Health spending projections through 2018: recession effects add uncertainty to the outlook. Health Aff (Millwood) 2009; 28:w346–57.

170. Birkmeyer JD, Dimick JB, Birkmeyer NJ. Measuring the quality of surgical care: structure, process, or outcomes? J Am Coll Surg 2004;198:626–32.

171. Barkun JS, Aronson JK, Feldman LS, et al. Evaluation and stages of surgical innovations. Lancet 2009;374:1089–96.

172. Ergina PL, Cook JA, Blazeby JM, et al. Challenges in evaluating surgical innovation. Lancet 2009;374:1097–104.

173. Vonlanthen R, Slankamenac K, Breitenstein S, et al. The impact of complications on costs of major surgical procedures: a cost analysis of 1200 patients. Ann Surg 2011;254:907–13.

174. Lucas DJ, Sweeney JF, Pawlik TM. The timing of complications impacts risk of readmission after hepatopancreatobiliary surgery. Surgery 2014;155:945–53.

Ablative Technologies for Hepatocellular, Cholangiocarcinoma, and Metastatic Colorectal Cancer of the Liver

Paul D. Hansen, MD*, Maria A. Cassera, BSc, Ronald F. Wolf, MD

KEYWORDS

- Liver • Ablation • Radiofrequency • Microwave • Cryotherapy
- Hepatocellular cancer • Colorectal liver metastasis

KEY POINTS

- When choosing an ablation technique or technology, the surgeon should not pit options against each other as a dichotomous choice. Rather, these options should be thought of as tools that the surgeon may select according to the needs of a particular clinical scenario.
- Benign and malignant, as well as primary and metastatic tumors may all be ablated in appropriately selected clinical scenarios.
- In general, ablation is limited to a few and small tumors and is favored over resection in patients who are poor candidates for major surgical interventions.
- Ablation technologies can generally be broken down into chemical and thermal. Each of these technologies can be applied using a percutaneous, laparoscopic, or open surgical approach.

INTRODUCTION

Surgical resection has historically been considered the gold standard for curative treatment in patients diagnosed with hepatocellular carcinoma (HCC), cholangiocarcinoma, colorectal cancer hepatic metastasis (CRLM), and selected patients with other types of primary and secondary tumors with liver-only disease. Nonetheless, only 5% to 15% of patients are candidates for liver resection because of

The authors have nothing to disclose.
Hepatobiliary and Pancreatic Surgery Program, Providence Cancer Center, Providence Portland Medical Center, 4805 NE Glisan St, Suite 6N60, Portland, OR 97213, USA
* Corresponding author.
E-mail address: phansen@orclinic.com

tumor size, location, volume, multifocality, or because of inadequate functional hepatic reserve or comorbid disease.[1] Ablative therapeutic techniques have been introduced as safe and effective treatment alternatives to hepatic resection. Recently, randomized trials and case-matched series[2,3] have indicated that results of ablative techniques can approach equivalence to results of resection in subsets of these patients.

A wide range of ablative technologies and techniques have been introduced over the last several decades, and each has specific advantages relative to the others, depending on the clinical situation. Ablative technologies generally fall into 2 categories: chemical and thermal. More recently, irreversible electroporation (IRE) has been introduced as an alternative form of electrically induced cellular destruction. In this article, a general overview is provided of liver tumor ablation technologies and techniques for use, as well as an overview of technology selection, patient selection, current ablation strategies, and overall outcomes.

ABLATION TECHNOLOGIES

Tumor ablation is not a new concept. Crude versions of tissue or tumor ablation have been reported over the centuries. With a better understanding of oncology and the advent of modern imaging and ablation technologies, we have developed the ability to evaluate tissues harboring cancers and accurately target tumors and safely ablate them. Although the usefulness and efficacy of using these strategies continues to be worked out, there is clear evidence that in selected cases, patients can be cured from lethal diseases with minimal morbidity.

Currently, the most common forms of tumor ablation use either chemical or thermal technologies. Specific details of each are reviewed later. In general, the interest in using nonresective techniques stems from several factors. Although resection has become significantly safer over the last 2 decades, and it is now possible to perform resection using minimally invasive approaches, the incidence of complications associated with ablation is substantially less than that described for surgical resection. In addition, because ablation can be targeted toward individual tumors, surrounding parenchyma is spared, an important factor in patients with extensive disease, limited liver reserve, or who may require repeated interventions.

Chemical Ablation

The most widely used form of chemical ablation is injection of ethanol, although some centers have reported using 5% acetic acid as an alternative.[4] Slow injection of 95% ethanol directly into a tumor induces local coagulation necrosis, thrombosis of tumor microvasculature, and tissue ischemia.

Benefits of chemical ablation include the simplicity of the procedure and the relatively lower cost of the procedure. The chemicals are inexpensive and if the target is easily identifiable, the procedure can be performed under ultrasonographic (US) guidance as an outpatient. A critical advantage of chemical ablation is the ability to limit the collateral damage by targeting tumors immediately adjacent to central biliary and vascular structures, which may be damaged by thermal ablation.

An important limitation of chemical ablation is that it depends on an equal distribution and exposure of the tumor to the chemical ablatant. Although HCC and neuroendocrine tumors (NETs) are relatively soft and often encapsulated, harder tumors such as metastatic adenocarcinoma, typically hard and fibrous, do not allow distribution of the ablatant within the tumor parenchyma.

As a result of relatively high recurrence rates, chemical ablation is typically considered only for patients with small HCCs (<2 cm), who are not resection or thermal ablation candidates (ie, adjacent to central biliary structures).

Thermal Ablation

Cryotherapy

Cryoablation is a technique that uses probe tips that are supercooled by the circulation of either liquid nitrogen or liquid argon. Supercooling to temperatures lower than −170°C induces cell death through the induction of ice crystal formation, cell wall disruption, and microvascular thrombosis.

The advantage of cryotherapy is primarily the ability to easily visualize the lead edge of the ice ball, and, therefore, the margin of the ablation. The lead edge is a bright echo reflector and easily seen on US.

There are several important limitations of cryotherapy. Probes range in diameter from 5 mm to 10 mm. The maximal size of ice ball created using a single probe is 5 cm. To create larger ablation zones, multiple probes are required. During the thaw cycle, ablations are prone to freeze fractures, akin to dropping an ice cube in a glass of warm water. Such freeze fracture can result in vascular injuries and significant hemorrhage. On removal of the probes, hemorrhage within the tract is not uncommon and is typically managed by packing the tract with thrombogenic agents. Both of these issues limit a minimally invasive approach. There are posttreatment systemic effects that are unique to cryotherapy, rarely seen with heat ablation. These effects include severe thrombocytopenia, coagulopathy, myoglobinuria, acute renal failure, as well as electrolyte disturbances and cardiac arrhythmia.[5–11] These potential problems require additional monitoring and fluid management and prolong postprocedure hospital stay (**Fig. 1**).

Heat therapy

There are a wide variety of technologies that induce tissue heating to temperatures higher than 50°C. At this temperature, proteins begin to denature, cell walls degrade, and microvascular thrombosis occurs. Higher than 60°C, cells die instantaneously. Thus, any technology that can be applied safely and accurately enough to induce 100% cellular necrosis of the target tumor and spare surrounding tissue may serve as an ablation technology. The most widely available technologies include radiofrequency ablation (RFA) and microwave ablation (MWA).

There are several limitations with current thermal ablation technologies. Thermal ablation depends on achieving lethal temperatures in the entire treatment region.

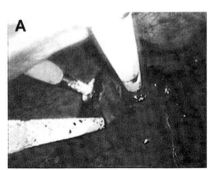
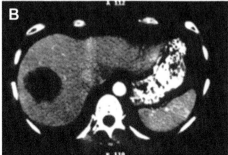

Fig. 1. (*A*) Three cryoprobes creating 5-cm ice ball in the liver. (*B*) CT scan showing the necrotic lesion 10 days postoperatively.

Although measurement of temperature at several points within the ablation zone is available for one of the clinically available thermal devices, others do so at a single point, or by using empirically determined ablation times, or impedance measurements. With tumors located close to central biliary structures, the thermal energy used to destroy the target tumor may also cause irreversible damage to the bile duct, which can lead to abscess or biliary stricture. Also, adjacent viscera, such as duodenum and colon, are easily damaged if near an ablation zone. Most surgeons avoid using thermal ablation within 1 to 2 cm of these structures and are careful to exclude colon and duodenum from the region being treated.

Radiofrequency ablation

RFA is the most commonly used technology for heat ablation. RFA uses a high-frequency alternating current to change the orientation of ions in the electrical field applied to the tumor and surrounding tissue. The agitation of ions creates frictional energy and heat, which are distributed via conduction. Ablation times for a single target depend on size and location, but range between 10 and 30 minutes, with an average of about 20 minutes for a 2-cm tumor. Advantages of RFA include the ease with which the technology can be applied percutaneously, laparoscopically, or in open surgery. The largest commercial probes allow the creation of a 6-cm to 7-cm zone of ablation with the placement of a single probe. This strategy facilitates the ablation of larger lesions with a single needle placement. The disadvantage of RFA is that it is slower than MWA and does not heat large vessels as well as MWA (**Fig. 2**).[12]

Microwave ablation

MWA uses dielectric hysteresis to produce heat. Tissue destruction occurs when tissues are heated as a result of the application of a magnetic field, typically 900 to 2500 MHz. The polar molecules present in tissue are forced to continuously realign with the oscillating electric field increasing their kinetic energy, increasing the

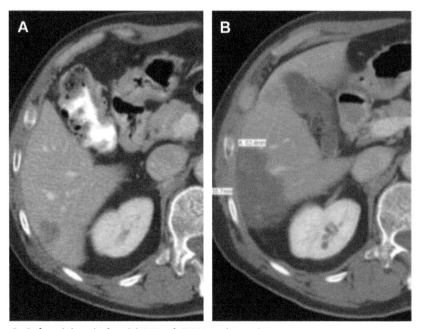

Fig. 2. Before (A) and after (B) RFA of CRLM and margin.

temperature of the tissue. Tissues with a high percentage of water, including tumors, are sensitive to this type of heating.

Microwaves are capable of propagating through and effectively heating many types of tissue, even those with low electrical conductivity, high impedance, or low thermal conductivity. Microwaves can readily penetrate the charred or desiccated tissues that tend to build up around other thermal ablation applicators, resulting in limited power delivery for non–microwave energy systems.

Advantages of MWA include the speed of ablation (range of 5–20 minutes and an average of 12 minutes for a 2-cm tumor) and the ability to treat tumors immediately adjacent to vasculature without the loss of heat as a result of the radiant cooling effect of blood flow. The main disadvantage of the currently available technologies is the size limitations of ablations using single probes. The maximal diameter of a single probe ablation is around 4.6 cm. Thus, the largest target tumor with a 1-cm margin that can be ablated with a single probe application is 2.6 cm. Larger ablations require multiple applications of a single probe or placement of multiple simultaneous probes, both of which may be problematic and raise the possibility of treatment failure, secondary to lack of overlap of concentric treatment zones (**Fig. 3**).

Irreversible electroporation

IRE is a newer, nonthermal ablation technique that uses pulsed direct current to induce cell death. IRE takes advantage of the electrical gradient that exists across cell membranes, and the application of high-voltage direct electrical current across the cell has the ability to alter the transmembrane potential and disrupt the lipid bilayer. This situation leads to the creation of small nanopores, which allow for an increased influx of extracellular ions. When the voltage applied is sufficiently high, these pores become permanent.[13] These ions are cleared by adenosine triphosphate (ATP)-dependent ion pumps, resulting in intracellular depletion of ATP, which subsequently leads to cell death by apoptosis, with tissues reaching a maximum apoptotic rate after 24 hours.[14] Although cell death is believed to occur via the formation of permanent nanopores in the cell membrane, the extracellular matrix, and thus, collagen structure of vessels and ducts, seem to remain intact.

Unlike thermal ablation techniques, IRE does not encounter the problem of a heat-sink effect, in which local flowing blood draws off the induced heat, with resultant reduced therapeutic effect. IRE is believed to be safe close to vital structures, because the proposed mechanism of action is nonthermal, although more recent articles have pointed out a thermal potential for IRE.[14]

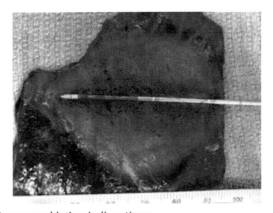

Fig. 3. Ex-vivo microwave ablation in liver tissue.

PATIENT SELECTION
Tumor Types

With the exception of extrahepatic bile duct tumors, essentially all primary and secondary tumor types in the liver are potential candidates for ablation. The indications for tumor ablation are varied and are based on clinical decision making similar to that used for liver tumor resection. Although the morbidity profile and traumatic impact of ablation are typically significantly less than those for resection, the clinical indications are not broadened.

In general, benign tumors of the liver are ablated only if they are symptomatic or growing. There are rarely indications to treat focal nodular hyperplasia and hemangiomas with resection or ablation. Adenomas do have a malignant potential and a propensity to bleed. If there are clinical indications to resect an adenoma, ablation may be considered as an alternative. When ablating a benign lesion, the requirement to ablate surrounding margin of normal tissue is typically relaxed, and thus, larger tumors may be treated with curative intent.

The indications to ablate malignant tumors of the liver are again similar to indications for resection. The advantage to the ablative approach is that the reduced traumatic impact, reduced morbidity profile, and parenchymal sparring with ablation, increase the patient pool in which a potentially curative procedure can be performed.

Hepatocellular carcinoma

There are unique features to treating patients with HCC. First is that most patients with HCC have cirrhosis. Limited hepatic reserve restricts a large percentage of these patients from undergoing curative treatments. The parenchymal sparring effect of ablation allows treatment with significantly less impact on hepatic reserve. HCC is often a soft and encapsulated tumor, thus allowing diffuse infiltration of the tumor with chemical ablatants. This situation makes the chemical ablation an option when treating HCC. HCC is often a multifocal tumor, with separate primaries, intrahepatic metastatic lesions, or satellite lesions near, but not a part of the primary tumor. This multifocality leads to a higher rate of treatment failure when using any form of ablation.

Colorectal cancer hepatic metastasis

CRLM are also amenable to an ablative approach. As a gastrointestinal adenocarcinoma, these tumors are firm, and thus, are not good candidates for chemical ablation. There is an increasing body of literature supporting the use of thermal ablation (primarily RFA and MWA) in patients with CRLM. Ablation can be used alone in patients who are not good candidates for surgical resection, or in combination in patients with extensive or bilobar disease.

Neuroendocrine tumors

Patients with NET are also potentially good candidates for ablation. Generally, liver NETs are metastatic tumors, because there are few primary liver NETs. Some are hormonally active and, therefore, symptomatic. NETs are typically slow growing, but persistent tumors, rarely cured once metastatic to the liver. These patients often require multiple interventions over the course of their disease. Because these are soft tumors, lesions abutting central biliary structures may be treated with chemical ablation.

Other

Ablation of a wide variety of other tumor types has been described in the literature. They include primary lesions such as intrahepatic cholangiocarcinoma, noncolorectal gastrointestinal malignancies, breast cancer, head and neck cancers, thoracic malignancies, and sarcomas. The clinical indications for ablating such lesions must be carefully considered. If there are indications to resect such a tumor, then, ablation may be considered.

General Health

One of the advantages of liver tumor ablation is that there are several approaches, including both percutaneous and surgical. Thus, selection of the appropriate ablation technique for a given patient includes not only consideration of the requirements of the tumor ablation but the ability of the patient to tolerate an intervention.

The percutaneous approach is generally believed to be the least traumatic. Both laparoscopic and open surgical approaches require general anesthesia. The laparoscopic approach is typically performed with only 2 10-mm ports. Although this approach is slightly more traumatic than a percutaneous approach, it is barely so. An open approach requires a laparotomy incision and, therefore, patients selected for such an approach must be able to tolerate this more maximally invasive intervention. Chemical ablations can be performed under sedation, although thermal ablations, because of pain, almost always require either deep sedation or general anesthesia.

Ablation Limitations

Although ablative technologies have opened the door to applying curative treatments to a wider array of patients, there are still clearly limitations on its use. All of the ablation technologies have size limitations. In all tumor types, and with all technologies, there is a higher likelihood of treatment failure in larger tumors. The bulk of the literature suggests that most technologies work well in tumors smaller than 3 cm. The likelihood of treatment failure is intermediate in tumors between 3 cm and 5 cm, and the likelihood of failure in tumors larger than 5 cm is high. Some clinical scenarios allow for multiple ablations of the same tumor to compensate for larger tumor size, but in practical terms, this almost always results in a poorer outcome.

Similarly, tumor number is a relative contraindication. Although no upper limit of tumor numbers has been established for any tumor type or technology, it is generally accepted that the more tumors requiring treatment, the higher the likelihood of both local and regional treatment failure. Challenges with ablations of multiple tumors include visualization of tumors, because most ablation technologies result in some obscuration of imaging of deeper structures. Keeping track of multiple ablations can be problematic both intraoperatively and postoperatively. Larger treatment volumes are associated with higher morbidity rates. Again, although no hard limits have been established, most practitioners do not ablate more than about 30% of the volume of the liver using any given technique. Treatment of larger volumes may require a combination of resection and ablation. Large volumes of ethanol injection result in acute hypotension and posttreatment intoxication.

As described earlier, thermal ablations within 1 to 2 cm of the central biliary structures (right, left, and common hepatic ducts) are fraught with danger. Thermal injury is nondiscriminating, and although larger central blood vessels remain patent because their, blood flow protects them by radiant cooling, the bile ducts are vulnerable. Some practitioners have described using cooling techniques, such as flushing the bile duct with cooled saline during the ablation.[15] The degree of heating is difficult to measure and control accurately. Most practitioners avoid aggressive thermal ablations in this area and instead opt for resection or chemical ablations where indicated (**Fig. 4**).

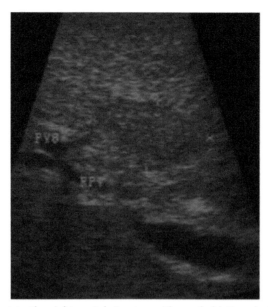

Fig. 4. NET adjacent to the right portal structures. Thermal ablation destroys the right hepatic duct. The tumor was injected with ethanol.

ABLATION APPROACHES
Percutaneous/Laparoscopic/Open Surgical

Each approach has theoretic and proven advantages and disadvantages. Percutaneous ablation has the advantage of providing a safe and the least invasive and least expensive approach to treating small hepatic tumors. Whether chemical or thermal, these approaches may be performed under sedation. This factor prevents costs and risks associated with general anesthesia.

The percutaneous approach also has the highest treatment failure rate. The reasons for this situation are multifactorial. The percutaneous approach does not include pretreatment staging with peritoneoscopy or intraoperative contact US. This situation leads to treatment failure because of additional undiagnosed hepatic lesions or extrahepatic disease. Further, tumor targeting is more problematic, because US imaging through the abdominal or chest wall limits the approach and degrades the quality of image relative to surface contact US with either a laparoscopic or open US approach.

Computed tomography (CT) or magnetic resonance imaging (MRI) guided ablations are limited because of the appearance of target tumors on these studies in the absence of contrast agents. Although CT and MRI are highly precise in defining tumor and liver anatomy with contrast, needle placement is performed without contrast when tumors are often not directly visible.

Whether using US, CT, or MRI, tumors that are high under the diaphragm may be difficult to reach percutaneously. Also, tumors on the surface of the liver near adjacent organs, which might be injured during thermal ablation, are at risk with nearby ablations. Both of these scenarios are better managed with laparoscopic or open surgical techniques, in which the dome of the liver can be accessed and surrounding viscera can be safely protected (**Fig. 5**).

The overall morbidity of a laparoscopic approach is not dissimilar to the percutaneous approach, but with the addition of 2 ports, 1 (5–10 mm) for the camera and a

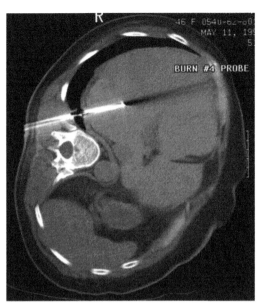

Fig. 5. CT-guided placement of an RFA probe high on the dome of the liver. Notice that the contrast has washed out during placement. Final probe position is determined via triangulation with other known anatomic landmarks.

10-mm port for the US device. However, laparoscopy requires general anesthesia and sometimes lysis of adhesions to gain access to the liver. Surgical incisions are sometimes a problem in cirrhotic patients who are at risk for the development of postprocedure liver decompensation and ascetic leaks.

An open approach involves a greater degree of trauma to the patient, with the associated physiologic stresses and recovery. Although there are no segments of the liver that cannot be accessed by a laparoscopic approach, an open approach may facilitate a concomitant procedure, such as a major resection. An open approach may also be useful if the surgeon does not have access to laparoscopic equipment or has not had training in the more technically challenging laparoscopic approach.

Targeting Techniques

Ultrasonographic tumor targeting
The basic technique involves locating the target tumor with the US. The US is aligned such that the ablation device courses parallel to the long axis of the US image as it approaches the tumor. This strategy allows the surgeon to adjust the angle (depth) of approach from top to bottom. By rolling the US slightly side to side, the surgeon can direct the ablation probe side to side to the center of the target.

With open surgical approaches, the entry point of the ablation probe is often close to the end of the US probe. The optimal angle of approach is about 45°. Too steep of an approach makes it difficult to see the approaching ablation probe. Using a laparoscopic technique, selecting the entry point on both the skin and the liver surface can be more challenging, because the surgeon needs to anticipate the thickness of the abdominal wall, the distance to the liver, and the depth of the target within the liver (**Fig. 6**).

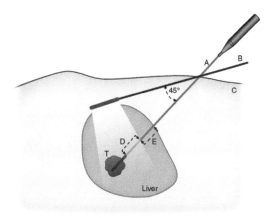

Fig. 6. Placement of the ablation needle under US guidance. The US and ablation probe are passed through the abdominal wall. The ablation probe is placed into the tumor under US guidance at a 45° degree angle. The angle can be adjusted by moving the entry point of the ablation probe through the abdominal wall. The US provides a longitudinal view directly below the head of the probe, and operators must take caution when placing the ablation needle through liver parenchyma outside the field of view. A, ablation probe; B, US probe; C, abdominal wall; D, within view of the US; E, out of view of the US; T, tumor.

PERIOPERATIVE PROCESS
Preoperative Evaluation

Treatment eligibility and screening generally involve routine history and physical, laboratory tests, and multiphasic cross-sectional imaging with either CT or MRI.

Patient Positioning

Percutaneous
The patient is positioned supine, and a sterile field is created. Heavy sedation or general anesthesia is often required, because thermal ablations can generate a strong pain and distress response. Placement of the ablation probe occurs under image guidance, ensuring that there is a safe pathway and nearby organs are not at risk for injury. After sedation or induction of general anesthesia, the ablation device is deployed into the tumor. Chemical ablatants are injected, monitoring the hypoechoic blush to ensure even disbursement throughout the target. If thermal ablation is being used, the probe is deployed into the tumor; precise placement within the target is required to ensure complete treatment. The ablation is performed, ensuring that the target tumor and a 1-cm margin of normal liver are ablated.

Laparoscopic
The patients is placed supine, general anesthesia is induced, and a sterile field is created. The surgeon stands on the patient's left, with the laparoscopic and US monitors near the right shoulder. This strategy allows the surgeon to stand in alignment with the target organ and the monitors. One 10-mm port is placed below the margin of the liver, lateral to rectus muscle. One port placed near the umbilicus is used for the camera (5–10 mm). After induction of general anesthesia, trocars are placed into the abdomen, and a staging laparoscopy is completed. In the absence of obvious unresectable extrahepatic disease, intraoperative US is performed to stage the current hepatic disease accurately and to direct treatment. Under US guidance, the RFA probe is deployed into the tumor, and a 1-cm margin of normal liver is ablated (**Fig. 7**).

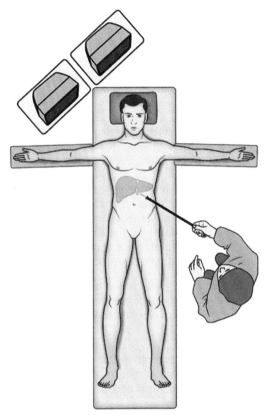

Fig. 7. Patient positioning for a liver tumor ablation procedure. (*Left monitor*) US; (*right monitor*) laparoscopic view.

Open surgical approach

Generally, a right subcostal or midline incision is made, with the surgeon standing on the patient's left for the RFA portion of the procedure. The US monitor is again placed near the patient's right shoulder to facilitate alignment of the surgeon, target tumor, and monitor. After the appropriate incision is made, exploration of the abdomen, and resection of other tumors if applicable, US of the liver is undertaken. Using direct contact US, the ablation device is passed into the liver and target and the ablation performed. Open RFA may facilitate access to the posterior aspects of the right lobe, segments 8 and 7, because ablation angles are more versatile, although experienced laparoscopists can generally reach all 8 segments.

Chemical ablation

The volume of ethanol required to ablate a tumor depends on the size of the tumor, the total dose being based on the results of imaging studies.[16,17] An injection volume equivalent to the estimated target volume is adequate. For spherical tumors, the formula $(4/3 * pi * r^2)$ is used. Although pure 95% ethanol is used for smaller volume injections, larger injections may require dilution with saline to as low as a 50% concentration. Large volume injections (>50 mL) must be performed with caution and under careful monitoring, because ethanol injections can cause transient hypotension and intoxication.

The injection is started on the deep aspect of the tumor, because the injectate creates a hyperechoic field, obscuring imaging of deeper structures. Injection may be performed with standard 15.2-cm (6 in), 20-gauge to 22-gauge spinal needle, or using a specially designed conical-tip needle with multiple side holes. The position of the needle is moved around inside the tumor during the injection to ensure an even distribution of injectate throughout the target.

Postoperative Concerns

Percutaneous and laparoscopic thermal ablation
Patients who undergo CT-guided ablations are typically discharged from the short-stay unit within 23 hours of the procedure, although some procedures are performed with same day discharge.

After laparoscopic RFA, patients are generally kept overnight for observation and discharged on postoperative day 1. Same day discharge is becoming more common. Before discharge, patients must be ambulatory, tolerate oral fluid intake, have adequate pain control, and be reliable and willing to return if problems arise. We recommend overnight observation of most patients with intrinsic liver function compromise, or patients with portal hypertension.

Open thermal ablation
Generally, length of hospital stay for patients with open RFA is determined by pain control and postlaparotomy factors. Liver function should be assessed.

Complications and Management

Complications after ablation are uncommon (1%–5%). Although large volume heat ablations can induce intermittent fevers related to volume of tissue destruction, the procedure is generally well tolerated. Most patients have pain in the epigastrium, right upper quadrant, and right flank, which can last 1 to 2 weeks. Liver abscesses can occur, primarily in patients who have had previous biliary manipulation. Bleeding and bile leak occur rarely. More rare, but more serious complications have been reported and include injury to bowel or bile-pleural fistulae (**Fig. 8**).

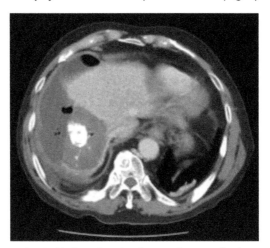

Fig. 8. Although some heat ablation sites develop small areas of entrapped gas, air bubbles may be a sign of abscess formation. Patients may show signs of infection and possibly sepsis. Treatment is antibiotics and possible percutaneous drainage. Surgical debridement is rarely necessary.

Liver failure may occur in patients with very large volume ablations or in those with compromised liver function caused by cirrhosis. Cirrhotic patients may be kept in hospital for a few days depending on the degree of liver dysfunction and the size of the ablation.

Long-Term Follow-Up

Contrast-enhanced, cross-sectional imaging is obtained 10 to 14 days after the procedure to evaluate the degree of ablation. Ablated tissue lacks perfusion. A nonperfused region should be seen incorporating the target tumor and a 1-cm margin of surrounding parenchyma. Persistent perfusion in or near the tumor suggests an incomplete ablation. Persistent disease may be retreated at this time. Over time, the ablated region may decrease in size, although the tumors rarely disappear.

OUTCOMES
Hepatocellular Carcinoma

Surgical resection and liver transplantation are the widely recognized curative options available for HCC, with 5-year survival rates reported in the literature ranging from 36% to 70% and 60% to 70%, respectively.[18] However, only 10% to 20% of patients diagnosed with HCC are deemed to have resectable disease, because of tumor burden, functional hepatic reserve, or comorbidities. Local ablative therapies such as percutaneous ethanol injection (PEI) and thermal ablation are of particular interest in this patient population and have potential for wider adoption. Prospective, randomized trials are impractical, because of the differences in the populations selected for each of the approaches.

Radiofrequency ablation for hepatocellular carcinoma
Of the thermal ablative technologies available, RFA has become the most widely used. Major complication rates reported in the literature range from 0% to 10%, with local failure rates between 1.7% and 29.4%.[19–31] Success rates are directly correlated with tumor size and approach. Higher success rates are seen in tumors smaller than 3 cm with surgical versus percutaneous approaches.

For the percutaneous and laparoscopic approaches, 1-year, 3-year, and 5-year survivals of 79% to 100%, 42% to 91%, and 20% to 72.8% have been reported, respectively.[19–31] These survivals compare with the reported survival results and improve on the complication rates for both resection and transplant (**Table 1**).

Percutaneous ethanol ablation for hepatocellular carcinoma
Major complications have been reported to range from 0% to 2.2% in the literature.[4,16,23,24,29,32–40] Local failure rates for PEI range from 0% to 34.5% in the published literature, and studies have shown that local failure for PEI is closely correlated to tumor size. Several studies have reported that a complete response can be obtained in 90% to 100% of tumors smaller than 2 to 3 cm, in 70% to 80% of tumors smaller than 3 cm, and in 50% to 60% of tumors larger than 3 cm.[41–43] Thus, PEI is generally not recommended for tumors larger than 5 cm.

One-year, 3-year, and 5-year survival rates as reported in the literature range from 88% to 97%, 62% to 81.6%, and 39% to 60.3%, respectively.[4,16,23,24,29,32–40]

Several randomized trials have shown that RFA significantly improved survival and reduced local recurrence rates over PEI for small HCC, and for this reason, thermal ablation techniques are preferred over chemical ablation (**Table 2**).[29,37,44,45]

Table 1
Outcomes for RFA of HCC

Author, Year	n	Approach	1-y Survival (%)	3-y Survival (%)	5-y Survival (%)	Complications (%)	Local Ablation Site Failures (%)
Cillo et al,[20] 2013	103	Lap	79	49	40	—	—
Wong et al,[30] 2013	76	Lap/open	87.3	61	48.6	4.7 (all diagnoses)	24.7
Shiina et al,[29] 2005	118	Perc	—	—	74 (4 y)	—	1.7
Guglielmi et al,[21] 2008	109	Perc	—	42	20	10	—
Wong et al,[30] 2013	100	Perc	92.8	68.7	47.2	4.7 (all diagnoses)	29.4
Chen et al,[19] 2006	71	Perc	95.8	71.4	64	4.2	4.2
Hong et al,[22] 2005	55	Perc	100	72.7	—	—	—
Lu et al,[27] 2006	51	Perc	93.5	87.1	—	7.8	—
Wong et al,[31] 2013	36	Perc	97.1	91	72.8	0	—

Abbreviations: Lap, laparoscopic; n, number of patients; Perc, percutaneous.

Cryoablation for hepatocellular carcinoma

Cryoablation has been used for treatment of small HCC; however, the only data currently in the literature that report cryoablation alone are data from smaller nonrandomized trials and retrospective review series. In addition, outcomes data for

Table 2
Outcomes for PEI of HCC

Author, Year	n	1-y Survival (%)	3-y Survival (%)	5-y Survival (%)	Complications (%)	Local Ablation Site Failures (%)
Ebara et al,[34] 2005	270	—	81.6	60.3	2.2	10
Shiina et al,[29] 2005	114	—	63	—	—	0
Pompili et al,[39] 2001	111	97	62	41	0	—
Fartoux et al,[35] 2005	102	—	70	—	0	24
Brunello et al,[33] 2008	69	—	57	—	—	—
Sung et al,[40] 2006	64	—	71	39	0	—
Lin et al,[37] 2005	62	88	81	—	0	34.5

Abbreviation: n, number of patients.

cryoablation in the setting of HCC are difficult to interpret, because almost all reports combine patients treated with cryoablation alone and cryoablation performed concomitantly with resection, or combine treatment outcomes for multiple diseases. The complication rates for cryoablation in the setting of HCC range from 0% to 59%, with a local failure rate of 13.6% to 27.3%, reported in the literature. One-year survival for HCC ranges from 63.9% to 66% in the literature (**Table 3**).[46–51]

Microwave ablation for hepatocellular carcinoma

MWA has been used in small series for HCC, with satisfactory results. Postoperative complication rates range from 0% to 15.9%, with local failure rates of 2.9% to 11.8%. One-year, 3-year, and 5-year survival rates range from 38% to 92.5%, 19% to 50.5%, and 36.8% to 70%, respectively (**Table 4**).[52–57]

Irreversible electroporation for hepatocellular carcinoma

Recently, IRE has been used as an alternative ablative therapy for unresectable HCC, and long-term outcomes data in the literature are sparse. In these small series, the complication rates ranged from 0% to 10%, with no local recurrences reported. The 1-year survivals were reported to be between 50% and 100%.[58–60]

A study by Cheung and colleagues[59] reported that IRE was both feasible and safe in treating unresectable HCC, with a 93% success rate for tumors smaller than 3 cm. For tumors greater than 3 cm, the success rate decreased to 72%. During the study follow-up period of 18 months, no recurrences or deaths were reported (**Table 5**).

Colorectal Liver Metastasis

Radiofrequency ablation for colorectal liver metastasis

Major complication rates reported in the literature range from 0% to 10.6%, with local failure rates between 2.6% and 37%.[2,61–74]

For the percutaneous approach, 1-year, 3-year, and 5-year survivals of 79% to 98%, 38% to 69%, and 19% to 25.5% have been reported, respectively. For the laparoscopic and open approaches, 1-year, 3-year, and 5-year survivals of 87% to 93.5%, 20.2% to 57%, and 18.4% to 33.1% have been reported, respectively.[2,61–74]

Table 3						
Outcomes for cryoablation of HCC						
Author, Year	**n**	**1-y Survival (%)**	**3-y Survival (%)**	**5-y Survival (%)**	**Complications (%)**	**Local Ablation Site Failures (%)**
Zhou & Tang,[51] 1998	78	63.9	40.3	26.9	0	—
Pearson et al,[48] 1999	54 all diagnosis (7 HCC)	—	—	—	40.7	13.6
Haddad et al,[47] 1998	31	59	22	—	59	—
Adam et al,[46] 2002	31	66	—	—	29	27.3
Wren et al,[50] 1997	12	64	—	—	8.3	—

Abbreviation: n, number of patients.

Table 4
Outcomes for MWA of HCC

Author, Year	n	1-y Survival (%)	3-y Survival (%)	5-y Survival (%)	Complications (%)	Local Ablation Site Failures (%)
Groeschl et al,[54] 2014	139	38	19	—	15.9 open 9.3 lap 11.1 perc	6
Dong et al,[53] 2003	82	92.5	75.3 (2 y)	—	—	—
Swan et al,[57] 2013	54	72.3	58.8 (2 y)	—	28.9	2.9
Lu et al,[55] 2005	49	81.6	50.5	36.8 (4 y)	8.2	11.8
Dong et al,[52] 1998	41	—	—	—	—	11
Seki et al,[56] 1999	23	—	—	70	0	8

Abbreviations: Lap, laparoscopic; n, number of patients; Perc, percutaneous.

A large meta-analysis conducted by Mulier and colleagues[75] found that on univariate analysis, factors associated with higher recurrence rates were larger size, subcapsular location of the tumor, proximity to large vessels, vascular occlusion, and a 1-cm margin. On multivariate analysis, tumor size smaller than 3 cm and surgical approach (open and laparoscopic) versus a percutaneous approach showed a statistically significant difference, with percutaneous ablation having a higher recurrence rate.

It is difficult to directly compare RFA and resection in patients treated with RFA, because of selection biases; however, a recent study by Hammill and colleagues[2] reported that in patients who underwent RFA and were deemed technically resectable, 5-year survival rate was 48%, which is comparable with that of hepatic resection. Difficulty in separating the end point of local failure (tumor recurrence in the ablation bed) versus overall survival makes interpretation of the efficacy of ablation confusing. In addition, defining the ablation as having curative intent compared with using it in the unresectable patient has complicated interpretation of the survival results (**Table 6**).

Microwave ablation for colorectal liver metastasis
Major complications for microwave in patients with CRLM range from 0% to 19%, with a 6% to 14% local recurrence rate. In the literature, 1-year, 3-year, and 5-year

Table 5
Outcomes for IRE of HCC

Author, Year	n	1-y Survival (%)	3-y Survival (%)	5-y Survival (%)	Complications (%)	Local Ablation Site Failures (%)
Cannon et al,[58] 2013	14	50	—	—	10 (all diagnoses)	0
Philips et al,[60] 2013	13	—	—	—	8.5 (all diagnoses)	0
Cheung et al,[59] 2013	11	100	—	—	0	0

Abbreviation: n, number of patients.

Table 6
Outcomes for RFA of CRLM

Author, Year	n	RFA Approach	1-y Survival (%)	3-y Survival (%)	5-y Survival (%)	Complications (%)	Local Ablation Site Failures (%)
Veltri et al,[73] 2008	122	Perc	79	38	22	1.1	26.3
Sorensen et al,[72] 2007	102	Perc	87	46	—	6.9	—
Solbiati et al,[70] 2012	99	Perc	98	69.3	25	2	6.9
Park et al,[68] 2008	30	Perc	—	—	19	—	23
White et al,[74] 2007	22	Perc	—	28	—	—	36
Hur et al,[65] 2009	25	Perc/lap	—	60	25.5	0	28
Siperstein et al,[69] 2007	234	Lap	—	20.2	18.4	—	—
Kennedy et al,[67] 2013	130	Lap	93.5	50.1	28.8	1.5	9.2 (3.6% <3 cm tumors)
Hammill et al,[2] 2011	113	Lap	87	52	33.1	1.8	2.6
Berber et al,[64] 2008	68	Lap	—	35	30	2.9	—
Aloia et al,[63] 2006	30	Open	—	57	27	—	37
Abitabile et al,[62] 2007	47	Open/perc	88	57	21	10.6	—

Abbreviations: Lap, laparoscopic; n, number of patients; Perc, percutaneous.

Table 7
Outcomes for MWA of CRLM

Author, Year	n	1-y Survival (%)	3-y Survival (%)	5-y Survival (%)	Complications (%)	Local Ablation Site Failures (%)
Tanaka et al,[80] 2006	16 (microwave + resection)	80	51	17	19	—
Groeschl et al,[54] 2014	198	45	17	—	—	6 (all diagnoses)
Ogata et al,[78] 2008	32	—	—	32	—	—
Liang et al,[77] 2003	21	91.4	46.4	—	0	14
Shibata et al,[79] 2000	14	71	57	14	14.3	—

Abbreviation: n, number of patients.

Table 8 RFA of NETs							
Author, Year	n	RFA Approach	1-y Survival (%)	3-y Survival (%)	5-y Survival (%)	Complications (%)	Local Ablation Site Failures (%)
Berber & Siperstein,[83] 2007	74	Lap	—	—	—	5	—
Karabulut et al,[84] 2011	69	Lap	—	—	—	10	22
Berber & Siperstein,[82] 2008	63	Lap	—	—	48	—	—
Mazzaglia et al,[85] 2007	63	Lap	98	—	57	—	6.3
Taner et al,[87] 2013	94	Hepatic resection + open ablation	100	93.6	80	1	3.8

Abbreviations: Lap, laparoscopic; n, number of patients; Perc, percutaneous.

survivals for MWA have been reported to range between 45% and 91.4%, 46.4% and 57%, and 14% and 32%, respectively.[54,76–80]

Shibata and colleagues[79] reported a microwave versus hepatic resection randomized trial. For the MWA group, 1-year, 3-year, and 5-year survival rates of 71%, 57% and 14% were reported, with a mean survival time of 25 months and local recurrence rate of 4.2% to 14%. These data were not found to be statistically different from the resection group. These results suggest that outcomes for MWA may be comparable with hepatic resection in treating CRLM; however, larger series are needed (**Table 7**).

Neuroendocrine

Radiofrequency ablation for neuroendocrine tumors
Several small series have reported complication rates of 1% to 10% in RFA for NETs of the liver, with a recurrence rate of 3.8% to 22%. Five-year survival has been reported to be as high as 80% in select patients.[81–87]

Data in the literature for NET are often difficult to interpret, because outcomes data are grouped with other diseases, or RFA is used in conjunction with hepatic resection. Five-year overall survival outcomes for patients who have undergone RFA in conjunction with hepatic resection range from 48% to 80% in the literature (**Table 8**).[88–90]

REFERENCES

1. Weng M, Zhang Y, Zhou D, et al. Radiofrequency ablation versus resection for colorectal cancer liver metastases: a meta-analysis. PLoS One 2012;7(9):21.
2. Hammill CW, Billingsley KG, Cassera MA, et al. Outcome after laparoscopic radiofrequency ablation of technically resectable colorectal liver metastases. Ann Surg Oncol 2011;18(7):1947–54.
3. Livraghi T, Meloni F, Di Stasi M, et al. Sustained complete response and complications rates after radiofrequency ablation of very early hepatocellular carcinoma in cirrhosis: is resection still the treatment of choice? Hepatology 2008;47(1):82–9.

4. Huo TI, Huang YH, Wu JC, et al. Comparison of percutaneous acetic acid injection and percutaneous ethanol injection for hepatocellular carcinoma in cirrhotic patients: a prospective study. Scand J Gastroenterol 2003;38(7):770–8.
5. McKinnon JG, Temple WJ, Wiseman DA, et al. Cryosurgery for malignant tumours of the liver. Can J Surg 1996;39(5):401–6.
6. Morris DL, Ross WB. Australian experience of cryoablation of liver tumors: metastases. Surg Oncol Clin N Am 1996;5(2):391–7.
7. Onik G, Rubinsky B, Zemel R, et al. Ultrasound-guided hepatic cryosurgery in the treatment of metastatic colon carcinoma. Preliminary results. Cancer 1991;67(4):901–7.
8. Onik GM, Atkinson D, Zemel R, et al. Cryosurgery of liver cancer. Semin Surg Oncol 1993;9(4):309–17.
9. Ravikumar TS, Kane R, Cady B, et al. A 5-year study of cryosurgery in the treatment of liver tumors. Arch Surg 1991;126(12):1520–3 [discussion: 1523–4].
10. Ross WB, Horton M, Bertolino P, et al. Cryotherapy of liver tumours–a practical guide. HPB Surg 1995;8(3):167–73.
11. Weaver ML, Atkinson D, Zemel R. Hepatic cryosurgery in treating colorectal metastases. Cancer 1995;76(2):210–4.
12. Hansen PD, Rogers S, Corless CL, et al. Radiofrequency ablation lesions in a pig liver model. J Surg Res 1999;87(1):114–21.
13. Rubinsky B. Irreversible electroporation in medicine. Technol Cancer Res Treat 2007;6(4):255–60.
14. Silk MT, Wimmer T, Lee KS, et al. Percutaneous ablation of peribiliary tumors with irreversible electroporation. J Vasc Interv Radiol 2014;25(1):112–8.
15. Stippel DL, Bangard C, Kasper HU, et al. Experimental bile duct protection by intraductal cooling during radiofrequency ablation. Br J Surg 2005;92(7):849–55.
16. Livraghi T, Giorgio A, Marin G, et al. Hepatocellular carcinoma and cirrhosis in 746 patients: long-term results of percutaneous ethanol injection. Radiology 1995;197(1):101–8.
17. Shiina S, Tagawa K, Unuma T, et al. Percutaneous ethanol injection therapy for hepatocellular carcinoma. A histopathologic study. Cancer 1991;68(7):1524–30.
18. Tiong L, Maddern GJ. Systematic review and meta-analysis of survival and disease recurrence after radiofrequency ablation for hepatocellular carcinoma. Br J Surg 2011;98(9):1210–24.
19. Chen MS, Li JQ, Zheng Y, et al. A prospective randomized trial comparing percutaneous local ablative therapy and partial hepatectomy for small hepatocellular carcinoma. Ann Surg 2006;243(3):321–8.
20. Cillo U, Vitale A, Dupuis D, et al. Laparoscopic ablation of hepatocellular carcinoma in cirrhotic patients unsuitable for liver resection or percutaneous treatment: a cohort study. PLoS One 2013;8(2):21.
21. Guglielmi A, Ruzzenente A, Valdegamberi A, et al. Radiofrequency ablation versus surgical resection for the treatment of hepatocellular carcinoma in cirrhosis. J Gastrointest Surg 2008;12(1):192–8.
22. Hong SN, Lee SY, Choi MS, et al. Comparing the outcomes of radiofrequency ablation and surgery in patients with a single small hepatocellular carcinoma and well-preserved hepatic function. J Clin Gastroenterol 2005;39(3):247–52.
23. Lencioni RA, Allgaier HP, Cioni D, et al. Small hepatocellular carcinoma in cirrhosis: randomized comparison of radio-frequency thermal ablation versus percutaneous ethanol injection. Radiology 2003;228(1):235–40.

24. Lin SM, Lin CJ, Lin CC, et al. Radiofrequency ablation improves prognosis compared with ethanol injection for hepatocellular carcinoma < or =4 cm. Gastroenterology 2004;127(6):1714–23.
25. Livraghi T, Goldberg SN, Lazzaroni S, et al. Small hepatocellular carcinoma: treatment with radio-frequency ablation versus ethanol injection. Radiology 1999; 210(3):655–61.
26. Llovet JM, Vilana R, Bru C, et al. Increased risk of tumor seeding after percutaneous radiofrequency ablation for single hepatocellular carcinoma. Hepatology 2001;33(5):1124–9.
27. Lu MD, Kuang M, Liang LJ, et al. Surgical resection versus percutaneous thermal ablation for early-stage hepatocellular carcinoma: a randomized clinical trial. Zhonghua Yi Xue Za Zhi 2006;86(12):801–5 [in Chinese].
28. Rossi S, Di Stasi M, Buscarini E, et al. Percutaneous RF interstitial thermal ablation in the treatment of hepatic cancer. AJR Am J Roentgenol 1996;167(3): 759–68.
29. Shiina S, Teratani T, Obi S, et al. A randomized controlled trial of radiofrequency ablation with ethanol injection for small hepatocellular carcinoma. Gastroenterology 2005;129(1):122–30.
30. Wong J, Lee KF, Yu SC, et al. Percutaneous radiofrequency ablation versus surgical radiofrequency ablation for malignant liver tumours: the long-term results. HPB (Oxford) 2013;15(8):595–601.
31. Wong KM, Yeh ML, Chuang SC, et al. Survival comparison between surgical resection and percutaneous radiofrequency ablation for patients in Barcelona Clinic Liver Cancer early stage hepatocellular carcinoma. Indian J Gastroenterol 2013;32(4):253–7.
32. Arii S, Yamaoka Y, Futagawa S, et al. Results of surgical and nonsurgical treatment for small-sized hepatocellular carcinomas: a retrospective and nationwide survey in Japan. The Liver Cancer Study Group of Japan. Hepatology 2000; 32(6):1224–9.
33. Brunello F, Veltri A, Carucci P, et al. Radiofrequency ablation versus ethanol injection for early hepatocellular carcinoma: a randomized controlled trial. Scand J Gastroenterol 2008;43(6):727–35. http://dx.doi.org/10.1080/00365520701885481.
34. Ebara M, Okabe S, Kita K, et al. Percutaneous ethanol injection for small hepatocellular carcinoma: therapeutic efficacy based on 20-year observation. J Hepatol 2005;43(3):458–64.
35. Fartoux L, Arrive L, Andreani T, et al. Treatment of small hepatocellular carcinoma with acetic acid percutaneous injection. Gastroenterol Clin Biol 2005;29(12): 1213–9.
36. Hasegawa S, Yamasaki N, Hiwaki T, et al. Factors that predict intrahepatic recurrence of hepatocellular carcinoma in 81 patients initially treated by percutaneous ethanol injection. Cancer 1999;86(9):1682–90.
37. Lin SM, Lin CJ, Lin CC, et al. Randomised controlled trial comparing percutaneous radiofrequency thermal ablation, percutaneous ethanol injection, and percutaneous acetic acid injection to treat hepatocellular carcinoma of 3 cm or less. Gut 2005;54(8):1151–6.
38. Livraghi T, Benedini V, Lazzaroni S, et al. Long term results of single session percutaneous ethanol injection in patients with large hepatocellular carcinoma. Cancer 1998;83(1):48–57.
39. Pompili M, Rapaccini GL, Covino M, et al. Prognostic factors for survival in patients with compensated cirrhosis and small hepatocellular carcinoma after percutaneous ethanol injection therapy. Cancer 2001;92(1):126–35.

40. Sung YM, Choi D, Lim HK, et al. Long-term results of percutaneous ethanol injection for the treatment of hepatocellular carcinoma in Korea. Korean J Radiol 2006; 7(3):187–92.
41. El-Serag HB, Marrero JA, Rudolph L, et al. Diagnosis and treatment of hepatocellular carcinoma. Gastroenterology 2008;134(6):1752–63. http://dx.doi.org/10.1053/j.gastro.2008.02.090.
42. Lencioni R, Llovet JM. Percutaneous ethanol injection for hepatocellular carcinoma: alive or dead? J Hepatol 2005;43(3):377–80.
43. Livraghi T, Bolondi L, Lazzaroni S, et al. Percutaneous ethanol injection in the treatment of hepatocellular carcinoma in cirrhosis. A study on 207 patients. Cancer 1992;69(4):925–9.
44. Bouza C, Lopez-Cuadrado T, Alcazar R, et al. Meta-analysis of percutaneous radiofrequency ablation versus ethanol injection in hepatocellular carcinoma. BMC Gastroenterol 2009;9:31. http://dx.doi.org/10.1186/1471-230X-9-31.
45. Orlando A, Leandro G, Olivo M, et al. Radiofrequency thermal ablation vs. percutaneous ethanol injection for small hepatocellular carcinoma in cirrhosis: meta-analysis of randomized controlled trials. Am J Gastroenterol 2009;104(2): 514–24. http://dx.doi.org/10.1038/ajg.2008.80.
46. Adam R, Hagopian EJ, Linhares M, et al. A comparison of percutaneous cryosurgery and percutaneous radiofrequency for unresectable hepatic malignancies. Arch Surg 2002;137(12):1332–9 [discussion: 1340].
47. Haddad FF, Chapman WC, Wright JK, et al. Clinical experience with cryosurgery for advanced hepatobiliary tumors. J Surg Res 1998;75(2):103–8.
48. Pearson AS, Izzo F, Fleming RY, et al. Intraoperative radiofrequency ablation or cryoablation for hepatic malignancies. Am J Surg 1999;178(6):592–9.
49. Tait IS, Yong SM, Cuschieri SA. Laparoscopic in situ ablation of liver cancer with cryotherapy and radiofrequency ablation. Br J Surg 2002;89(12):1613–9.
50. Wren SM, Coburn MM, Tan M, et al. Is cryosurgical ablation appropriate for treating hepatocellular cancer? Arch Surg 1997;132(6):599–603 [discussion: 603–4].
51. Zhou XD, Tang ZY. Cryotherapy for primary liver cancer. Semin Surg Oncol 1998; 14(2):171–4.
52. Dong BW, Liang P, Yu XL, et al. Sonographically guided microwave coagulation treatment of liver cancer: an experimental and clinical study. AJR Am J Roentgenol 1998;171(2):449–54.
53. Dong BW, Zhang J, Liang P, et al. Sequential pathological and immunologic analysis of percutaneous microwave coagulation therapy of hepatocellular carcinoma. Int J Hyperthermia 2003;19(2):119–33.
54. Groeschl RT, Pilgrim CH, Hanna EM, et al. Microwave ablation for hepatic malignancies: a multiinstitutional analysis. Ann Surg 2014;259(6):1195–200.
55. Lu MD, Xu HX, Xie XY, et al. Percutaneous microwave and radiofrequency ablation for hepatocellular carcinoma: a retrospective comparative study. J Gastroenterol 2005;40(11):1054–60.
56. Seki T, Wakabayashi M, Nakagawa T, et al. Percutaneous microwave coagulation therapy for patients with small hepatocellular carcinoma: comparison with percutaneous ethanol injection therapy. Cancer 1999;85(8):1694–702.
57. Swan RZ, Sindram D, Martinie JB, et al. Operative microwave ablation for hepatocellular carcinoma: complications, recurrence, and long-term outcomes. J Gastrointest Surg 2013;17(4):719–29.
58. Cannon R, Ellis S, Hayes D, et al. Safety and early efficacy of irreversible electroporation for hepatic tumors in proximity to vital structures. J Surg Oncol 2013; 107(5):544–9.

59. Cheung W, Kavnoudias H, Roberts S, et al. Irreversible electroporation for unresectable hepatocellular carcinoma: initial experience and review of safety and outcomes. Technol Cancer Res Treat 2013;12(3):233–41. http://dx.doi.org/10.7785/tcrt.2012.500317.

60. Philips P, Hays D, Martin RC. Irreversible electroporation ablation (IRE) of unresectable soft tissue tumors: learning curve evaluation in the first 150 patients treated. PLoS One 2013;8(11):e76260.

61. Abdalla EK, Vauthey JN, Ellis LM, et al. Recurrence and outcomes following hepatic resection, radiofrequency ablation, and combined resection/ablation for colorectal liver metastases. Ann Surg 2004;239(6):818–25 [discussion: 825–7].

62. Abitabile P, Hartl U, Lange J, et al. Radiofrequency ablation permits an effective treatment for colorectal liver metastasis. Eur J Surg Oncol 2007;33(1): 67–71.

63. Aloia TA, Vauthey JN, Loyer EM, et al. Solitary colorectal liver metastasis: resection determines outcome. Arch Surg 2006;141(5):460–6 [discussion: 466–7].

64. Berber E, Tsinberg M, Tellioglu G, et al. Resection versus laparoscopic radiofrequency thermal ablation of solitary colorectal liver metastasis. J Gastrointest Surg 2008;12(11):1967–72. http://dx.doi.org/10.1007/s11605-008-0622-8.

65. Hur H, Ko YT, Min BS, et al. Comparative study of resection and radiofrequency ablation in the treatment of solitary colorectal liver metastases. Am J Surg 2009; 197(6):728–36. http://dx.doi.org/10.1016/j.amjsurg.2008.04.013.

66. Iannitti DA, Dupuy DE, Mayo-Smith WW, et al. Hepatic radiofrequency ablation. Arch Surg 2002;137(4):422–6 [discussion: 427].

67. Kennedy TJ, Cassera MA, Khajanchee YS, et al. Laparoscopic radiofrequency ablation for the management of colorectal liver metastases: 10-year experience. J Surg Oncol 2013;107(4):324–8.

68. Park IJ, Kim HC, Yu CS, et al. Radiofrequency ablation for metachronous liver metastasis from colorectal cancer after curative surgery. Ann Surg Oncol 2008; 15(1):227–32.

69. Siperstein AE, Berber E, Ballem N, et al. Survival after radiofrequency ablation of colorectal liver metastases: 10-year experience. Ann Surg 2007;246(4):559–65 [discussion: 565–7].

70. Solbiati L, Ahmed M, Cova L, et al. Small liver colorectal metastases treated with percutaneous radiofrequency ablation: local response rate and long-term survival with up to 10-year follow-up. Radiology 2012;265(3):958–68.

71. Solbiati L, Livraghi T, Goldberg SN, et al. Percutaneous radio-frequency ablation of hepatic metastases from colorectal cancer: long-term results in 117 patients. Radiology 2001;221(1):159–66.

72. Sorensen SM, Mortensen FV, Nielsen DT. Radiofrequency ablation of colorectal liver metastases: long-term survival. Acta Radiol 2007;48(3):253–8.

73. Veltri A, Sacchetto P, Tosetti I, et al. Radiofrequency ablation of colorectal liver metastases: small size favorably predicts technique effectiveness and survival. Cardiovasc Intervent Radiol 2008;31(5):948–56. http://dx.doi.org/10.1007/s00270-008-9362-0.

74. White RR, Avital I, Sofocleous CT, et al. Rates and patterns of recurrence for percutaneous radiofrequency ablation and open wedge resection for solitary colorectal liver metastasis. J Gastrointest Surg 2007;11(3):256–63.

75. Mulier S, Ni Y, Jamart J, et al. Local recurrence after hepatic radiofrequency coagulation: multivariate meta-analysis and review of contributing factors. Ann Surg 2005;242(2):158–71.

76. Bhardwaj N, Strickland AD, Ahmad F, et al. Microwave ablation for unresectable hepatic tumours: clinical results using a novel microwave probe and generator. Eur J Surg Oncol 2010;36(3):264–8.
77. Liang P, Dong B, Yu X, et al. Prognostic factors for percutaneous microwave coagulation therapy of hepatic metastases. AJR Am J Roentgenol 2003;181(5):1319–25.
78. Ogata Y, Uchida S, Hisaka T, et al. Intraoperative thermal ablation therapy for small colorectal metastases to the liver. Hepatogastroenterology 2008;55(82–83):550–6.
79. Shibata T, Niinobu T, Ogata N, et al. Microwave coagulation therapy for multiple hepatic metastases from colorectal carcinoma. Cancer 2000;89(2):276–84.
80. Tanaka K, Shimada H, Nagano Y, et al. Outcome after hepatic resection versus combined resection and microwave ablation for multiple bilobar colorectal metastases to the liver. Surgery 2006;139(2):263–73.
81. Berber E, Flesher N, Siperstein AE. Laparoscopic radiofrequency ablation of neuroendocrine liver metastases. World J Surg 2002;26(8):985–90.
82. Berber E, Siperstein A. Local recurrence after laparoscopic radiofrequency ablation of liver tumors: an analysis of 1032 tumors. Ann Surg Oncol 2008;15(10):2757–64. http://dx.doi.org/10.1245/s10434-008-0043-7.
83. Berber E, Siperstein AE. Perioperative outcome after laparoscopic radiofrequency ablation of liver tumors: an analysis of 521 cases. Surg Endosc 2007;21(4):613–8.
84. Karabulut K, Akyildiz HY, Lance C, et al. Multimodality treatment of neuroendocrine liver metastases. Surgery 2011;150(2):316–25.
85. Mazzaglia PJ, Berber E, Milas M, et al. Laparoscopic radiofrequency ablation of neuroendocrine liver metastases: a 10-year experience evaluating predictors of survival. Surgery 2007;142(1):10–9.
86. Siperstein A, Garland A, Engle K, et al. Local recurrence after laparoscopic radiofrequency thermal ablation of hepatic tumors. Ann Surg Oncol 2000;7(2):106–13.
87. Taner T, Atwell TD, Zhang L, et al. Adjunctive radiofrequency ablation of metastatic neuroendocrine cancer to the liver complements surgical resection. HPB (Oxford) 2013;15(3):190–5.
88. Landry CS, McMasters KM, Scoggins CR, et al. Proposed staging system for gastrointestinal carcinoid tumors. Am Surg 2008;74(5):418–22.
89. Musunuru S, Chen H, Rajpal S, et al. Metastatic neuroendocrine hepatic tumors: resection improves survival. Arch Surg 2006;141(10):1000–4 [discussion: 1005].
90. Touzios JG, Kiely JM, Pitt SC, et al. Neuroendocrine hepatic metastases: does aggressive management improve survival? Ann Surg 2005;241(5):776–83 [discussion: 783–5].

Hepatic Artery Infusion Chemotherapy for Liver Malignancy

Julie N. Leal, MD, FRCSC, T. Peter Kingham, MD*

KEYWORDS

- Regional therapy • Liver-directed therapy • Primary liver cancer • Liver metastases

KEY POINTS

- The predominant blood supply of primary and metastatic tumors of the liver is the hepatic artery.
- Administration of chemotherapeutic agents via the hepatic artery allows preferential delivery of cytotoxic drugs to tumor cells with a relative sparing of normal hepatocytes.
- Optimal drug delivery via surgically inserted hepatic artery catheters and implantable pumps is technically feasible, and in experienced centers is associated with acceptable morbidity.
- Evidence suggests that hepatic artery infusion (HAI) chemotherapy has a role in the treatment of both unresectable colorectal cancer liver metastasis (CRLM) and as adjuvant therapy in resectable CRLM.
- Trials of HAI chemotherapy for the treatment of primary liver cancer and non-CRLM are few, and its use in this setting requires further study.

INTRODUCTION

The liver is unique in that it receives blood from the systemic arterial circulation and the enterohepatic circulation. Most blood flow to normal hepatocytes is derived from the portal venous system; alternatively, liver tumors obtain their nutrient blood supply almost exclusively from the hepatic artery (HA).[1] For decades, attempts to take advantage of this dual blood supply to selectively deliver regional therapy to tumors isolated to the liver have been made. In the early 1960s, initial trials of continuous hepatic artery infusion (HAI) chemotherapy for the treatment of liver cancers were reported by Sullivan and colleagues.[2] Though small and inclusive of multiple tumor types, these seminal investigations indicated that HAI chemotherapy was

Financial Disclosures/Conflicts of Interest: None.
Department of Surgery, Division of Hepatopancreatobiliary Surgery, Memorial Sloan Kettering Cancer Center, 1275 York Avenue, New York, NY 10065, USA
* Corresponding author.
E-mail address: kinghamt@mskcc.org

feasible, and that there appeared to be a quantifiable tumor response. Unfortunately, general applicability was limited owing to a lack of standardized chemotherapeutic regimens and tumor response measurements. Furthermore, clinical implementation was hampered by unacceptably high complication rates related to catheter insertion, prolonged infusions, and cumbersome external infusion pumps.[3] Despite the limitations of these early investigations, 3 essential components for safe and effective implementation of HAI chemotherapy were identified: (1) insertion of a durable arterial catheter that allows prolonged use; (2) identification of appropriate drugs; and (3) a delivery system that allows protracted, reliable, and convenient drug administration.[4]

The primary goal of HAI chemotherapy is to selectively deliver high concentrations of drugs to cancer cells while limiting drug exposure to normal hepatocytes. To achieve this, drugs used for HAI chemotherapy must have quantifiable antitumor activity and an optimal pharmacokinetic profile characterized by: (1) high first-pass hepatic extraction; (2) short plasma half-life; and (3) first-order kinetics with steep dose-response curves.[5] To date, several suitable agents with activity against primary and metastatic liver cancers have been evaluated in the setting of HAI chemotherapy.[6–11] Pharmacokinetic profiles of these commonly used drugs are provided in **Table 1**. Relative to other agents, delivery of floxuridine (FUDR) via the HA is most favorable. HAI chemotherapy with FUDR results in 100- to 400-fold greater exposure within the liver and a 15-fold higher drug concentration within tumor cells in comparison with normal hepatocytes. Up to 92% is extracted by the liver on first pass, limiting systemic exposure, and it is rapidly eliminated from the body.[4,12]

Successful HAI chemotherapy is contingent on both the use of an effective drug and the ability to place a durable HA catheter, allowing safe, long-term drug delivery. At present HA catheters are primarily inserted via open laparotomy.[13] In efforts to combat the morbidity of a major abdominal operation, percutaneous techniques have also been used. A recent study by Arru and colleagues[14] compared transaxillary percutaneous (PCT) HA catheter insertion with insertion via laparotomy (LPT). Length of hospitalization and analgesia requirement was greater in the LPT. However, catheter-related complications resulting in delay or cessation of treatment were seen in 43% of the PCT group, compared with 7% of the LPT group ($P = .005$). This finding translated into significantly fewer HAI chemotherapy cycles in the PCT

Table 1 Pharmacokinetics of chemotherapeutics delivered via the hepatic artery				
Drug	Hepatic Extraction (%)	Plasma Half-Life (min)	Fold Increase Exposure with HA Infusion	Retained Systemic Exposure Relative to IV Administration (%)
5-Fluorouracil (5-FU)	22–45	10	5–10	60–70
Floxuridine (FUDR)	69–92	<10	100–400	<5
Mitomycin C (MMC)	22	≤10	6–8	80–90
Cisplatin (CDDP)	—	20–30	4–7	100
Doxorubicin	45–50	60	2	40–50

Abbreviations: HA, hepatic artery; IV, intravenous.
Data from Ensminger WD, Gyves JW. Clinical pharmacology of hepatic arterial chemotherapy. Semin Oncol 1983;10(2):176–82.

group than in the LPT group (4.3 vs 6.5, P = .038). It seems that despite the initial morbidity of a major abdominal procedure, LPT-placed catheters are more durable and allow for more consistent long-term drug delivery. More recently, minimally invasive techniques for HA catheter insertion have been described.[15,16] In a single-center review of 27 patients undergoing laparoscopic placement of HA catheters, correct catheter placement was observed in 100% of cases, average operative time was 45 to 55 minutes, and overall catheter-related complications were seen in 11% of patients.[17] Use of laparoscopic techniques for HA catheter insertion is feasible, and appears to be associated with an acceptable complication rate in specialized centers. More recently, robotic-assisted procedures have also been documented.[18]

Early HAI chemotherapy drug delivery systems included HA port systems and percutaneous catheters connected to external pumps. These devices were cumbersome, inconvenient, and associated with significant complications. Such device-related limitations contributed considerably to the slow evolution of HAI chemotherapy. In 1979, the first totally implantable pump system for continuous long-term drug delivery was introduced for clinical use.[19] Subsequent evaluation of the pumps for HAI chemotherapy revealed the feasibility and safety of insertion in addition to acceptable device-related morbidity.[20] In a series of more than 180 patients, Heinrich and colleagues[21] compared totally implantable pumps with HA port systems for HAI chemotherapy. Complications that could not be salvaged and required cessation of treatment occurred in 47% of patients in the port group compared with 30% in the pump group. Complication-free survival was 12.2 months in the pump group compared with 7.3 months in the port group (P = .002). A second study found that patients with implantable pumps had a 3-fold decrease in the number of treatment interruptions when compared with those with ports (P = .003).[22] Furthermore, a recent systematic review of more than 3000 patients reported complication rates of more than 30% for port systems, compared with 16% with implantable pumps.[23] In this review, the number studies reporting on chemotherapy cycles delivered were few; however, among these, the median number of cycles delivered in the pump group was 12 versus 8 in the port group, suggesting increased durability and reliability of implanted pumps over HA port systems for HAI chemotherapy.

For completeness, it must be noted that liver-directed chemotherapy via the portal vein (PVI) has been described and evaluated extensively. PVI catheters may be placed into a convenient venous tributary (ileocolic, colic, inferior mesenteric, or gastroepiploic) and used for local drug delivery. A meta-analysis of PVI chemotherapy trials completed before 1987 (10 trials of PVI in more than 4000 patients) suggested an absolute survival benefit of 4.7%.[24] However, this finding was not supported by more recent prospective trials of 5-fluorouracil (5-FU)-based PVI chemotherapy,[25–28] all of which suggest no significant benefit of PVI in terms of recurrence-free survival (RFS) or overall survival (OS). At present, liver-directed chemotherapy via the portal vein seems to provide little, if any, benefit and is rarely used in the clinical setting.

TECHNICAL ASPECTS
The Pump

Totally implantable infusion pumps are advantageous in that they allow for long-term, reliable, and continuous drug delivery in the outpatient setting. Several models have been produced. Some rely on a chemical power source while others are battery powered. One of the most commonly used continuous pumps is a titanium disk approximately 7 cm in diameter with volume capacitance varying from 20 to 50 mL (**Fig. 1**). It consists of 2 chambers separated by a welded bellows. The inner infusate chamber

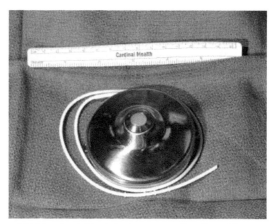

Fig. 1. The Codman 3000 implantable infusion pump. (Implantable Constant-Flow Infusion Pump. Codman Corporation, Johnson & Johnson Company, Raynham, MA.)

contains the drug to be administered while the outer charging fluid chamber contains the volatile liquid/vapor mixture used as the chemical power source. The pump is designed such that the process of filling the infusate chamber "recharges" the chemical power source, and the only energy source required for continuous function and flow is that provided by periodic refill injections.[19,20]

The Patient

All patients being considered for HAI chemotherapy require an extensive search for radiographic, endoscopic, and/or clinical evidence of extrahepatic disease (EHD).[29] **Table 2** outlines patient and tumor characteristics that are considered relative contraindications to HAI chemotherapy. In general, patients with no obvious EHD, good performance status, and preserved liver function may be considered for HAI chemotherapy.[30] In those deemed suitable, evaluation of the celiac and superior mesenteric arteries is requisite to delineate HA anatomy.[31] Direct angiography has long been the gold standard for evaluation of hepatic arterial anatomy. However, recent development of faster, better quality computed tomography (CT) scanners has significantly improved noninvasive arterial imagining. CT angiography, performed using the latest technology, allows rapid imagine acquisition and 3-dimensional volume rendering such that detection of aberrant/replaced HA anatomy is conducted similarly to traditional angiography techniques and the morbidity of an arterial puncture is avoided.[32] Consequently, CT angiography is the preferred method for initial surgical evaluation of HA anatomy at most centers.

Table 2	
Relative contraindications to continuous hepatic arterial infusional chemotherapy	
Patient Factors	**Tumor/Anatomic Factors**
Poor performance status (Karnofsky <60%)	Extrahepatic disease
Liver insufficiency (total bilirubin ≥1.5 mg/dL)	Extensive hepatic metastasis (>70% hepatic replacement)
	Portal vein thrombosis

The Procedure

Careful review of the preoperative hepatic arterial anatomy is essential for successful insertion of implantable pumps. The technical goals of pump placement are outlined in **Box 1**. Laparotomy is typically performed via a midline incision unless a concomitant liver resection necessitates a subcostal or hockey-stick incision. On entering the abdomen a thorough search for EHD is completed. If the pump is being placed in the setting of unresectable disease, upfront staging laparoscopy is valuable to rule out EHD before committing patients to open exploration.[33] Once EHD is ruled out, a cholecystectomy is performed to avoid the development of chemical cholecystitis. In patients with normal hepatic anatomy (**Fig. 2**) the common hepatic artery (CHA) and gastroduodenal artery (GDA) are palpable within the porta hepatis. Once the CHA is localized, dissection is initiated 1 cm proximal to the takeoff of the GDA. The distal CHA, GDA, and proper hepatic artery (PHA) are mobilized circumferentially, and the right gastric artery is ligated. All collateral branches arising from the dissected CHA, GDA, and PHA are ligated to prevent extrahepatic perfusion. The pump pocket is then created at a convenient location, typically in the left abdomen. An 8-cm transverse incision is created in a location that prevents the pump from touching the costal margin and anterior superior iliac spine. The pocket is created superficial to the abdominal wall fascia so that the pump can be easily filled with a needle placed through the abdominal wall. Only when the pocket is complete and the GDA is ready for cannulation should the pump be brought to the surgical field. The pump is filled with heparinized saline and the catheter flushed, an aperture is created in fascia at the center of the pocket, and the catheter is passed into the abdominal cavity. The pump, with the catheter positioned behind it, is then secured in the pocket with stay sutures (**Fig. 3**). Proximal and distal vascular control of the GDA is achieved through ligation of the distal GDA with nonabsorbable suture and placement of vascular bulldogs/clamps on the CHA and PHA. Alternatively isolated GDA control can be obtained by placing the vascular clamp on the GDA at its takeoff from the CHA. This latter approach facilitates proper catheter placement in that inadvertent advancement into the CHA is prevented. After appropriate vascular control is confirmed, an arteriotomy is made in the GDA and the catheter advanced such that the tip lies at the junction of the CHA and GDA (**Fig. 4**). Placement of the catheter into the CHA may result in turbulent flow and thrombosis, whereas a catheter placed distally in the GDA leaves a segment of this vessel directly exposed to cytotoxic drugs with minimal flow. This malpositioning can result in sclerosis, thrombosis, or pseudoaneurysm. The catheter is then secured in place with 2 to 3 nonabsorbable ties, as outlined in **Fig. 4B**.

Once the catheter is secured in the GDA, catheter placement and hepatic perfusion are assessed. Methylene blue (using visible light) or fluorescein (using Wood lamp and black light) is injected via the pump and the liver is assessed for uniform dye

---

Box 1
Primary technical goals of HAI chemotherapy pump insertion

Technical goals:

Catheter placement allowing uniform bilobar hepatic perfusion

Ligation of all collateral branches distal to the catheter and proximal to the liver to avoid extrahepatic perfusion

Strategic catheter placement with tip at the gastroduodenal artery/common hepatic artery junction to avoid thrombosis

Identification and ligation of any accessory/replaced hepatic arteries

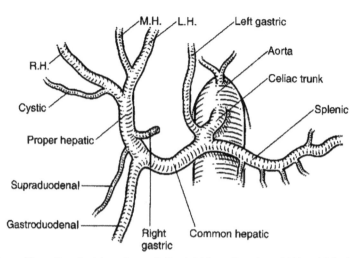

Fig. 2. Normal hepatic arterial anatomy. R.H., right hepatic artery; M.H., middle hepatic artery; L.H., left hepatic artery. (*From* Chamberlain RS. Essential functional hepatic and biliary anatomy for the surgeon. In: Abdeldayem H, editor. Hepatic surgery. 2013. (Figure 5). Available at: http://www.intechopen.com/books/hepatic-surgery. Accessed September 5, 2014; with permission.)

distribution. Evaluation for evidence of extravasation of dye or inadvertent extrahepatic perfusion is also completed (**Fig. 5**). In the event of abnormal liver perfusion and/or extrahepatic perfusion, the angiogram is rereviewed to identify potential accessory hepatic arteries or collateral vessels. When found, the vessel(s) should be localized and ligated. Following satisfactory completion of the perfusion test the catheter is flushed, the wounds are closed, and the procedure completed.

MANAGEMENT OF VARIANT HEPATIC ARTERIAL ANATOMY

Autopsy series suggest that normal HA anatomy, as depicted in **Fig. 2**, is present in only 50% to 60% of humans. In his original autopsy series, Michels[34] defined 10 different categories of anomalous hepatic circulation. In essence, these can be divided into variant right or variant left anatomy, and further subcategorized as

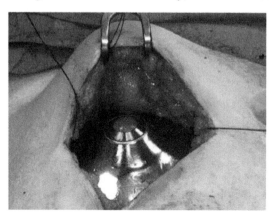

Fig. 3. Totally implantable hepatic arterial infusion pump within subcutaneous pocket on anterior aspect of lower abdominal wall.

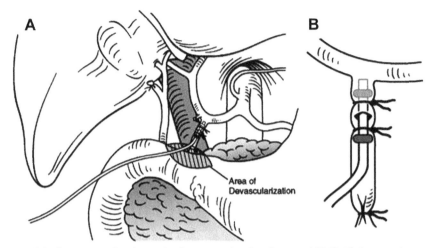

Fig. 4. (*A*) Placement of catheter in the gastroduodenal artery (GDA). Right gastric artery is shown adjacent to the GDA and is ligated. (*B*) Technique for placement and securing infusion catheter in the GDA. (*Adapted from* Skitzki JJ, Chang AE. Hepatic artery chemotherapy for colorectal liver metastases: technical considerations and review of clinical trials. Surg Oncol 2002;11(3):126; with permission.)

accessory (in addition to a normal branch) or replaced (in place of a normal branch). One review of more than 1900 patients found that a replaced or accessory right hepatic artery (RHA) off the superior mesenteric artery is the most common variant (14.9%). The second most frequent anomaly is an accessory or replaced left hepatic artery (LHA) originating from the left gastric artery (11.3%).[30]

The presence of aberrant HA anatomy does not usually preclude placement of an HAI pump. Previously dual-lumen pumps were used, whereby both the GDA and the aberrant vessel could be cannulated to achieve uniform drug delivery to the whole liver.[35] These pumps, however, are no longer produced. In general, the optimal means of managing aberrant HA anatomy is to ligate the anomalous vessel and place the pump catheter in the GDA (**Fig. 6**A, B). The safety of this ligation was described in a study of liver perfusion in patients with ligated hepatic lobar arteries that demonstrated uniform bilobar hepatic perfusion in 100% of patients on postoperative day 5.[36] This method, for the most part, also avoids cannulation of a vessel other than the GDA, which in a review of 544 patients undergoing HAI pump insertion was associated with increased risk of pump related complications and failure.[37] Although relatively unusual, variation in the origin of the GDA may be encountered, and includes trifurcation of the LHA/RHA/GDA off the CHA. As depicted in **Fig. 6**C, this may be managed in a similar fashion to accessory of replaced LHA/RHA, with ligation of the smaller lobar vessel and catheter insertion into the GDA. On rare occasion the nonaberrant vessel is very small and requires the use of specialized microcatheters for cannulation. In patients with a GDA that cannot be used for a catheter or in patients with no GDA and completely replaced hepatic arteries, advanced techniques using autologous vein or synthetic grafts to construct a conduit for the pump catheter have been described.[38]

POSTOPERATIVE MANAGEMENT AND TREATMENT SURVEILLANCE

Before initiating HAI chemotherapy, a radionuclide pump-flow study is completed to assess hepatic perfusion. Radiolabeled sulfur-colloid (SC) is injected intravenously,

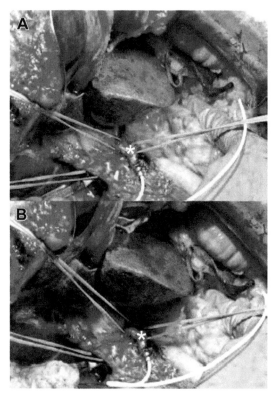

Fig. 5. Post–methylene blue dye injection for assessment of arterial catheter placement and hepatic perfusion. (*A*) Early phase post injection. (*B*) Late phase post injection, with evidence of adequate bilobar perfusion and no evidence of extrahepatic perfusion. Asterisk indicates GDA with catheter secured in place.

followed by technetium-labeled macroaggregated albumin (MAA) injected via the HAI pump. The perfusion scans are then overlaid and compared to determine uniformity of hepatic perfusion and assess for evidence of extrahepatic perfusion. In the setting of a normal MAA scan, HAI chemotherapy may be initiated, typically 1 to 4 weeks following pump placement.[13] Patients undergoing HAI chemotherapy require fastidious clinical, laboratory, and radiographic follow-up to monitor for treatment related complications and assess disease status. In general, follow-up consists of biochemical laboratory screening (aspartate aminotransferase [AST], alanine aminotransferase, alkaline phosphatase [ALP], total bilirubin) every 2 weeks, and formal clinical examination and toxicity assessment every 4 weeks. Routine radiographic disease surveillance with CT scans of the chest, abdomen, and pelvis may be obtained on a 3- to 4-month basis.[39]

COMPLICATIONS

Early observations of HAI chemotherapy in patients with primary and metastatic liver cancers suggested significant tumor response rates (RR). However, major concerns surrounding high rates of complications limited the use and widespread acceptance of HAI chemotherapy. Depending on the study, complication rates were reported to range anywhere from 30% to 79%.[40–42] These high rates in part reflect that unlike

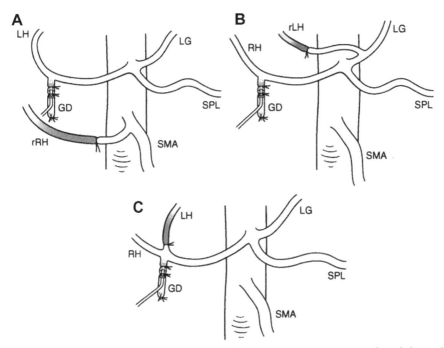

Fig. 6. (*A*) Replaced right hepatic artery (RHA) off superior mesenteric artery (SMA), ligated and catheter inserted into GDA off left hepatic artery (LHA). (*B*) Replaced LHA off left gastric (LG), ligated and catheter inserted into the GDA off RHA. (*C*) Trifurcation of the common hepatic artery with ligation of the LHA and catheter insertion into the GDA. GD, gastroduodenal; LH, left hepatic; RH, right hepatic; rLH, replaced left hepatic; rRH, replaced right hepatic; SPL, splenic artery. (*Adapted from* Skitzki JJ, Chang AE. Hepatic artery chemotherapy for colorectal liver metastases: technical considerations and review of clinical trials. Surg Oncol 2002;11(3):126; with permission.)

systemic cancer therapies, HAI chemotherapy is subject to both chemotherapy-related toxicities and potential technical complications related to surgery, the HA infusion catheter, and the implanted pump.

Technical Complications

Over the past 40 years multiple studies have sought to evaluate the incidence of, risk factors for, and clinical impact of technical complications of HAI chemotherapy. The most comprehensive review of these complications, published by Allen and colleagues[37] in 2005, included 544 patients undergoing pump placement over a 15-year period. In this study, the overall pump-related complication rate was 22%. Complications related to the HA system (thrombosis, incomplete perfusion, extrahepatic perfusion, hemorrhage) were most common (51%). **Table 3** summarizes complication and salvage rates stratified by timing of complication. The overall pump salvage rate for all complications was 45%. Stratification of complications into those occurring early (<30 days) versus late (>30 days) revealed late complications to be more common and less likely to be salvaged compared with early complications (30% vs 70% respectively; $P < .001$). In total, 12% of patients had a complication that resulted in pump failure and cessation of therapy. Independent risk factors for pump-related complications in this study were non-GDA cannulation and surgeon experience.

Table 3
Specific types of complications, timing of their occurrence (<30 days or >30 days from operation), and the ability to salvage pump function by the timing of the complications

Type of Complication	n	Early (<30 d) n	Early (<30 d) % Salvaged	Late (>30 d) n	Late (>30 d) % Salvaged
Pump malfunction	6	6	100	—	—
Pocket					
Infection	14	4	50	10	40
Hematoma	1	1	100	—	—
Pump migration	4	1	100	3	33
Catheter					
Occlusion	11	—	—	11	36
Dislodgment	18	—	—	18	11
Erosion	4	—	—	4	0
Arterial					
Hemorrhage	1	1	100	—	—
Thrombosis	33	13	31	20	30
Extrahepatic perfusion	16	9	100	7	57
Incomplete perfusion	12	9	78	3	67
Overall	120	44	70	76	30

From Allen PJ, et al. Technical complications and durability of hepatic artery infusion pumps for unresectable colorectal liver metastases: an institutional experience of 544 consecutive cases. J Am Coll Surg 2005;201(1):60; with permission.

Arterial Thrombosis

Acute intraoperative thrombosis and intimal dissection of the GDA or CHA have been reported during pump insertion. A systematic review of more than 17 studies of implantable pumps revealed a thrombosis rate of 6.6%.[23] Thrombosis can occur early (<30 days) or late (>30 days) following pump insertion; the latter is more common and related to chronic exposure to cytotoxic drugs, sclerosis, and subsequent thromboses. Comparatively, early thrombosis is usually related to catheter malposition and flow disturbance. Regardless of timing, the use of thrombolytics and/or anticoagulants results in salvage rates of approximately 30%.

Extrahepatic/Incomplete Perfusion

Incomplete hepatic perfusion (IHP) occurs in 2% of cases, and typically results from failure to ligate an unrecognized aberrant HA or from failure of collaterals to develop following ligation of a lobar artery. Although IHP presents no danger to the patient or to liver function, the concern is that the oncologic effectiveness of HAI chemotherapy will be diminished. In general, most patients with IHP in the setting of a ligated lobar artery can be followed; repeat imaging scans in 2 to 4 weeks have been associated with near 100% resolution of perfusion abnormality.[21,38] Alternatively, IHP secondary to a patent accessory artery may be managed with embolization.

Extrahepatic perfusion (EHP) occurs in 2% to 9% of cases. EHP may be related to catheter malposition or collateral vessels arising distal to the catheter tip, leading to perfusion of the stomach, duodenum, or pancreas. These complications may be detected early with a postoperative MAA scan, or later with chemotherapy infusion.

EHP is commonly associated with signs and symptoms such as severe epigastric pain or diarrhea with infusion. These symptoms can be caused by ulcers or pancreatitis. In this setting the infusion is discontinued, the drug is emptied from the pump, and investigations including pump flow studies and endoscopy are completed.[12] Embolization of culprit vessel(s) allows for pump salvage in most cases. **Fig. 7** depicts an abnormal MAA scan in which EHP is evident in the area of the porta hepatis, and subsequent embolization and repeat scan reveals complete resolution of EHP. Sofocleous and colleagues[43] evaluated the use of embolization for pump salvage in 473 patients with implantable pumps, 45 (9.5%) of whom had MAA scans suggestive of EHP. Of the patients with EHP, 32 (7%) were found to have concomitant angiographic abnormalities. In 8 of 32 (25%) patients, HA thrombosis or catheter-tip migration precluded embolization. In the remaining 24 patients embolization was performed and was technically successful in 21 (87.5%), and resulted in clinical pump salvage in 79% of patients.

Pump Pocket Complications

Pump pocket complications are relatively uncommon but can significantly affect the ability to deliver therapy. Infection of the pocket occurs in 2% to 3%[44] of patients and can lead to skin necrosis, dehiscence, and pump extrusion (**Fig. 8**). Simple cellulitis over the pump pocket may be managed with oral antibiotics; however, more aggressive infections or collections require washout and intravenous antibiotics, given the presence of a foreign body (the pump). Failure to resolve the infection, evidence of dehiscence, or pump extrusion warrants reoperation. This approach requires a

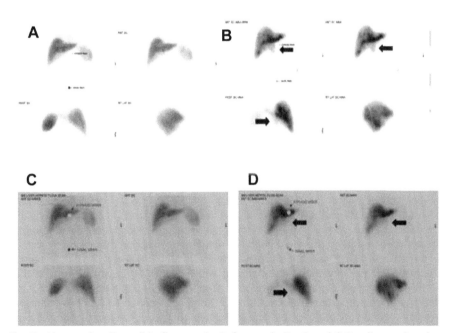

Fig. 7. Abnormal radionuclide flow study. Before embolization: (A) Baseline technetium-labeled sulfur-colloid scan. (B) Technetium-labeled macroaggregated albumin (MAA) scan; arrows indicate site of perfusion abnormality. After embolization: (C) Baseline technetium-labeled sulfur-colloid scan. (D) Technetium-labeled MAA scan showing resolution of perfusion abnormality. Arrows indicate site of resolution.

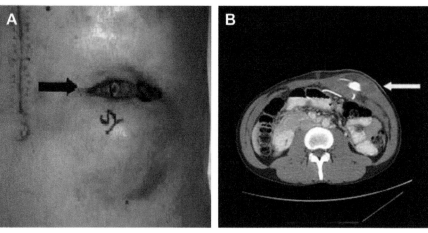

Fig. 8. (*A*) Pump pocket infection and skin dehiscence (*black arrow* indicates skin dehiscence with pump extrusion). (*B*) Pump pocket hematoma (*white arrow*).

laparotomy, cutting the catheter, splicing the old catheter and new pump catheter together, and creating a new pump pocket. Pump pocket hematomas occur in less than 1% of cases, and management depends on the timing of development. Early postoperative hematomas that are rapidly expanding should be immediately reexplored and a bleeding source sought. In those that occur late, it is reasonable to assess the hematoma radiographically. Small lesions may be needle aspirated; however, larger hematomas typically require formal clot evacuation.

Toxic Complications

Drug-related complications observed with HAI chemotherapy depend on the type and dose of drug, the dosing schedule, the degree of first-pass liver metabolism, and subsequent systemic exposure. **Table 1** lists some of the pharmacokinetic characteristics of commonly used HAI chemotherapeutics. Toxicity profiles of the most frequently used fluoropyrimidine-based therapies, 5-FU or FUDR, differ in direct relation to their degree of hepatic versus systemic exposure. Hepatic extraction rate of 5-FU is 20% to 40%; consequently, complications related to its use in HAI chemotherapy are similar to those observed with systemic administration. Gastrointestinal distress, including nausea, vomiting, and diarrhea, are the most common and reportedly occur in more than 30% of patients. Mucositis/stomatitis is less frequent, occurring in approximately 3% of patients treated with HAI 5-FU.[45] In the case of severe toxicity that fails to respond to supportive therapy, dose reductions or treatment interruption may be necessary.

Alternatively, FUDR is almost entirely extracted by the liver, limiting systemic exposure. The primary toxicities observed with HAI FUDR are therefore local hepatobiliary toxicities. Chemically induced hepatitis is common with HAI FUDR, and rates have been reported anywhere from 30% to 70% depending on the definition. Typically this complication is mild and manifests only as biochemical abnormalities. **Table 4** outlines an FUDR dose-reduction schedule based on laboratory evaluation of AST, ALP, and total bilirubin. Most patients will have resolution of their enzyme abnormalities with careful adherence to dose-reduction schedules.

Biliary sclerosis is the most feared complication of HAI chemotherapy, and is reported to occur in 1% to 26% of patients. Unlike in normal hepatocytes, the blood

Table 4
Dose reductions for hepatic arterial infusion (HAI) floxuridine (FUDR)

Liver Blood Test				FUDR Dose
AST	Reference range	≤50 U/L	>50 U/L	
	Current value	0 to <3 × ref	0 to <2 × ref	100%
		3 to <4 × ref	2 to <3 × ref	80%
		4 to <5 × ref	3 to <4 × ref	50%
		≥5 × ref	≥4 × ref	Hold
	If held, restart when	<4 × ref	<3 × ref	50% of last dose
ALP	Reference	≤90 U/L	>90 U/L	
	Current value	0 to <1.5 × ref	0 to <1.2 × ref	100%
		1.5 to <2 × ref	1.2 to <1.5 × ref	80%
		≥2 × ref	≥1.5 × ref	Hold
	If held, restart when	<1.5 × ref	<1.2 × ref	25% of last dose
Total bilirubin	Reference	≤1.2 mg/dL	>1.2 mg/dL	
	Current value	0 to <1.5 × ref	0 to <1.2 × ref	100%
		1.5 to <2 × ref	1.2 to <1.5 × ref	50%
		≥2 × ref	≥1.5 × ref	Hold
	If held, restart when	<1.5 × ref	<1.2 × ref	25% of last dose

Abbreviations: ALP, alkaline phosphatase; AST, aspartate aminotransferase; ref, reference.
   From Power DG, Kemeny NE. The role of floxuridine in metastatic liver disease. Mol Cancer Ther 2009;8(5):1021; with permission.

supply to the bile duct is the HA and GDA collaterals; consequently, placement of a catheter into the GDA and infusion of high concentrations of cytotoxic agents puts the bile duct at significant risk for injury. The presumed mechanism of biliary sclerosis associated with HAI chemotherapy is a result of both ischemic injury and direct drug toxicity.[46] It occurs almost exclusively with FUDR infusion, and is more common in the adjuvant setting.[46] The addition of dexamethasone (DEX) to FUDR has been shown to decrease rates of biliary toxicity. In a prospective trial of FUDR alone versus FUDR/DEX, rates of biliary toxicity were 30% and 9%, respectively ($P = .07$). Following this study all HAI FUDR is administered with DEX. More recently it has been reported that the use of systemic bevacizumab (BEV) in conjunction with HAI FUDR significantly increases the risk of biliary sclerosis, and is contraindicated.[47] Early recognition is essential in managing biliary sclerosis. Failure of biochemical abnormalities to resolve with dose reduction/cessation and/or the presence of an isolated elevation in total bilirubin require prompt CT evaluation for evidence of external compression suggesting potential recurrent disease. In the absence of radiographic evidence of external biliary compression, magnetic resonance cholangiopancreatography is completed, and any discrete stricture may be treated with endoscopic retrograde cholangiopancreatography stent/dilation. Despite the need for dose reductions or cessation, survival in patients with isolated strictures, in whom biliary stenting/dilation is feasible, is not compromised.[46]

CLINICAL OUTCOMES WITH HEPATIC ARTERY INFUSION CHEMOTHERAPY
Adjuvant Hepatic Artery Infusion Chemotherapy and Resectable Colorectal Cancer Metastases

Unfortunately, 70% to 80% of patients undergoing resection of colorectal cancer liver metastasis (CRLM) will develop recurrence, 50% of which will be in the liver. In efforts to improve outcomes, adjuvant systemic therapy following hepatic resection has been considered. Use of HAI chemotherapy in this setting is attractive given the high rates of local recurrence observed. To date multiple randomized controlled trials (RCTs) and retrospective reviews have evaluated the use of HAI chemotherapy following resection of CRLM.

One of the first trials of HAI chemotherapy in the postoperative setting was conducted by Lorenz and colleagues.[48] In this trial patients were randomly assigned to surgery (Sx) alone or Sx + HAI 5-FU/leucovorin (LV). Overall disease-free survival (DFS) was not different between groups (14.2 months Sx + HAI 5-FU vs 13.7 months Sx alone) nor was liver-specific DFS (21.6 months Sx + HAI 5-FU vs 24 months Sx alone). For OS, no difference was observed between the 2 groups; however, only 30% of patients in the HAI chemotherapy arm actually received planned therapy, limiting interpretation of these findings. Furthermore, the trial was stopped early because of safety/futility concerns. A second smaller trial from Germany enrolled 42 patients and randomized to HAI mitomycin C (MMC) + Sx or Sx alone. No differences in terms of 5-year OS (25% in the HAI chemotherapy arm vs 31% Sx alone) or DFS (15% in HAI chemotherapy vs 23% Sx alone) were observed between groups. In the HAI MMC group, there appeared to be a trend toward greater extrahepatic recurrences, but this was not significant.[49]

In 1999, Kemeny and colleagues[12] completed a trial in which patients with resected CRLM were randomized at the time of operation to HAI FUDR/DEX + 5-FU/LV or 5-FU/LV alone. Randomization was stratified according to previous treatment and number of metastases. In the treatment arm, median OS was 73 months compared with 60 months in the control arm, and cumulative 2-year OS was 86% in the HAI chemotherapy group compared with 74% in the systemic group ($P = .03$). At 2 years, survival free of hepatic recurrence was significantly higher in the HAI chemotherapy group than in the systemic group (90% vs 60%, $P<.001$). The 2-year DFS was 57% and 42% for the HAI arm and the systemic arm, respectively, and was not significantly different ($P = .07$). The major limitation of this trial was the high rate of treatment modifications. Only 26% of patients in the treatment arm received more the half of the planned dose of FUDR, owing to toxicity-related dose reductions. Despite these limitations it appeared that HAI FUDR/DEX + 5-FU/LV improved disease control in the liver as well as cumulative 2-year OS. In 2005, follow-up results from this trial were published. At that time, data from this trial had matured such that the median follow-up time was 10 years.[50] Median DFS was 31.3 months in the combined therapy group compared with 17.2 months in the systemic alone group ($P = .02$). Similarly, survival free of liver recurrence in the combination group where the median had not yet been reached was significantly improved in comparison with the systemic group (median 32.5 months). Median OS in the HAI chemotherapy was 68 months in the combination group and 59 months in the systemic only group ($P = .10$). Cumulative 10-year OS rates were 41% in the HAI chemotherapy group and 27% in controls.

In another RCT from a group in Greece, HAI chemotherapy + systemic chemo-immunotherapy (HAI MMC/FU + MMC + interleukin [IL]-2) was compared with systemic MMC + IL-2 alone following curative intent surgery for CRLM. In this trial, overall DFS was 46 months in the HAI chemotherapy arm versus 19 months in the systemic arm ($P = .006$), and survival free of disease in the liver was 79 months in the HAI chemotherapy compared with 45 months in the systemic group ($P<.0001$). Median OS was also significantly improved in the HAI chemotherapy group (79 months vs 66 months, $P = .05$). These data suggest that combined locoregional therapy in conjunction with systemic chemo-immunotherapy improves both DFS and OS.

In 2002, Kemeny and colleagues[51] reported on a multicenter adjuvant trial of HAI FUDR + 5-FU/LV versus surgery alone, in low-risk patients (1–3 tumors). In the HAI arm, overall 4-year DFS and survival free of liver recurrence was improved (46% vs 25% DFS and 67% vs 43%, DFS-liver, respectively). In terms of OS no differences were observed in either cumulative 4-year OS or median OS between the groups. Accrual into this trial was slow, with only 109 patients recruited over a 9-year period at 25 different centers. Changes in surgical techniques and subsequent therapies over time may limit interpretation of these results. Furthermore, randomization occurred preoperatively, which resulted in 29 patients being taken off study at the time of operation (18 in the HAI arm and 11 in the surgery only arm); 80 patients were included in the final analysis and, as such, the study lacked power to address survival.

More recently 2 single-arm phase I/II trials of modern systemic chemotherapy in conjunction with HAI chemotherapy were completed. In the first, HAI FUDR/DEX was combined with irinotecan in escalating doses in the safety/toxicity phase of the trial. Once the maximum tolerated dose (MTD) was identified, 24 patients were added to the study at the MTD. The MTD of combination therapy was 200 mg/m^2 irinotecan and 0.12 mg/kg FUDR $\times$ pump volume/flow rate. Dose-limiting toxicities were diarrhea and neutropenia. In the entire cohort (N = 96) 18-month DFS was 47%, survival free of liver recurrence at 2 years was 88%, and cumulative 2-year OS was 89%. Of the patients who were treated at the MTD (n = 27), 1 liver recurrence was reported at 16 months. Overall, 4 recurrences (1 liver + 3 extrahepatic) were observed in this group and 1-year DFS was 91%.[52] In a similarly designed phase I trial a regimen of combination FOLFOX (5-FU/LV/oxaliplatin [Ox]) + FUDR/DEX was evaluated. MTD was established, and dose-limiting toxicities included diarrhea and hyperbilirubinemia. Four-year OS was 88% and DFS 50%.[53] These 2 trials identified the safety of combining HAI FUDR/DEX with modern chemotherapy regimens in patients with resected CRLM. Although not large enough to draw conclusions regarding clinical outcomes, they provided stimulus for further evaluation of these combination locoregional/systemic treatments in larger phase III trials.

To date, no large randomized phase III trials of modern adjuvant systemic chemotherapy with HAI chemotherapy exist; however, multiple phase II trials have been reported. Kemeny and colleagues[54] compared outcomes of 73 patients randomized to HAI FUDR/DEX + systemic therapy with and without BEV. In this trial randomization was appropriately stratified by clinical risk. Reported 4-year DFS and OS were 37% and 81% in the BEV group, and 46% and 85% in the no BEV group, and were not significantly different. Biliary toxicity was significantly increased in the BEV arm, with 5 patients developing bilirubin elevation greater than 3 mg/dL and 4 patients requiring biliary stents; no patients who did not receive BEV developed either complication. Concerns regarding these toxicities resulted in removal of BEV from the trial. However, it is reasonable to conclude that the addition of BEV to HAI FUDR/DEX + systemic therapy following liver resection for CRLM did not improve DFS or OS, but appears to increase biliary complications and should be avoided.

A single-arm phase II trial of alternating HAI FUDR/DEX + systemic Ox and capecitabine following liver resection or ablation enrolled 76 patients. Twenty-one patients were unable to begin protocol-directed therapy; as such, 55 patients were evaluable. DFS at 2 years was 60%, survival free of liver recurrence was 76%, and OS was 89%. In terms of treatment delivery, 67% of patients received all 6 cycles of therapy, which indicates the tolerability and feasibility of this treatment.[55] Although the phase II nature of the trial limits generalized conclusions, this combination of therapy seems safe and may be associated with favorable recurrence and survival outcomes.

Several retrospective reviews have been reported. Tomlinson and colleagues[56] reviewed 612 patients who underwent liver resection for CRLM. In patients receiving adjuvant HAI FUDR, 10-year OS was 38% compared with 15% in those who did not (P<.0001). Furthermore, Ito and colleagues[57] reviewed more than 1000 patients undergoing hepatectomy. In this cohort, multivariate analysis revealed adjuvant HAI FUDR as an independent factor associated with improved survival (68 months HAI FUDR vs 50 months no HAI chemotherapy, P<.0001). A third review from Memorial Sloan Kettering Cancer Center (MSKCC) by House and colleagues[58] retrospectively evaluated 250 patients who had liver resection for CRLM and modern adjuvant systemic chemotherapy (Ox, irinotecan); 125 also had adjuvant HAI FUDR. Survival free of liver recurrence was 79% in the HAI group versus 55% in modern chemotherapy alone group (P<.001); 5-year RFS was 48% in the HAI group and 25% in controls (P = .01), and disease-specific survival (DSS) was 75% in the HAI group versus 55% in controls at 5 years (P = .01). Most recently a review by Goere and colleagues[59] evaluated 98 high-risk patients (>4 tumors), and compared those treated with HAI Ox + systemic 5-FU/LV (n = 44) with those treated with systemic therapy alone (n = 54). Significant differences between the groups were observed in overall DFS (3-year DFS HAI Ox 33% vs 5% for controls, P<.0001) and survival free of liver recurrence at 3 years (49% HAI Ox vs 21% for controls, P = .0008). OS among the groups was not different, 3-year OS 75% versus 62% for HAI Ox and controls, respectively.

The accumulation of multiple small trials of HAI chemotherapy in the adjuvant setting highlights some of the issues that have impaired the ability to conduct any large phase III randomized trials. First, the rapid emergence of newer systemic therapies makes identification of appropriate control arms difficult. Furthermore, use of FUDR, the most extensively studied drug for adjuvant HAI, is limited outside of the United States, making large multinational trials problematic and limiting generalizability. In addition, accrual to trials is often slow, and what is considered standard at the initiation of a trial may no longer be at the time of closure. Finally, advancements in surgical technologies and adjuncts such as ablative techniques continue to redefine resectable CRLM, often making identification of the treatment group difficult. However, despite a lack of large randomized phase III trials, it seems that HAI chemotherapy in the adjuvant setting may improve DFS and survival free of liver recurrence. Whether a significant OS advantage exists remains to be seen.

UNRESECTABLE COLORECTAL CANCER METASTASES
First Line: Hepatic Artery Infusion Chemotherapy Alone

To date, 10 RCTs have investigated the use of HAI chemotherapy as first-line treatment of unresectable colorectal cancer liver metastases (UR-CRLM). Significant heterogeneity exists among the trials in terms of design and implementation, which has led to discrepant and somewhat inconclusive results. **Table 5** outlines these trials and contrasts their outcomes.

Five RCTs of HAI chemotherapy for UR-CRLM were published between 1987 and 1990. Chang and colleagues[60] evaluated HAI FUDR versus systemic FUDR in 64 patients with UR-CRLM. RR were 62% in the HAI FUDR arm, compared with 17% in the systemic arm (P<.003). This finding did not translate into an OS benefit; median OS was 17 months with HAI FUDR, compared with 12 months with systemic chemotherapy (P = .27). This trial was criticized for including patients with positive portal nodes in the HAI FUDR arm. Subgroup analysis of patients without nodal involvement revealed a 2-year OS of 47% in the HAI FUDR group compared with 13% in the systemic arm (P = .03). A larger trial from MSKCC randomized 162 patients to HAI FUDR or systemic FUDR. At the time of laparotomy, 63 patients were excluded because of the presence of EHD or evidence of resectable disease. Crossover from systemic

Table 5
Randomized control trials of HAI chemotherapy alone for unresectable colorectal cancer liver metastases

Authors,[Ref.] Year (Group)	N	Treatment	Response Rate (%)	P Value	Progression-Free Survival (mo)	P Value	Overall Survival (mo)	P Value
Chang et al,[60] 1987 (NCI)	64	HAIC FUDR	62	**<.003**	—	—	17	.72
		Systemic FUDR	17		—		12	
Kemeny et al,[61] 1987 (MSKCC)	99	HAIC FUDR	50	**.001**	—	—	17	.42
		Systemic FUDR	20		—		12	
Hohn et al,[62] 1989 (NCOG)	143	HAIC FUDR	42	**.0001**	13.2	**.009**	16.6	NS
		Systemic FUDR	6		6.6		16.1	
Wagman et al,[63] 1990	56	HAI FUDR	55	NR	8.8	.94	13.8	.55
		Systemic 5FU/LV	20		7.5		11.6	
Martin et al,[64] 1990 (NCCTG)	74	HAIC FUDR	48	**.02**	6.0	.31	12.6	.53
		Systemic 5-FU	21		5.0		10.5	
Rougier et al,[65] 1992 (France)	163	HAIC FUDR	43	NR	—	—	15	**.02**
		BSC or 5-FU	9		—		11	
Allen-Mersh et al,[66] 1994 (UK-HAPT)	100	HAIC FUDR	—	—	—	—	13.5	**.03**
		BSC	—		—		7.5	
Lorenz et al,[67] 2000 (German cooperative group)	168	HAIC 5-FU/LV			9.2	**.03**	18.7	.09 (HAIC 5-FU vs HAIC FUDR)
		HAIC FUDR			5.9		12.7	
		Systemic 5-FU			6.6		17.6	
Kerr et al,[68] 2003 (EORTC)	290	HAIC 5-FU/LV	—	—	7.7	.27	14.7	.79
		Systemic 5-FU	—		6.7		14.8	
Kemeny et al,[69] 2006 (CALGB)	135	HAIC/FUDR/DEX/LV	47	**.012**	5.3	.95	24.4	**.003**
		Systemic 5-FU/LV	24		6.8		20.0	

Numbers in bold are significant values.

Abbreviations: BSC, best supportive care; CALGB, Cancer and Leukemia Group B; DEX, dexamethasone; EORTC, European Organization for Research and Treatment of Cancer; HAIC, hepatic artery infusion chemotherapy; LV, leucovorin; MSKCC, Memorial Sloan Kettering Cancer Center; NCCTG, North Central Cancer Treatment Group; NCI, National Cancer Institute; NCOG, Northern California Oncology Group; NR, not reported; NS, not significant; UK-HAPT, Hepatic Artery Pump Trial (United Kingdom).

FUDR to HAI FUDR was permitted in the setting of tumor progression. In the HAI FUDR group, RR was 50% compared with 20% in the systemic arm (P = .001). This increased RR did not translate into a survival benefit; however, a 60% crossover rate was observed, making survival analysis difficult to interpret. If patients who crossed over were excluded from analysis, median OS in the HAI chemotherapy arm was 18 months, versus 8 months in the systemic arm.[61] A third trial from the Northern California Oncology Group randomized 143 patients to HAI FUDR or systemic FUDR with primary end points of RR and time to disease progression (TTP). In the HAI FUDR group RR was 42%, compared with 6% in the systemic FUDR group (P = .0001). TTP was longer in the HAI chemotherapy group (13.2 vs 6.6 months, P = .009) but median OS was not different between the groups (16.6 vs 16.1 months).[62] Significant toxicity was noted in this trial, and more than 50% of the treatment arm received less than half of the intended therapy. As with the MSKCC trial, crossover from systemic to HAI chemotherapy was permitted and interpretation of survival data are limited.

A study by Wagman and colleagues[63] randomized 56 patients with UR-CRLM to receive HAI FUDR or systemic 5-FU/LV. No differences were found between the groups in terms of RR (HAI FUDR 55% vs 20% 5-FU/LV), time to failure (8.8 months HAI FUDR vs 7.5 months 5-FU/LV), or OS (13.8 months HAI FUDR vs 11.6 months). It is noteworthy that the systemic therapy used in this trial, in comparison with previous trials, was 5-FU/LV and not FUDR, the latter of which, when delivered systemically, has been shown to have decreased RR compared with 5-FU/LV. Similarly, a study from the Mayo clinic randomized 74 patients to HAI FUDR versus systemic 5-FU/LV, and found no difference in TTP (6.0 months HAI FUDR vs 5.0 months 5-FU/LV, P = .31) or OS (12.6 months HAI FUDR vs 10.5 months 5-FU/LV, 0.53) despite improved RR (48% vs 21%, HAI FUDR and 5-FU/LV).[64]

Rougier and colleagues[65] evaluated HAI FUDR in comparison with best supportive care (BSC) or systemic 5-FU. The trial permitted crossover from HAI to systemic therapy or BSC in the advent of disease progression. RR in the FUDR group was 43%, compared with 9% for the 5-FU/BSC group. OS was found to be significantly different between the 2 arms, with median OS of 15 months in the FUDR group compared with 11 months in the 5-FU/BSC group (P = .02). The crossover rate in this study was 30%, and management of the control was not standardized; limiting the interpretation of these results. A similar randomized study of treatment-naïve patients with UR-CRLM comparing HAI FUDR with BSC also reported significant improvement in median OS in the HAI FUDR arm (13.5 months) compared with BSC (7.5 months, P = .03).[66]

In 2000, the German Cooperative group published the results of 168 patients with UR-CRLM randomized to 1 of 3 arms: HAI 5-FU/LV, HAI FUDR, or systemic 5-FU/LV. TTP was 9.2, 6.6, and 5.9 months for the HAI 5-FU/LV, HAI FUDR, and 5-FU/LV groups, respectively. This result was statistically different between the HAI 5-FU/LV group and the HAI FUDR group (P = .033). No differences were seen in OS, although a trend favoring HAI 5-FU/LV was observed. Similarly to other reported trials, this study allowed treatment crossover from HAI chemotherapy to systemic therapy, again making survival analysis suspect.[67]

The largest RCT evaluating HAI chemotherapy in UR-CRLM was published in 2003 and consisted of 290 patients randomized to either HAI 5-FU/LV or systemic 5-FU/LV. No differences were observed in progression-free survival (PFS) or OS between the 2 groups. However, 37% of patients assigned to the HAI 5-FU/LV arm received no treatment and 29% had treatment stopped owing to catheter failure, and crossed over to the systemic arm. The median number of cycles in the HAI chemotherapy group was

2, compared with 8.5 in the systemic arm. The investigators concluded that the increased risk of complication with HAI chemotherapy was not offset by any significant survival advantage, and that HAI chemotherapy should not be used in the treatment of UR-CRLM.[68]

The CALGB 9481 trial, published in 2006, randomized 135 patients with UR-CRLM to receive HAI FUDR/LV/DEX or systemic 5-FU/LV. It was designed with primary end point of survival, and no crossover between arms was permitted. RRs were significantly different between treatment arms (47% HAI chemotherapy vs 24% systemic, $P = .012$). Overall, TTP was not different between groups. Hepatic TTP, however, was significantly longer in the HAI chemotherapy group, 9.8 months compared with 7.3 months in the systemic group ($P = .03$). In terms of OS, in the HAI chemotherapy group median OS was 24.4 months compared with 20 months in the systemic group, which was significantly different ($P = .003$.).[69] This trial was the first to observe an OS benefit of HAI chemotherapy when compared with the best available systemic therapy, 5-FU/LV.

The first meta-analysis of these trials was published in 1996 by the Meta-Analysis Group in Cancer, and included RCTs published up to 1994 (see **Table 5**). Tumor RR of pooled data was significantly different between treatment types. HAI chemotherapy (5-FU or FUDR) RR was 41% compared with 14% in the systemic therapy arms (5-FU or FUDR) (odds ratio 0.25, 95% confidence interval [CI] 0.16–0.40). Survival analysis of all trials seemed to suggest benefit of HAI chemotherapy over systemic therapy ($P = .0009$); however, when the trials with no therapeutic control arm (BSC) were excluded, the benefit was no longer apparent ($P = .14$).[70] An updated meta-analysis was published in 2007 and included all the RCTs presented in **Table 5**.[71] Pooling of the data suggested RR similar to the initial meta-analysis, 42.9% HAI chemotherapy compared with 18.4% systemic ($P<.0001$). The small OS advantage observed in the initial evaluation was not appreciated, mean OS of HAI chemotherapy being 15.9 months, versus 12.4 months systemic (hazard ratio 0.90, 95% CI 0.76–1.07; $P = 0.24$). Cumulative evaluation of these data suggest that HAI chemotherapy alone (without systemic therapy) for the treatment of UR-CRLM results in improved tumor RR, but this improvement does not appear to translate into a survival advantage.

Second Line: Hepatic Artery Infusion Chemotherapy + Systemic Therapy

Outcomes of patients with UR-CRLM who fail first-line chemotherapy are poor. Even with modern chemotherapy regimens RR are 20% at best, and median OS is in the realm of 9 to 12 months.[72] Despite a lack of survival benefit, early HAI trials indicated that progression of disease in the liver was significantly delayed, and disease failure tended to be systemic. In efforts to address this, multiple investigations of HAI chemotherapy in combination with systemic therapy were initiated.

In a study of 84 patients randomized to HAI FUDR + systemic 5-FU/LV or systemic 5-FU/LV alone, no significant difference in survival was observed: 1-year OS was 46% HAI FUDR + 5-FU/LV versus 53% 5-FU/LV. Increased toxicity was observed in the combination HAI FUDR + 5-FU/LV arm, suggesting a lack of benefit, and a potential for harm with HAI FUDR + systemic 5-FU/LV.[73] Since that time, evidence of improved RR with newer chemotherapy regimens (Ox, irinotecan) over standard 5-FU/LV prompted several phase I trials evaluating HAI FUDR in combination with modern chemotherapy. A phase I trial of systemic irinotecan with HAI FUDR in 46 previously treated patients found no increase in toxicity with concomitant administration of the drugs. Furthermore, RR was 74%; median overall TTP was 8.1 months, and TTP in the liver was 8.5 months. Median OS was 17.2 months.[74] A second phase I trial of dual-agent systemic Ox therapy—(a) Ox + irinotecan or (b) Ox + 5-FU/LV

(FOLFOX)—in combination with HAI FUDR similarly found impressive RR and OS. In the FOLFOX + HAI FUDR group, RR was 87% and in the Ox + irinotecan + HAI FUDR, RR was 90%. Median OS was 22 and 36 months, respectively.[75] From these trials, data on HAI chemotherapy/FUDR + irinotecan in 39 patients previously treated with systemic Ox was reviewed retrospectively. Most patients had failed 1 or 2 previous treatment regimens (33 of 39). TTP in the liver was 8.6 months and TTP anywhere was 6.5 months. RR for this heavily treated cohort was 44% and median OS was 20 months. Rate of conversion to resectable disease was 18%.

Given that FUDR is not approved for use in many countries, HAI chemotherapy with Ox (HAI Ox) has been used as an alternative. A phase I trial from France evaluated the use of HAI Ox + systemic 5-FU/LV in 44 patients with UR-CRLM who had failed first-line chemotherapy. The number of previously failed treatments ranged from 1 to 5 with a median of 2. Median OS was 16 months, PFS was 7 months, and overall RR was 55%. Partial response (PR) was seen in 17 patients who previously failed FOLFIRI (5-FU/LV/irinotecan) and 12 patients who failed FOLFOX. Seven of 44 patients (18%) were converted from unresectable to resectable disease and underwent surgical intervention.[76] A second trial by the same group looked at the same regimen (HAI Ox + 5-FU/LV) in 28 patients who had no previous exposure to Ox. In this select cohort RR was 64%, median OS 27 months, and PFS 27 months.[77] Although from small phase I trials and retrospective reviews, these results are impressive and suggest a potential benefit of HAI chemotherapy + modern systemic chemotherapy in terms of RR and survival in patients with UR-CRLM who fail first-line therapy.

Conversion from Unresectable to Resectable

Despite the advent of newer more active chemotherapies for use in CRLM, RR remains around 30% to 40% and median OS 20 months.[78] Surgery is the only potentially curative treatment of CRLM. Consequently, the focus of several recent studies has been on the ability to convert patients from unresectable to resectable disease. A recent trial from MSKCC evaluated HAI FUDR + irinotecan/Ox in 49 patients with technically UR-CRLM (73% >5 tumors, 98% bilobar disease). Overall RR was 92%, with complete response observed in 8% and PR in 84%. In terms of conversion, 23 of the 49 patients were converted to resectable (47%). Of the patients who went on to resection, median DFS was 7.6 months. A second study from MSKCC reported on 39 patients who received HAI FUDR/DEX + irinotecan in the unresectable setting and found 44% RR, and 7 of 39 (18%) patients were converted to resectable disease. Furthermore, in a retrospective review of patients with UR-CRLM treated with HAI FUDR + systemic chemotherapy at MSKCC, 373 patients were identified. Two hundred ninety-six of these patients (79%) had been previously treated with systemic chemotherapy. Ninety-three (25%) patients were converted and went on to surgical resection with or without ablation. Median OS was 59 months in patients who underwent resection, compared with 16 months in those who did not ($P<.001$).[79] Despite extensive burden of disease and significant pretreatment in this cohort, conversion to resection was achieved in 25% of patients, suggesting that combination FUDR + modern systemic therapy is an effective treatment strategy.

HAI Ox has been used extensively in France, where FUDR is not available. Small trials, already mentioned, of HAI Ox + systemic therapy in the unresectable setting revealed conversion rates of around 18%. A retrospective review of these trials included 87 patients who were treated with HAI Ox+ systemic 5-FU/LV. In total, 21 patients (24%) went on to curative-intent resection. Median follow-up for the entire cohort was 63 months and 5-year OS was 56% in the group that was resected, compared with 0% in the patients who did not undergo resection ($P<.0001$).[80] These results suggest that similarly to HAI FUDR + systemic therapy, HAI Ox + systemic therapy offers a greater than 20% chance of conversion to resection, and may impart a long-term survival benefit.

HEPATIC ARTERY INFUSION CHEMOTHERAPY AND PRIMARY LIVER TUMORS

Primary cancer of the liver (PLC), including intrahepatic cholangiocarcinoma (ICC) and hepatocellular carcinoma (HCC), often present late with advanced disease, for which few good treatment options exist. Median OS in this setting is less than 12 months. To date, few trials of HAI chemotherapy for the treatment of PLC have been completed within North America. In 2009, Jarnagin and colleagues[81] reported a single-arm phase II trial of HAI FUDR/DEX in 34 patients with PLC (26 unresectable ICC, 8 advanced HCC). Toxicity was observed in 14.7% of patients and pump-related complications occurred in 24%. PR was observed in 16 (47%) patients and duration of response in the liver was 24 months. Stable disease (SD) was present in 14 patients (41%), and 3 patients (9%) had progressive disease (PD). Disease control rate (PR + SD) was 88%. Overall RR for ICC was 54% and for HCC RR, 25%. At 25 months' follow-up, 33 of 34 patients had disease progression and 21 (61.8%) had progression in the liver (18 liver only, 3 liver + extrahepatic). The initial site of disease progression was extrahepatic in 21 of the 33 patients. DSS stratified by response was as follows: PR 35.1 months, SD 28.6 months, and PD 9.8 months. Overall PFS was 7.4 months and liver-specific PFS was 10.3 months. A second study from MSKCC included 22 patients with PLC (18 ICC, 4 HCC) treated with HAI FUDR/DEX + BEV, and compared these with 34 patients treated with HAI FUDR/DEX without BEV. In patients with ICC, PR was observed in 7 (39%) and SD in 11 (61%) patients, and median duration of response was 11 months in the PR group and 6 months in the SD group. All patients with HCC had SD, with median duration of response being 9 months. Median PFS in the BEV group was 8.5 months compared with 7.5 months in the control group; hepatic PFS was 11 months for the BEV group versus 10 months for controls. In the BEV group, median OS was 31 months compared with 30 months in controls. In this trial, excessive biliary toxicity was observed in patients treated with BEV; 5 of 22 (23%) developed toxicity, 3 (14%) of whom required stent placement, compared with 2 of 34 (6%) with biliary toxicity without BEV and no stent placement.[82] Based on these findings, BEV was removed from the trial for safety reasons. Recently an update of these trials was published, focusing on those patients with ICC. In total, 44 patients with ICC treated with HAI chemotherapy were included: 22 with HAI FUDR/DEX and 18 with HAI FUDR/DEX + BEV. Median follow-up was 29 months, at which time 93% of patients had died of disease. In the entire cohort 48% had PR, 50% had SD, and after response 3 patients went on to resection. The first site of disease progression was the liver in 55% of patients, extrahepatic 43%, and 2% at both sites concomitantly. Median OS was 29 months in the FUDR alone group and 28 months in the FUDR + BEV group. There were 10 patients who survived at least 3 years and 5 who survived at least 5 years. In these long-term survivors (≥3 years) liver-specific PFS was longer, 13 months compared with 9 months in those surviving less than 3 years,[83] suggesting that disease control in the liver may be of benefit regarding OS. Treatment of patients with unresectable PLC, most specifically ICC, with HAI FUDR/DEX is safe, and in some may result in long-term survival. Many trials of HAI chemotherapy for the treatment of PLC, mainly HCC, have been completed in Japan and Asia where the incidence of HCC is significantly higher and the primary underlying etiology differs markedly from North America. Application of these results in the non-Asian setting is difficult.

HEPATIC ARTERY INFUSION CHEMOTHERAPY AND NONCOLORECTAL LIVER METASTASES

The use of HAI chemotherapy in the setting of noncolorectal liver metastases (non-CRLM) has been poorly studied; however, a few small trials of HAI chemotherapy in aggressive cancers have been completed. At present no good treatment for ocular melanoma metastatic to the liver exists, and median OS is less than 5 months, HAI chemotherapy has been suggested as a treatment in this setting, and has been evaluated in a few small trials. A group from France reported a single-arm prospective evaluation of fotemustine delivered via HAI for the treatment of liver metastases from ocular melanoma following surgical debulking. In terms of treatment tolerability, 2 patients had hepatic toxicity mandating cessation of therapy, and 9 patients had catheter complications precluding delivery after a median of 10 cycles. Four patients (13%) had complete response and 8 (27%) PR. Overall, RR was 40% and duration of response was 11 months. Median OS was 14 months, with 7 patients surviving longer than 2 years. In patients who showed an objective response, median OS was 20 months compared with 10 months in nonresponders.[84] Melichar and colleagues[85] also reported a small retrospective series of 10 patients with liver metastases from ocular melanoma treated with HAI chemotherapy using a multidrug regimen, in addition to systemic therapies. In terms of RR, 2 patients had PR, 4 had SD, and 4 had PD. Median OS was 16 months, and all patients with PD were dead by 1 year. HAI chemotherapy is attractive in ocular melanoma liver metastases; because of the miliary distribution of these metastases, other liver-directed therapies theoretically would be less effective. To date no evidence to support its routine use exists.

Recently, a phase I trial of HAI cisplatin + systemic liposomal doxorubicin was evaluated in a heterogeneous group of patients with metastatic cancer with dominant liver involvement.[86] A total of 30 patients were included (11 breast cancer, 8 CRLM, 4 ocular melanoma, and 7 other: HCC/gastric/pancreatic/head and neck/neuroendocrine/cutaneous melanoma/leiomyosarcoma). The trial was designed to evaluate safety and toxicity but also reported on outcomes. In terms of disease control (PR + SD), 4 (17%) patients had PR and 7 (29%) SD. In the patients with breast cancer, 3 (27%) had PR and 5 (45%) had SD. Median OS was 7.5 months. In patients with breast cancer the median OS was 8.5 months, compared with 5.3 months for all other tumor types.[86] The use of this regimen seems to be safe and potentially has benefits in terms of RR, but more data are required before any judgment of a potential survival benefit can be made.

SUMMARY

HAI chemotherapy is a locoregional cancer therapy that has been used for decades in the treatment of both primary and metastatic cancers of the liver. Techniques for catheter insertion and convenient drug delivery via implantable pumps have evolved, and in experienced centers complications are minimized. HAI chemotherapy in the setting of both UR-CRLM and the adjuvant setting appears to be associated with improved RR; however, OS benefits have yet to be observed. Promising results of HAI chemotherapy in combination with modern systemic chemotherapy as a method of converting UR-CRLM to resectable CRLM have been observed. However, significant toxicity remains a concern, and further study in this setting is warranted. Few North American trials evaluating HAI chemotherapy in PLC have been completed; however, HAI chemotherapy may be deemed safe, and some evidence exists to suggest improvement in RR and survival. Larger trials with longer follow-up times, and comparisons with modern chemotherapeutic and/or targeted agents, are required to make definitive conclusions. Few studies of HAI chemotherapy for non-CRLM exist. The small number and heterogeneity of these trials in terms of type of therapy and tumor do not allow for formal conclusion as to the utility of HAI chemotherapy for non-CRLM. Concern still exists regarding the risk of complications associated with HAI chemotherapy, and skepticism regarding the overall benefits is common; consequently, the use of HAI chemotherapy in the treatment of primary and metastatic liver cancers remains controversial.

REFERENCES

1. Breedis C, Young G. The blood supply of neoplasms in the liver. Am J Pathol 1954;30(5):969–77.
2. Sullivan RD, Norcross JW, Watkins E Jr. Chemotherapy of metastatic liver cancer by prolonged hepatic-artery infusion. N Engl J Med 1964;270:321–7.
3. Cady B. Hepatic arterial patency and complications after catheterization for infusion chemotherapy. Ann Surg 1973;178(2):156–61.
4. Ensminger WD, Gyves JW. Clinical pharmacology of hepatic arterial chemotherapy. Semin Oncol 1983;10(2):176–82.
5. Ensminger WD. Regional chemotherapy. Semin Oncol 1993;20(1):3–11.
6. Burrows JH, Talley RW, Drake EH, et al. Infusion of fluorinated pyrimidines into hepatic artery for treatment of metastatic carcinoma of liver. Cancer 1967;20(11):1886–92.
7. Clarkson B, Young C, Dierick W, et al. Effects of continuous hepatic artery infusion of antimetabolites on primary and metastatic cancer of the liver. Cancer 1962;15:472–88.
8. Ensminger WD, et al. A clinical-pharmacological evaluation of hepatic arterial infusions of 5-fluoro-2′-deoxyuridine and 5-fluorouracil. Cancer Res 1978;38(11 Pt 1):3784–92.
9. Ensminger WD, Rosowsky A, Raso V, et al. Hepatic arterial BCNU: a pilot clinical-pharmacologic study in patients with liver tumors. Cancer Treat Rep 1978;62(10):1509–12.
10. Kelsen DP, Hoffman J, Alcock N, et al. Pharmacokinetics of cisplatin regional hepatic infusions. Am J Clin Oncol 1982;5(2):173–8.
11. Garnick MB, Ensminger WD, Israel M. A clinical-pharmacological evaluation of hepatic arterial infusion of adriamycin. Cancer Res 1979;39(10):4105–10.
12. Kemeny N, Huang Y, Cohen AM, et al. Hepatic arterial infusion of chemotherapy after resection of hepatic metastases from colorectal cancer. N Engl J Med 1999;341(27):2039–48.
13. Kingham TP, D'Angelica M, Kemeny NE. Role of intra-arterial hepatic chemotherapy in the treatment of colorectal cancer metastases. J Surg Oncol 2010;102(8):988–95.
14. Arru M, Aldrighetti L, Gremmo F, et al. Arterial devices for regional hepatic chemotherapy: transaxillary versus laparotomic access. J Vasc Access 2000;1(3):93–9.
15. Urbach DR, Herron DM, Khajanchee YS, et al. Laparoscopic hepatic artery infusion pump placement. Arch Surg 2001;136(6):700–4.
16. Franklin ME Jr, Gonzalez JJ Jr. Laparoscopic placement of hepatic artery catheter for regional chemotherapy infusion: technique, benefits, and complications. Surg Laparosc Endosc Percutan Tech 2002;12(6):398–407.
17. Franklin M, Trevino J, Hernandez-Oaknin H, et al. Laparoscopic hepatic artery catheterization for regional chemotherapy: is this the best current option for liver metastatic disease? Surg Endosc 2006;20(4):554–8.

18. Hellan M, Pigazzi A. Robotic-assisted placement of a hepatic artery infusion catheter for regional chemotherapy. Surg Endosc 2008;22(2):548–51.

19. Blackshear PJ, Rohde TD, Dorman FD, et al. An implantable pump for long-term intravascular drug infusion. Med Instrum 1981;15(4):226–8.

20. Buchwald H, Grage TB, Vassilopoulos PP, et al. Intraarterial infusion chemotherapy for hepatic carcinoma using a totally implantable infusion pump. Cancer 1980;45(5):866–9.

21. Heinrich S, Petrowsky H, Schwinnen I, et al. Technical complications of continuous intra-arterial chemotherapy with 5-fluorodeoxyuridine and 5-fluorouracil for colorectal liver metastases. Surgery 2003;133(1):40–8.

22. Fordy C, Burke D, Earlam S, et al. Treatment interruptions and complications with two continuous hepatic artery floxuridine infusion systems in colorectal liver metastases. Br J Cancer 1995;72(4):1023–5.

23. Bacchetti S, Pasqual E, Crozzolo E, et al. Intra-arterial hepatic chemotherapy for unresectable colorectal liver metastases: a review of medical devices complications in 3172 patients. Med Devices (Auckl) 2009;2:31–40.

24. Portal vein chemotherapy for colorectal cancer: a meta-analysis of 4000 patients in 10 studies. Liver Infusion Meta-analysis Group. J Natl Cancer Inst 1997;89(7): 497–505.

25. James RD, on behalf of the AXIS collaborators. Intraportal 5FU (PVI) and perioperative radiotherapy (RT) in the adjuvant treatment of colorectal cancer (CRCa)—3681 patients randomised in the UK Coordinating Committee on Cancer Research (UKCCCR) AXIS trial. Proc Am Soc Clin Oncol 1999;18:1013 [abstract].

26. Labianca R, Boffi L, Marsoni S, et al. A randomized trial of intraportal (IP) versus systemic (SY) versus IP + SY adjuvant chemotherapy in patients (pts) with resected Dukes B-C colon carcinoma (CC). Proc Am Soc Clin Oncol 1999;18: 1014 [abstract].

27. Rougier P, Sahmoud T, Nitti D, et al. Adjuvant portal-vein infusion of fluorouracil and heparin in colorectal cancer: a randomised trial. European Organisation for Research and Treatment of Cancer Gastrointestinal Tract Cancer Cooperative Group, the Gruppo Interdisciplinare Valutazione Interventi in Oncologia, and the Japanese Foundation for Cancer Research. Lancet 1998;351(9117): 1677–81.

28. Laffer U, Maibach R, Metzger U, et al. Randomized trial of adjuvant perioperative chemotherapy in radically resected colorectal cancer (SAKK 40/87). Proc Am Soc Clin Oncol 17:983, [abstract].

29. Cohen AD, Kemeny NE. An update on hepatic arterial infusion chemotherapy for colorectal cancer. Oncologist 2003;8(6):553–66.

30. Skitzki JJ, Chang AE. Hepatic artery chemotherapy for colorectal liver metastases: technical considerations and review of clinical trials. Surg Oncol 2002; 11(3):123–35.

31. Kemeny MM. The surgical aspects of the totally implantable hepatic artery infusion pump. Arch Surg 2001;136(3):348–52.

32. Saba L, Mallarini G. Multidetector row CT angiography in the evaluation of the hepatic artery and its anatomical variants. Clin Radiol 2008;63(3):312–21.

33. Grobmyer SR, Fong Y, D'Angelica M, et al. Diagnostic laparoscopy prior to planned hepatic resection for colorectal metastases. Arch Surg 2004;139(12): 1326–30.

34. Michels NA. Newer anatomy of the liver and its variant blood supply and collateral circulation. Am J Surg 1966;112(3):337–47.

35. Kemeny MM, Hogan JM, Goldberg DA, et al. Continuous hepatic artery infusion with an implantable pump: problems with hepatic artery anomalies. Surgery 1986;99(4):501–4.
36. Rayner AA, Kerlan RK, Stagg RJ, et al. Total hepatic arterial perfusion after occlusion of variant lobar vessels: implications for hepatic arterial chemotherapy. Surgery 1986;99(6):708–15.
37. Allen PJ, Nissan A, Picon AI, et al. Technical complications and durability of hepatic artery infusion pumps for unresectable colorectal liver metastases: an institutional experience of 544 consecutive cases. J Am Coll Surg 2005;201(1):57–65.
38. Curley SA, Chase JL, Roh MS, et al. Technical considerations and complications associated with the placement of 180 implantable hepatic arterial infusion devices. Surgery 1993;114(5):928–35.
39. Kemeny N, Seiter K, Niedzwiecki D, et al. A randomized trial of intrahepatic infusion of fluorodeoxyuridine with dexamethasone versus fluorodeoxyuridine alone in the treatment of metastatic colorectal cancer. Cancer 1992;69(2):327–34.
40. Patt YZ, Mavligit GM, Chuang VP, et al. Percutaneous hepatic arterial infusion (HAI) of mitomycin C and floxuridine (FUDR): an effective treatment for metastatic colorectal carcinoma in the liver. Cancer 1980;46(2):261–5.
41. Kemeny N, Daly J, Oderman P, et al. Hepatic artery pump infusion: toxicity and results in patients with metastatic colorectal carcinoma. J Clin Oncol 1984;2(6):595–600.
42. Niederhuber JE, Ensminger W, Gyves J, et al. Regional chemotherapy of colorectal cancer metastatic to the liver. Cancer 1984;53(6):1336–43.
43. Sofocleous CT, Schubert J, Kemeny N, et al. Arterial embolization for salvage of hepatic artery infusion pumps. J Vasc Interv Radiol 2006;17(5):801–6.
44. Roybal JJ, Feliberti EC, Rouse L, et al. Pump removal in infected patients with hepatic chemotherapy pumps: when is it necessary? Am Surg 2006;72(10):880–4.
45. Barnett KT, Malafa MP. Complications of hepatic artery infusion: a review of 4580 reported cases. Int J Gastrointest Cancer 2001;30(3):147–60.
46. Ito K, Ito H, Kemeny NE, et al. Biliary sclerosis after hepatic arterial infusion pump chemotherapy for patients with colorectal cancer liver metastasis: incidence, clinical features, and risk factors. Ann Surg Oncol 2012;19(5):1609–17.
47. Cercek A, D'Angelica M, Power D, et al. Floxuridine hepatic arterial infusion associated biliary toxicity is increased by concurrent administration of systemic bevacizumab. Ann Surg Oncol 2014;21(2):479–86.
48. Lorenz M, Muller HH, Schramm H, et al. Randomized trial of surgery versus surgery followed by adjuvant hepatic arterial infusion with 5-fluorouracil and folinic acid for liver metastases of colorectal cancer. German Cooperative on Liver Metastases (Arbeitsgruppe Lebermetastasen). Ann Surg 1998;228(6):756–62.
49. Rudroff C, Altendorf-Hoffmann A, Stangl R, et al. Prospective randomised trial on adjuvant hepatic-artery infusion chemotherapy after R0 resection of colorectal liver metastases. Langenbecks Arch Surg 1999;384(3):243–9.
50. Kemeny NE, Gonen M. Hepatic arterial infusion after liver resection. N Engl J Med 2005;352(7):734–5.
51. Kemeny MM, Adak S, Gray B, et al. Combined-modality treatment for resectable metastatic colorectal carcinoma to the liver: surgical resection of hepatic metastases in combination with continuous infusion of chemotherapy–an intergroup study. J Clin Oncol 2002;20(6):1499–505.
52. Kemeny N, Jarnagin W, Gonen M, et al. Phase I/II study of hepatic arterial therapy with floxuridine and dexamethasone in combination with intravenous irinotecan

as adjuvant treatment after resection of hepatic metastases from colorectal cancer. J Clin Oncol 2003;21(17):3303–9.

53. Kemeny N, Capanu M, D'Angelica M, et al. Phase I trial of adjuvant hepatic arterial infusion (HAI) with floxuridine (FUDR) and dexamethasone plus systemic oxaliplatin, 5-fluorouracil and leucovorin in patients with resected liver metastases from colorectal cancer. Ann Oncol 2009;20(7):1236–41.

54. Kemeny NE, Jarnagin WR, Capanu M, et al. Randomized phase II trial of adjuvant hepatic arterial infusion and systemic chemotherapy with or without bevacizumab in patients with resected hepatic metastases from colorectal cancer. J Clin Oncol 2011;29(7):884–9.

55. Alberts SR, Roh MS, Mahoney MR, et al. Alternating systemic and hepatic artery infusion therapy for resected liver metastases from colorectal cancer: a North Central Cancer Treatment Group (NCCTG)/National Surgical Adjuvant Breast and Bowel Project (NSABP) phase II intergroup trial, N9945/CI-66. J Clin Oncol 2010;28(5):853–8.

56. Tomlinson J, Jarnagin W, DeMatteo R, et al. Actual 10-year survival after resection of colorectal liver metastases. J Clin Oncol 2007;25:4575–82.

57. Ito H, Are C, Gonen M, et al. Effect of postoperative morbidity on long-term survival after hepatic resection for metastatic colorectal cancer. Ann Surg 2008; 247(6):994–1002.

58. House MG, Kemeny NE, Gonen M, et al. Comparison of adjuvant systemic chemotherapy with or without hepatic arterial infusional chemotherapy after hepatic resection for metastatic colorectal cancer. Ann Surg 2011;254(6):851–6.

59. Goere D, Benhaim L, Bonnet S, et al. Adjuvant chemotherapy after resection of colorectal liver metastases in patients at high risk of hepatic recurrence: a comparative study between hepatic arterial infusion of oxaliplatin and modern systemic chemotherapy. Ann Surg 2013;257(1):114–20.

60. Chang AE, Schneider PD, Sugarbaker PH, et al. A prospective randomized trial of regional versus systemic continuous 5-fluorodeoxyuridine chemotherapy in the treatment of colorectal liver metastases. Ann Surg 1987;206(6):685–93.

61. Kemeny N, Daly J, Reichman B, et al. Intrahepatic or systemic infusion of fluorodeoxyuridine in patients with liver metastases from colorectal carcinoma. A randomized trial. Ann Intern Med 1987;107(4):459–65.

62. Hohn DC, Stagg RJ, Friedman MA, et al. A randomized trial of continuous intravenous versus hepatic intraarterial floxuridine in patients with colorectal cancer metastatic to the liver: the Northern California Oncology Group trial. J Clin Oncol 1989;7(11):1646–54.

63. Wagman LD, Kemeny MM, Leong L, et al. A prospective, randomized evaluation of the treatment of colorectal cancer metastatic to the liver. J Clin Oncol 1990; 8(11):1885–93.

64. Martin JK Jr, O'Connell MJ, Wieand HS, et al. Intra-arterial floxuridine vs systemic fluorouracil for hepatic metastases from colorectal cancer. A randomized trial. Arch Surg 1990;125(8):1022–7.

65. Rougier P, Laplanche A, Huguier M, et al. Hepatic arterial infusion of floxuridine in patients with liver metastases from colorectal carcinoma: long-term results of a prospective randomized trial. J Clin Oncol 1992;10(7):1112–8.

66. Allen-Mersh TG, Earlam S, Fordy C, et al. Quality of life and survival with continuous hepatic-artery floxuridine infusion for colorectal liver metastases. Lancet 1994;344(8932):1255–60.

67. Lorenz M, Muller HH. Randomized, multicenter trial of fluorouracil plus leucovorin administered either via hepatic arterial or intravenous infusion versus

fluorodeoxyuridine administered via hepatic arterial infusion in patients with non-resectable liver metastases from colorectal carcinoma. J Clin Oncol 2000;18(2): 243–54.

68. Kerr DJ, McArdle CS, Ledermann J, et al. Intrahepatic arterial versus intravenous fluorouracil and folinic acid for colorectal cancer liver metastases: a multicentre randomised trial. Lancet 2003;361(9355):368–73.

69. Kemeny NE, Niedzwiecki D, Hollis DR, et al. Hepatic arterial infusion versus systemic therapy for hepatic metastases from colorectal cancer: a randomized trial of efficacy, quality of life, and molecular markers (CALGB 9481). J Clin Oncol 2006;24(9):1395–403.

70. Reappraisal of hepatic arterial infusion in the treatment of nonresectable liver metastases from colorectal cancer. Meta-Analysis Group in Cancer. J Natl Cancer Inst 1996;88(5):252–8.

71. Mocellin S, Pilati P, Lise M, et al. Meta-analysis of hepatic arterial infusion for unresectable liver metastases from colorectal cancer: the end of an era? J Clin Oncol 2007;25(35):5649–54.

72. Kemeny N. The management of resectable and unresectable liver metastases from colorectal cancer. Curr Opin Oncol 2010;22(4):364–73.

73. Allen-Mersh TG, Glover C, Fordy C, et al. Randomized trial of regional plus systemic fluorinated pyrimidine compared with systemic fluorinated pyrimidine in treatment of colorectal liver metastases. Eur J Surg Oncol 2000;26(5):468–73.

74. Kemeny N, Gonen M, Sullivan D, et al. Phase I study of hepatic arterial infusion of floxuridine and dexamethasone with systemic irinotecan for unresectable hepatic metastases from colorectal cancer. J Clin Oncol 2001;19(10):2687–95.

75. Kemeny N, Jarnagin W, Paty P, et al. Phase I trial of systemic oxaliplatin combination chemotherapy with hepatic arterial infusion in patients with unresectable liver metastases from colorectal cancer. J Clin Oncol 2005;23(22):4888–96.

76. Boige V, Malka D, Elias D, et al. Hepatic arterial infusion of oxaliplatin and intravenous LV5FU2 in unresectable liver metastases from colorectal cancer after systemic chemotherapy failure. Ann Surg Oncol 2008;15(1):219–26.

77. Ducreux M, Ychou M, Laplanche A, et al. Hepatic arterial oxaliplatin infusion plus intravenous chemotherapy in colorectal cancer with inoperable hepatic metastases: a trial of the gastrointestinal group of the Federation Nationale des Centres de Lutte Contre le Cancer. J Clin Oncol 2005;23(22):4881–7.

78. Power DG, Kemeny NE. Chemotherapy for the conversion of unresectable colorectal cancer liver metastases to resection. Crit Rev Oncol Hematol 2011;79(3): 251–64.

79. Ammori JB, Kemeny NE, Fong Y, et al. Conversion to complete resection and/or ablation using hepatic artery infusional chemotherapy in patients with unresectable liver metastases from colorectal cancer: a decade of experience at a single institution. Ann Surg Oncol 2013;20(9):2901–7.

80. Goere D, Deshaies I, de Baere T, et al. Prolonged survival of initially unresectable hepatic colorectal cancer patients treated with hepatic arterial infusion of oxaliplatin followed by radical surgery of metastases. Ann Surg 2010;251(4): 686–91.

81. Jarnagin WR, Schwartz LH, Gultekin DH, et al. Regional chemotherapy for unresectable primary liver cancer: results of a phase II clinical trial and assessment of DCE-MRI as a biomarker of survival. Ann Oncol 2009;20(9):1589–95.

82. Kemeny NE, Schwartz L, Gonen M, et al. Treating primary liver cancer with hepatic arterial infusion of floxuridine and dexamethasone: does the addition of systemic bevacizumab improve results? Oncology 2011;80(3–4):153–9.

83. Konstantinidis IT, Do RK, Gultekin DH, et al. Regional chemotherapy for unresectable intrahepatic cholangiocarcinoma: a potential role for dynamic magnetic resonance imaging as an imaging biomarker and a survival update from two prospective clinical trials. Ann Surg Oncol 2014;21(8):2675–83.
84. Leyvraz S, Spataro V, Bauer J, et al. Treatment of ocular melanoma metastatic to the liver by hepatic arterial chemotherapy. J Clin Oncol 1997;15(7):2589–95.
85. Melichar B, Voboril Z, Lojik M, et al. Liver metastases from uveal melanoma: clinical experience of hepatic arterial infusion of cisplatin, vinblastine and dacarbazine. Hepatogastroenterology 2009;56(93):1157–62.
86. Tsimberidou AM, Moulder S, Fu S, et al. Phase I clinical trial of hepatic arterial infusion of cisplatin in combination with intravenous liposomal doxorubicin in patients with advanced cancer and dominant liver involvement. Cancer Chemother Pharmacol 2010;66(6):1087–93.

Transarterial Chemoembolization for Primary Liver Malignancies and Colorectal Liver Metastasis

CrossMark

John T. Miura, MD[a], T. Clark Gamblin, MD, MS[b],*

KEYWORDS

- Liver • Hepatocellular carcinoma • Intrahepatic cholangiocarcinoma
- Colorectal liver metastasis • Transarterial chemoembolization
- Drug-eluting bead transarterial chemoembolization • Transarterial therapies
- Locoregional therapies

KEY POINTS

- Transarterial chemoembolization is a viable treatment option for unresectable liver tumors or tumors refractory to other therapies.
- Current chemoembolization techniques are being performed with greater safety and efficacy when compared with transarterial therapies performed in the past.
- Chemoembolization remains an acceptable approach for unresectable tumors with preserved liver function.
- Optimal chemoembolization strategies require further prospective studies.

INTRODUCTION

Over the past 2 decades, novel treatment modalities for primary and metastatic liver tumors have been developed. Although surgical resection continues to offer the best chance for long-term survival, up to 70% of patients with hepatic malignancies are deemed unresectable, thereby precluding many from a durable treatment approach. Liver transplantation remains an additional curative treatment; however, the scarcity of available organs continues to be the primary limitation of this modality. Instead, most patients rely on alternative therapies, often considered palliative, which attempt to maintain similar tenets to surgery: improve quality of life

Disclosures: none.
[a] Division of Surgical Oncology, Medical College of Wisconsin, 9200 West Wisconsin Avenue, Milwaukee, WI 53226, USA; [b] Division of Surgical Oncology, Department of Surgery, Medical College of Wisconsin, 9200 West Wisconsin Avenue, Milwaukee, WI 53226, USA
* Corresponding author.
E-mail address: tcgamblin@mcw.edu

Surg Oncol Clin N Am 24 (2015) 149–166
http://dx.doi.org/10.1016/j.soc.2014.09.004
1055-3207/15/$ – see front matter © 2015 Elsevier Inc. All rights reserved.

and prolong survival. Taking advantage of the unique dual blood supply of the liver, hepatic artery–based locoregional therapies have emerged as a treatment strategy for liver malignancies. In contrast to the normal liver parenchyma, which is supplied predominantly by the portal venous system, liver tumors are supplied almost exclusively by the hepatic arterial system, which provides the rationale for transarterial therapies.[1,2]

First described in the late 1970s for the treatment of hepatocellular carcinoma (HCC), transarterial therapies continue to evolve and are essential for the management of HCC and other malignancies, which include intrahepatic cholangiocarcinoma (ICC) and colorectal liver metastases (CRLM).[3–5] Although a variety of techniques such as bland embolization (TAE), transarterial chemoinfusion, and yttrium-90 radioembolization also use a transarterial approach, transarterial chemoembolization (TACE) remains the most widely performed and accepted locoregional therapy for inoperable liver malignancies. In this article, current evidence regarding the role of TACE and drug-eluting bead (DEB) TACE for HCC, ICC, and CRLM are examined and summarized.

PRINCIPLES OF TRANSARTERIAL CHEMOEMBOLIZATION

The advantage of TACE therapy rests in its ability to deliver high concentrations of cytotoxic agents to hypervascular liver tumors by selective disruption of feeding arteries and to minimize damage to the surrounding liver parenchyma.[6,7] Combining chemotherapeutic drugs with embolic material results in a synergistic treatment effect; ischemic tumor necrosis and extended exposure of the tumor to the chemotherapeutic agent are the major treatment-related benefits of this approach. Moreover, the use of the embolizing agents facilitates lower systemic drug levels, thereby reducing toxicity.

Patient Selection

General indications for transarterial therapy for hepatic malignancies continue to evolve. Standard assessment of patients being considered for TACE generally involve evaluation of liver function, severity of portal hypertension, hepatic arterial anatomy, tumor size and distribution, comorbidities, and functional status. Although generally contraindicated in the setting of portal vein thrombosis, limited TACE therapy can be performed in the presence of hepatopetal flow via collateral vessels.[8,9] Among the different hepatic malignancies, established guidelines currently exist for HCC. According to the American Association for Study of Liver Diseases (AASLD), TACE is recommended as a first line noncurative therapy for patients with large or multinodular tumors without vascular invasion, absence of extrahepatic disease, compensated liver disease (Child-Pugh A/B), and overall good performance status (Eastern Cooperative Oncology Group [ECOG] Performance Status 0).[10] Although not in formal guidelines, additional variables described as contraindications to TACE have included age greater than 70/80 years, bilirubin levels greater than 3 mg/dL, tumor size 10 cm or larger, bile duct occlusion or incompetent papilla secondary to surgical manipulation, and greater than 50% replacement of the liver by tumor.[11–14] Technical contraindications include untreatable arteriovenous fistula.[11] TACE therapy necessitates prerequisites for the treatment of other unresectable liver malignancies similar to those indications for HCC. However, TACE has also been applied as a treatment adjunct in other clinical settings. Additional uses for TACE have included preoperative neoadjuvant therapy, tumor downstaging for potential resection/liver transplantation, and as salvage therapy for chemorefractory tumors.[15]

Transarterial Chemoembolization

TACE remains the most widely performed transarterial therapy. Traditionally performed under moderate sedation, the procedure consists of selectively delivering via catheter injection a mix of a chemotherapeutic agent and embolic material to the tumor arterial supply (**Fig. 1**). A variety of cytotoxic agents have been used. However, doxorubicin, cisplatin, epirubicin, mitoxantrone, mitomycin, and SMANCS (styrene maleic acid neocarzinostatin) remain the most common single agents for TACE.[16] A triple-agent TACE regimen consisting of cisplatin, doxorubicin, and mitomycin C has also been described.[17]

Delivery of the cytotoxic agent(s) to the tumor is aided by the use of Lipiodol (iodized oil, Guerbet, France) an oily contrast medium, which serves as a vehicle to carry and localize the drug inside the tumor.[18] This procedure is generally followed by mechanical embolization by either spherical or nonspherical embolic agents. Although temporary, Gelfoam particles are the most commonly used embolizing agent. Other materials used to achieve arterial obstruction include polyvinyl alcohol (PVA), starch microspheres, trisacryl gelatin, or metallic coils.[16] Successful embolization is usually defined as stasis in either the second-order or third-order lobar hepatic artery branches.[19]

Drug-Eluting Bead Transarterial Chemoembolization

Similar to conventional TACE therapies, DEB TACE is an alternative technique that consists of highly absorbent PVA microspheres that have been modified with sulfonate groups, enabling active sequestering of cytotoxic compounds in their salt form when mixed together. After transarterial embolization (TAE), the DEB release the cytotoxic agent in a controlled fashion over several days. The most common cytotoxic agents used with the DEB platform include doxorubicin, oxaliplatin, and irinotecan. With DEB-TACE, studies[20] have reported more favorable pharmacokinetics along with reduced systemic toxicity when compared with traditional TACE.

Assessment of Response to Therapy

Although the primary end point of cancer research and therapy development is overall survival, time to progression and tumor response continue to serve as important

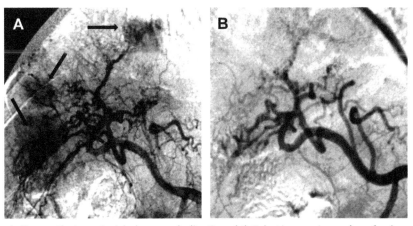

Fig. 1. Transcatheter arterial chemoembolization. (*A*) Selective angiography of a hepatic arterial branch showing 3 hypervascular tumor nodules (*arrows*). (*B*) After delivery of doxorubicin-Lipiodol emulsion and Gelfoam embolization, completion angiogram shows absence of tumor vascularity. (*Courtesy of* D. Geller, MD, Pittsburgh, PA.)

surrogate measures of treatment efficacy.[21] The World Health Organization criteria and Response Evaluation Criteria in Solid Tumors (RECIST) guidelines were originally designed to evaluate tumor response to chemotherapeutic agents.[22,23] These measures were subsequently applied to assess locoregional therapies; however, the results were misleading because of the inability of the guidelines to assess tumor viability beyond anatomic size.[24] In 2008, amendments to the RECIST guidelines, referred to as the modified RECIST assessment (mRECIST), included tumor enhancement on arterial phase during contrast-enhanced radiologic imaging as an additional criterion to assess the extent of tumor response to therapy.[25]

According to the recent guidelines issued by the European Association for the Study of the Liver and the European Organization for Research and Treatment of Cancer, response to therapy should be based on contrast-enhanced radiologic imaging using mRECIST criteria (**Fig. 2**).[26] Furthermore, it is recommended that the initial radiographic assessment after therapy be performed 4 weeks after initial treatment. The direct tumor necrosis caused by TACE and DEB-TACE can be accurately characterized by mRECIST criteria and have been validated by recent studies showing its correlation with survival outcomes.[27,28]

Toxicity/Complications

The overall rate and severity of treatment-related complications are variable for TACE and DEB-TACE therapies. Postembolization syndrome, which consists of transient abdominal pain, nausea, fever, fatigue, and increased hepatic transaminases, occurs most commonly (60%–80% of patients); however, it is not considered a complication but an expected side effect of the procedure.[29] In contrast, major complications occur in up to 10% of patients, with 30-day mortality ranging from 2% to 4% for TACE.[8,30,31] Development of hepatic abscesses and biliary sclerosis is the most common major complication.[32,33] Other complications include liver failure, biloma, ischemic cholecystitits, gastrointestinal hemorrhage/ulceration, vascular injury, and pulmonary embolism, but these are less common (<1%).[31,34]

Although the toxicity profile for DEB-TACE and TACE are similar, drug-related adverse events have been reported less often with DEB-TACE.[35–37] In a recent series by Malagari and colleagues,[36] complications associated with doxorubicin DEB-TACE (DEBDOX) therapy were evaluated in 237 patients. Using the National Cancer Institute Common Terminology Criteria for Adverse Events, grade 4 and 5 complications occurred in 5.48% and 1.26% of the cohort, respectively. Moreover, there were no periprocedural deaths, and the 30-day mortality was only 1.26%. Despite being a

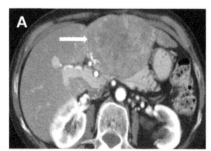
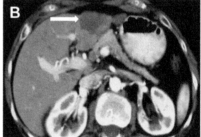

Fig. 2. mRECIST complete response in a patient with HCC treated with TACE. (*A*) Pretreatment contrast-enhanced computed tomography (CT) scan showing a large hypervascular tumor involving segments II/III (*arrow*). (*B*) CT scan at 3 months after TACE shows absence in tumor enhancement and reduction in size (*arrow*). (*Courtesy of* D. Geller, MD, Pittsburgh, PA.)

newer and evolving technology, the safety profile associated with DEB-TACE remains promising.

HEPATOCELLULAR CARCINOMA

Currently the third leading cause of cancer-related mortality worldwide, HCC remains a complex disease, which continues to pose challenges to the medical community.[10,38] Factors leading to the development of HCC are well established (eg, viral hepatitis, alcohol consumption, and metabolic disorders, including nonalcoholic steatohepatitis); however, attempts at identifying early stage disease through the implementation of surveillance programs have resulted in suboptimal results.[39] As a result, curative treatments (surgical resection, transplantation, or image-guided ablation), which are generally limited to early stage disease, are available to only a small percentage of patients with newly diagnosed HCC. Up to 70% of patients present with intermediate or advanced disease (Barcelona Clinic Liver Cancer (BCLC) classification: B and C, respectively), limiting the available treatment options.[40]

Transarterial Chemoembolization for Hepatocellular Carcinoma

TACE therapy is the standard of care for intermediate stage (BCLC-B), multifocal HCC, without vascular invasion, or extrahepatic disease.[10,26] However, initial studies evaluating the role of TACE compared with conservative management resulted in equivocal outcomes (**Table 1**).[41–43] It was not until 2002, when 2 seminal randomized controlled trials (RCTs) were published, that significant improvement in overall survival in patients with HCC treated with TACE was shown. In the study by Llovet and colleagues,[44] 112 patients with unresectable HCC and compensated liver disease (Child-Pugh class A/B) were randomized to receive either doxorubicin-based TACE or conservative management only (symptom management). The investigators reported that patients who received TACE had a significant improvement in survival rates at 1 and 2 years (82% and 63%, respectively) compared with those who underwent conservative treatment (63% and 27%, $P = .009$). Moreover, in multivariate models, treatment allocation was independently associated with survival (odds ratio [OR] 0.45; 95% confidence interval [CI] 0.25–0.81; $P = .02$). Similarly, improved survival after cisplatin-based TACE compared with symptomatic treatment of patients with unresectable HCC was reported by Lo and colleagues.[45] A total of 40 patients underwent TACE and experienced significant improvement in survival at 1 and 2 years (57% and 31%, respectively) compared with the control group (32% and 11%, $P = .002$). Although both studies reported a benefit after TACE, the relative superior survival in the trial by Llovet and colleagues compared with the trial by Lo and colleagues has been attributed to their strict enrollment criteria. Most patients recruited by Llovet and colleagues had compensated liver disease (70% Child-Pugh class A), with an overall good performance status (80% ECOG performance status 0), which likely contributed to the 27% 2-year survival experience by patients in the untreated control group. In contrast, broader enrollment criteria by Lo and colleagues resulted in patients with advanced disease being included in the cohort (57% with ECOG performance status 1/2/3, 27% with limited portal vein involvement). Despite the variable outcomes reported by the 2 studies, these trials were the first to show the potential survival benefit achieved with TACE and were pivotal in how patients with unresectable HCC were treated.

Multiple prospective and retrospective trials[17,46] have since been published that have supported the role of TACE for HCC treatment. In a large retrospective analysis, Brown and colleagues[46] recently reported their experience with TACE over a 15-year

Table 1
Summary of selected series on survival after TACE or DEB-TACE for unresectable HCC

Author, Year	No. of Patients	Study Design	Treatment Regimen	Median Survival (mo)	Overall Survival		
					1 y (%)	2 y (%)	3 y (%)
TACE							
Pelletier et al,[41] 1990	42	RCT	Doxorubicin	NR	24	NR	NR
Trinchet et al,[42] 1995	96	RCT	Cisplatin	NR	62	37.8	NR
Llovet et al,[44] 2002	112	RCT	Doxorubicin	28.7[a]	82	63	29
Lo et al,[45] 2002	80	RCT	Cisplatin	NR	57	31	26
Brown et al,[46] 2008	209	RC	Cisplatin, Doxorubicin, mitomycin C	15.5	NR	NR	NR
Georgiades et al,[17] 2006	172	PC	Cisplatin, doxorubicin, mitomycin C	18.3	NR	NR	NR
Sahara et al,[51] 2012	51	RCT	Epirubicin vs ECMF	21 / 19	85 / 95	76 / 65	NR
DEB-TACE							
Burrel et al,[55] 2012	104	RC	Doxorubicin	48.6	89.9	66.3	54.2
Malagari et al,[56] 2013	45	RC	Doxorubicin	NR	NR	NR	62.2[b]

Abbreviations: 5-FU, 5-fluorouracil; ECMF, epirubicin, cisplatin, mitomycin C; NR, not reported; PC, prospective cohort; RC, retrospective cohort; RCT, randomized controlled trial.
[a] Mean overall survival.
[b] 5-year overall survival.

period. Of the 209 patients included in the study, the investigators reported a median overall survival of 15.5 months. In addition, the efficacy of TACE has been further bolstered by 2 meta-analyses. In 2003, a study by Llovet and Bruix[47] evaluated 14 randomized clinical trials comparing TACE/TAE with either best supportive care or tamoxifen therapy (control). When compared with the control group, TACE/TAE resulted in a significant improvement in 2-year survival (41% vs 27%, OR 0.53; 95% CI 0.32–0.89; $P = .17$). Moreover, sensitivity analysis comparing TACE with best supportive care showed a significant benefit favoring TACE (OR 0.42; 95% CI 0.20–0.88). A second meta-analysis conducted by Marelli and colleagues[16] reported similar results showing a significant decrease in mortality favoring TACE/TAE compared with nonoperative management (OR 0.705; 95% C: 0.499–0.994; $P = .0026$). As a result of these investigations, TACE has become the standard of care for patients with intermediate stage HCC (BCLC-B).

Although TACE has been established in the treatment algorithm for HCC, information regarding the optimal chemotherapeutic agent(s) remains equivocal. Multiple studies have failed to show a significant difference in survival when comparing doxorubicin with either epirubicin or cisplatin.[48–50] In addition, a recent RCT[51] of 63 patients comparing epirubicin versus multiagent (epirubicin, cisplatin, mitomycin C, and 5-fluorouracil) TACE was unable to identify a survival benefit between either regimen. In contrast, a retrospective study evaluating patients with HCC treated with doxorubicin or cisplatin/doxorubicin/mitomycin C (CDM), reported that patients treated with CDM-TACE experienced a higher tumor response rate and longer interval in progression-free survival.[52] As a result, the variability in chemotherapy agent–related outcomes has resulted in a lack of uniform approach regarding the optimal type of cytotoxic therapy for TACE.

Drug-Eluting Bead Transarterial Chemoembolization for Hepatocellular Carcinoma

Compared with TACE, DEB-TACE is an emerging innovation in chemoembolization techniques. In earlier clinical trials, DEB-TACE was shown to maintain a favorable pharmacokinetic profile along with a low peak plasma concentration, which resulted in reduced rates of treatment-related toxicity.[20,53] This finding subsequently led to the execution of the phase 2 randomized control study, PRECISION V, which compared the safety and efficacy of doxorubicin DEB-TACE with conventional TACE.[54] Although the study was unable to show an overall survival difference or objective response between treatment arms in the collective cohort, subgroup analysis of patients with Child-Pugh B, ECOG 1, bilobar disease treated with DEB-TACE experienced a significant increase in objective response rate compared with TACE ($P = .038$). Moreover, the DEB-TACE cohort versus the conventional TACE cohort reported a significant reduction in serious liver toxicity, resulting in improved patient tolerance to treatment ($P<.001$).

Multiple retrospective studies have since been conducted that have supported the role of DEB-TACE for the treatment of HCC. In 2012, Burrel and colleagues[55] evaluated the survival of patients with intermediate stage, unresectable HCC (BCLC-A/B) treated with DEB-TACE. Of the 104 patients treated, median and 5-year overall survival was 48.6 months and 38.3%, respectively, which was double the survival expectancy previously reported. Likewise, a smaller retrospective study conducted by Malagari and colleagues[56] reported a 5-year overall survival of 62.2% among patients with intermediate stage HCC treated with DEB-TACE. Therefore, the improved treatment-related toxicity profile along with similar, or perhaps superior, survival benefit, suggest DEB-TACE as a better approach compared with conventional TACE for HCC treatment.

Combination Strategies

A common challenge faced by all TACE regimens is the durability of treatment. High rates of tumor recurrence or disease progression continue to limit the overall efficacy of TACE.[44,45] The 2002 RCT conducted by Llovet and colleagues reported a sustained objective response of greater than 6 months after TACE in only 35% of their cohort. A potential cause of the high incidence of tumor recurrence that has been proposed relates to the derangement of the tumor microenvironment after TACE. It has been well documented that the hypoxia caused by TACE results in upregulation of inducible factor 1α, which in turn increases expression of vascular endothelial growth factor (VEGF) and platelet-derived growth factor receptor, leading to tumor angiogenesis.[57,58] As a result, there has been recent enthusiasm toward combining antiangiogenic targeted agents with TACE in attempts to improve the overall efficacy of therapeutic strategies.

Sorafenib, a multikinase inhibitor that inhibits angiogenesis by targeting the VEGF receptor 2, has been shown to improve overall survival (10.7 months) compared with placebo for advanced stage HCC.[59] In 2011, the first of several phase 2 trials was published,[60] which sought to evaluate the safety and efficacy of combining DEB-TACE with sorafenib for patients with advanced HCC. Although most patients in the series experienced at least 1 grade 3 to 4 toxicity, most toxicities were minor (grade 1–2, 83% vs grade 3–4, 17%). Moreover, preliminary efficacy data were promising, with a 95% reported disease control rate by RECIST criteria.

Multiple retrospective and phase 2/3 trials combining TACE with sorafenib have since been conducted, with mixed results.[61–64] As a result, a recent meta-analysis was performed by Liu and colleagues,[65] which sought to assess the safety and efficacy of the combination therapy. In total, 17 studies were included in the analysis, of which only 3 were RCTs. The investigators reported that time to progression was improved when TACE was combined with sorafenib (hazard ratio [HR] 0.76; 95% CI 0.66–0.89; $P<.001$) when compared with TACE alone. However, overall survival was not improved with combination therapy (HR 0.81; 95% CI 0.65–1.01; $P = .061$). Although the study was unable to show a survival benefit when sorafenib was combined with TACE, there was a wide variation in both treatment protocol and inclusion criteria among trials, which limited the ability of the study to fully assess the survival benefit of a combined approach. Despite the equivocal results surrounding the current literature regarding combined sorafenib and TACE therapy, well-designed phase 3 studies are ongoing and it is hoped will bring solace to this ongoing debate.[66]

Expanding the Treatment Pool/Future Directions

According to the guidelines by the AASLD, HCC lesions with concomitant portal vein thrombosis are a contraindication to TACE. However, in recent years, attempts to expand the treatment pool have resulted in studies evaluating TACE in the setting of portal thrombus.[9,67] In a single-institution prospective study by Georgiades and colleagues,[9] 32 consecutive patients with unresectable HCC and portal vein thrombus were treated with TACE. The study reported an acceptable safety profile along with survival outcomes superior to historical best supportive care controls. The investigators concluded that in appropriately selected patients, portal thrombus should not be an absolute contraindication for TACE.

Understanding that resection and transplantation offer the best chance for long-term survival, TACE has also been used as a treatment adjunct for these modalities. A prospective study conducted by Luo and colleagues[68] evaluated TACE in a neoadjuvant setting before resection. A total of 168 patients with large (>5 cm) or multinodular resectable HCC tumors received either TACE plus resection or resection alone. Patients who responded to TACE and subsequently underwent resection experienced 1-year, 3-year, and 5-year overall survival rates of 92%, 67%, and 50%, respectively. These results were significantly higher than the survival rates experienced by the resection alone cohort, suggesting that a combined approach is more effective in patients with large, or multifocal, resectable HCC tumors.

In addition, TACE has been used as a technique to downstage tumors to allow for transplantation.[69] A case series in 2008 reported that 23.7% of patients in the study cohort were able to be successfully downstaged by TACE to qualify for liver transplantation under the Milan criteria.[70] At a median follow-up of 19.6 months, 94.1% of patients who underwent successful liver transplantation were alive. The investigators reported that patients successfully downstaged with TACE can achieve similar survival outcomes to American Joint Commission on Cancer stage II patients.

INTRAHEPATIC CHOLANGIOCARCINOMA

Second to HCC as the most common primary liver malignancy, ICC remains a rare, but aggressive malignancy, which carries an overall poor prognosis (median overall survival in untreated patients: 3–8 months).[71] Surgical resection offers the best chance for a cure. However, similar to HCC, most patients when initially diagnosed present at advanced stages (50%–70%), precluding surgery.[72] As a result, alternative pallia-tive approaches have been investigated, which include systemic chemotherapy and external beam radiation, but with reported limited efficacy.[73,74] In recent years, TACE has been proposed as an additional treatment modality for ICC, because of its favorable safety profile and outcomes.[75] Most of the TACE literature has focused primarily on HCC, with only a few series investigating its use for ICC treatment (**Table 2**).

Transarterial Chemoembolization for Intrahepatic Cholangiocarcinoma

In 2005, Burger and colleagues[76] published one of the first series that reported the safety and efficacy of TACE in patients with unresectable ICC. A total of 17 patients were included in the study, of whom all underwent a TACE regimen that consisted of cisplatin, doxorubicin, and mitomycin-C. Compared with historical best supportive care controls, patients who received TACE experienced a significant improvement in median overall survival of 23 months. Furthermore, the procedure was well tolerated by most of the cohort, with preservation of both liver function and performance status in 88% and 82% of the cohort, respectively.

The largest series evaluating the effectiveness of TACE for ICC was conducted by Vogl and colleagues[77] in 2012. The primary aim of the study was to compare the

Table 2
Summary of selected series on survival after TACE or DEB-TACE for unresectable intrahepatic cholangiocarcinoma

Author, Year	No. of Patients	Study Design	Treatment Regimen	Median Survival (mo)	Overall Survival 1 y (%)	2 y (%)	3 y (%)
TACE							
Burger et al,[76] 2005	17	PC	Cis, doxorubicin, mito	23	NR	NR	NR
Gusani et al,[92] 2008	42	PC	Gem, cis, ox, or gem/cis combo	9.1	NR	NR	NR
Kiefer et al,[93] 2011	62	PC	Cis, doxorubicin, mito	15	61	27	8
Park et al,[94] 2011	72	RC	Cis	12.2	51	12	NR
Vogl et al,[77] 2012	115	RC	Mito or gem or mito-cis or gem-cis	13	52	29	10
DEB-TACE							
Aliberti et al,[78] 2008	11	RC	Doxorubicin	13	NR	NR	NR
Poggi et al,[95] 2009	9	RC	Ox DEB-TACE + systemic gem-ox	30	NR	NR	NR
Kuhlman et al,[79] 2012	36	PC	Irinotecan DEB-TACE vs Mito TACE	11.7 5.7	NR	NR	NR

Abbreviations: cis, cisplatin; gem, gemcitabine; mito, mitomycin C; NR, not reported; ox, oxalipla-tin; PC, prospective cohort; RC, retrospective cohort.

efficacy of 4 TACE regimens: (1) mitomycin C only, (2) gemcitabine only, (3) mitomycin C with gemcitabine, (4) mitomycin C, gemcitabine, and cisplatin. Of the 115 patients treated, median survival was 13 months from the start of TACE. Moreover, the investigators reported no statistically significant difference between treatment cohorts. Despite the inability to identify a TACE regiment that resulted in superior outcomes when compared with other agents, current studies have confirmed that TACE is an effective treatment option for unresectable ICC.

Drug-Eluting Bead Transarterial Chemoembolization for Intrahepatic Cholangiocarcinoma

The role of DEB-TACE for ICC was first described by Aliberti and colleagues[78] in 2008. In the study, 11 patients with unresectable ICC were treated with doxorubicin DEB-TACE. The investigators reported a response rate of 100% by RECIST criteria, with a median overall survival of 13 months. DEB-TACE was also shown to be well tolerated in the cohort, with no major complications occurring during the study.

However, comparisons of DEB-TACE with conventional TACE remain limited and with mixed results. A recent prospective single-center study by Kuhlman and colleagues[79] evaluated the efficacy of mitomycin C TACE and irinotecan DEB-TACE and compared the 2 treatments with a historical systemic chemotherapy regimen consisting of gemcitabine and oxaliplatin. Median overall survival was 11.7 months in the DEB-TACE group, 5.7 months for TACE, and 11.7 months in the systemic chemotherapy group. Although the investigators concluded that the outcomes associated with DEB-TACE were favorable and similar to systemic chemotherapy, the heterogeneity in tumor characteristics in the treatment cohorts likely contributed to differences in survival.

Literature on TACE and DEB-TACE for ICC continues to evolve, but current evidence suggests that either therapy results in improved outcomes when compared with best supportive care. Further studies are needed before the true efficacy of these developing techniques can be fully assessed.

METASTATIC COLORECTAL CARCINOMA TO THE LIVER

The liver remains the most common site of CRLM. Current evidence indicates that despite having metastatic disease, resection of isolated CRLM can result in 5-year overall survival rates of 50%.[80] However, only 25% of patients with CRLM are amendable to surgical resection, thereby creating a greater impetus toward the development of other viable treatment options, such as TACE and DEB-TACE.[81]

Transarterial Chemoembolization for Colorectal Liver Metastases

Initial experiences with chemoembolization for CRLM were first described in the early 1990s, with encouraging results.[82,83] However, multiple subsequent studies have since been published with equivocal outcomes (**Table 3**). According to a recent expert consensus statement,[84] current evidence assessing the efficacy of TACE for CRLM remains limited, because of the lack of standardization in treatment protocols between studies.

The largest series that examined the role of TACE for CRLM was conducted by Vogl and colleagues[85] in 2009. The study design was a phase 1/2 trial that examined the efficacy of different TACE drug combinations in the treatment of unresectable CRLM. The local chemotherapy protocol consisted of mitomycin C alone, mitomycin C plus gemcitabine, or mitomycin C plus irinotecan. A total of 463 patients with unresectable CRLM were included in the study and received repeated TACE treatments

Table 3
Summary of selected series on survival after TACE or DEB-TACE for unresectable colorectal liver metastasis

Author, Year	No. of Patients	Study Design	Treatment Regimen	Median Survival (mo)[a]	Overall Survival 1 y (%)	2 y (%)	3 y (%)
TACE							
Lang and Brown,[82] 1993	46	PC	Doxorubicin	NR	65	22	15
Sanz-Altamira et al,[96] 1997	40	PC	5-Fluorouracil, mitomycin C	10	NR	NR	NR
Tellez et al,[97] 1998	30	PC	Cisplatin, doxorubicin, mitomycin C	8.6	20	NR	NR
Hong et al,[98] 2009	21	RC	Cisplatin, doxorubicin, mitomycin C	7.7	43	10	NR
Vogl et al,[85] 2009	463	PC	Mitomycin C; mitomycin C+ gemcitabine; mitomycin C + irinotecan	14	62	28	NR
Albert et al,[86] 2011	121	RC	Cisplatin, doxorubicin, mitomycin C	9	36	13	4
DEB-TACE							
Bower et al,[99] 2010	55	PC	Irinotecan	12	NR	NR	NR
Martin et al,[90] 2011	55	PC	Irinotecan	19	75	NR	NR
Fiorentini et al,[91] 2012	36	RCT	Irinotecan	22	NR	NR	NR
Narayanan et al,[100] 2013	28	RC	Irinotecan	13.3	NR	NR	NR

Abbreviations: NR, not reported; PC, prospective cohort; RC, retrospective cohort.
[a] From first TACE treatment.

over 4-week intervals. Local tumor control was achieved in 62.9% of the cohort (partial response: 14.7%, stable disease: 48.2%). The 1-year and 2-year survival rates were 62% and 28%, respectively, with a median survival of 38 months from the date of liver metastasis diagnosis. Similarly, a retrospective study by Albert and colleagues[86] of 121 patients treated with cisplatin, doxorubicin, mitomycin C–based TACE reported 1-year and 2-year survival rates of 85% and 55%, respectively. Compared with published reports that used systemic chemotherapy regimens of either FOLFOX (5-fluorouracil, leucovorin, and oxaliplatin) or FOLFIRI (folinic acid, fluorouracil, and irinotecan), with reported 1-year and 2-year survival of 55% and 33% respectively, available data evaluating TACE for CRLM highlight its potential efficacy.[87–89]

Drug-Eluting Bead Transarterial Chemoembolization for Colorectal Liver Metastases

Similar to other malignancies, the role of DEB-TACE for CRLM is limited and continues to evolve. Several phase 2 trials have reported favorable safety profiles along with high tumor response rates after DEB-TACE. In a recent prospective study[90] of 55 patients with CRLM who failed systemic chemotherapy and went on to receive irinotecan DEB-TACE, tumor response was achieved in 75% of the cohort. Median overall survival was 19 months, with 75% of the patients alive at 1 year. Although complications occurred in 28% of the patients, most were minor, highlighting the advantage of DEB-TACE therapy.

In a comparative study,[91] and the only phase 3 RCT, 74 patients with unresectable CRLM were randomly assigned to receive irinotecan DEB-TACE versus systemic FOLFIRI. Patients treated with DEB-TACE experienced a significant improvement in overall survival (22 months) when compared with those treated with FOLFIRI (15 months, $P = .031$). Tumor response was also achieved in 68.6% of those treated with DEB-TACE versus only 20% in the FOLFIRI arm. Quality of life was sustained for a longer time interval in the DEB-TACE group compared with those in the FOLFIRI group (8 vs 3 months, $P<.001$). Further prospective studies are needed; however, available evidence suggests DEB-TACE to be an effective therapy and an alternative to standard chemotherapy for patients with unresectable CRLM.

SUMMARY

TACE remains the most widely performed transarterial locoregional therapy for unresectable liver tumors. Advancements in TACE therapies have further improved its safety and efficacy, resulting in the expansion in treatment indications. Although initially used for palliation, TACE has proved to be a viable treatment option. Durability in treatment response continues to be a major limitation of TACE. Therefore, further prospective studies are needed that assess different TACE regimens and combination treatment strategies if improvements in survival and quality of life are to occur.

REFERENCES

1. Breedis C, Young G. The blood supply of neoplasms in the liver. Am J Pathol 1954;30(5):969–77.
2. Lucke B, Breedis C, Woo ZP, et al. Differential growth of metastatic tumors in liver and lung; experiments with rabbit V2 carcinoma. Cancer Res 1952; 12(10):734–8.
3. Tadavarthy SM, Knight L, Ovitt TW, et al. Therapeutic transcatheter arterial embolization. Radiology 1974;112(1):13–6.
4. Yamada R, Nakatsuka H, Nakamura K, et al. Hepatic artery embolization in 32 patients with unresectable hepatoma. Osaka City Med J 1980;26(2):81–96.
5. Wheeler PG, Melia W, Dubbins P, et al. Non-operative arterial embolisation in primary liver tumours. Br Med J 1979;2(6184):242–4.
6. Bruix J, Sala M, Llovet JM. Chemoembolization for hepatocellular carcinoma. Gastroenterology 2004;127(5 Suppl 1):S179–88.
7. Vogl TJ, Naguib NN, Nour-Eldin NE, et al. Review on transarterial chemoembolization in hepatocellular carcinoma: palliative, combined, neoadjuvant, bridging, and symptomatic indications. Eur J Radiol 2009;72(3):505–16.
8. Brown DB, Nikolic B, Covey AM, et al. Quality improvement guidelines for transhepatic arterial chemoembolization, embolization, and chemotherapeutic infusion for hepatic malignancy. J Vasc Interv Radiol 2012;23(3):287–94.
9. Georgiades CS, Hong K, D'Angelo M, et al. Safety and efficacy of transarterial chemoembolization in patients with unresectable hepatocellular carcinoma and portal vein thrombosis. J Vasc Interv Radiol 2005;16(12):1653–9.

10. Bruix J, Sherman M, American Association for the Study of Liver Diseases. Management of hepatocellular carcinoma: an update. Hepatology 2011;53(3): 1020–2.

11. Raoul JL, Sangro B, Forner A, et al. Evolving strategies for the management of intermediate-stage hepatocellular carcinoma: available evidence and expert opinion on the use of transarterial chemoembolization. Cancer Treat Rev 2011;37(3):212–20.

12. Befeler AS. Chemoembolization and bland embolization: a critical appraisal. Clin Liver Dis 2005;9(2):287–300, vii.

13. Kettenbach J, Stadler A, Katzler IV, et al. Drug-loaded microspheres for the treatment of liver cancer: review of current results. Cardiovasc Intervent Radiol 2008;31(3):468–76.

14. Lau WY, Yu SC, Lai EC, et al. Transarterial chemoembolization for hepatocellular carcinoma. J Am Coll Surg 2006;202(1):155–68.

15. Xing M, Kooby DA, El-Rayes BF, et al. Locoregional therapies for metastatic colorectal carcinoma to the liver–an evidence-based review. J Surg Oncol 2014;110(2):182–96.

16. Marelli L, Stigliano R, Triantos C, et al. Transarterial therapy for hepatocellular carcinoma: which technique is more effective? A systematic review of cohort and randomized studies. Cardiovasc Intervent Radiol 2007;30(1):6–25.

17. Georgiades CS, Liapi E, Frangakis C, et al. Prognostic accuracy of 12 liver staging systems in patients with unresectable hepatocellular carcinoma treated with transarterial chemoembolization. J Vasc Interv Radiol 2006;17(10): 1619–24.

18. Nakakuma K, Tashiro S, Hiraoka T, et al. Studies on anticancer treatment with an oily anticancer drug injected into the ligated feeding hepatic artery for liver cancer. Cancer 1983;52(12):2193–200.

19. Lencioni R, Petruzzi P, Crocetti L. Chemoembolization of hepatocellular carcinoma. Semin Intervent Radiol 2013;30(1):3–11.

20. Varela M, Real MI, Burrel M, et al. Chemoembolization of hepatocellular carcinoma with drug eluting beads: efficacy and doxorubicin pharmacokinetics. J Hepatol 2007;46(3):474–81.

21. Lencioni R, Llovet JM. Modified RECIST (mRECIST) assessment for hepatocellular carcinoma. Semin Liver Dis 2010;30(1):52–60.

22. Miller AB, Hoogstraten B, Staquet M, et al. Reporting results of cancer treatment. Cancer 1981;47(1):207–14.

23. Therasse P, Arbuck SG, Eisenhauer EA, et al. New guidelines to evaluate the response to treatment in solid tumors. European Organization for Research and Treatment of Cancer, National Cancer Institute of the United States, National Cancer Institute of Canada. J Natl Cancer Inst 2000;92(3):205–16.

24. Forner A, Ayuso C, Varela M, et al. Evaluation of tumor response after locoregional therapies in hepatocellular carcinoma: are response evaluation criteria in solid tumors reliable? Cancer 2009;115(3):616–23.

25. Llovet JM, Di Bisceglie AM, Bruix J, et al. Design and endpoints of clinical trials in hepatocellular carcinoma. J Natl Cancer Inst 2008;100(10):698–711.

26. European Association for the Study of The Liver, European Organisation for Research and Treatment of Cancer. EASL-EORTC clinical practice guidelines: management of hepatocellular carcinoma. J Hepatol 2012;56(4):908–43.

27. Gillmore R, Stuart S, Kirkwood A, et al. EASL and mRECIST responses are independent prognostic factors for survival in hepatocellular cancer patients treated with transarterial embolization. J Hepatol 2011;55(6):1309–16.

28. Shim JH, Lee HC, Kim SO, et al. Which response criteria best help predict survival of patients with hepatocellular carcinoma following chemoembolization? A validation study of old and new models. Radiology 2012;262(2):708–18.
29. Leung DA, Goin JE, Sickles C, et al. Determinants of postembolization syndrome after hepatic chemoembolization. J Vasc Interv Radiol 2001;12(3):321–6.
30. Sakamoto I, Aso N, Nagaoki K, et al. Complications associated with transcatheter arterial embolization for hepatic tumors. Radiographics 1998;18(3):605–19.
31. Chung JW, Park JH, Han JK, et al. Hepatic tumors: predisposing factors for complications of transcatheter oily chemoembolization. Radiology 1996;198(1): 33–40.
32. Yu JS, Kim KW, Jeong MG, et al. Predisposing factors of bile duct injury after transcatheter arterial chemoembolization (TACE) for hepatic malignancy. Cardiovasc Intervent Radiol 2002;25(4):270–4.
33. Kim HK, Chung YH, Song BC, et al. Ischemic bile duct injury as a serious complication after transarterial chemoembolization in patients with hepatocellular carcinoma. J Clin Gastroenterol 2001;32(5):423–7.
34. Xia J, Ren Z, Ye S, et al. Study of severe and rare complications of transarterial chemoembolization (TACE) for liver cancer. Eur J Radiol 2006;59(3):407–12.
35. Vogl TJ, Lammer J, Lencioni R, et al. Liver, gastrointestinal, and cardiac toxicity in intermediate hepatocellular carcinoma treated with PRECISION TACE with drug-eluting beads: results from the PRECISION V randomized trial. AJR Am J Roentgenol 2011;197(4):W562–70.
36. Malagari K, Pomoni M, Spyridopoulos TN, et al. Safety profile of sequential transcatheter chemoembolization with DC Bead™: results of 237 hepatocellular carcinoma (HCC) patients. Cardiovasc Intervent Radiol 2011;34(4):774–85.
37. Prajapati HJ, Dhanasekaran R, El-Rayes BF, et al. Safety and efficacy of doxorubicin drug-eluting bead transarterial chemoembolization in patients with advanced hepatocellular carcinoma. J Vasc Interv Radiol 2013;24(3):307–15.
38. Ferlay J, Shin HR, Bray F, et al. Estimates of worldwide burden of cancer in 2008: GLOBOCAN 2008. Int J Cancer 2010;127(12):2893–917.
39. Lencioni R. Chemoembolization for hepatocellular carcinoma. Semin Oncol 2012;39(4):503–9.
40. Llovet JM, Burroughs A, Bruix J. Hepatocellular carcinoma. Lancet 2003; 362(9399):1907–17.
41. Pelletier G, Roche A, Ink O, et al. A randomized trial of hepatic arterial chemoembolization in patients with unresectable hepatocellular carcinoma. J Hepatol 1990;11(2):181–4.
42. Trinchet JC, Rached AA, Beaugrand M, et al. A comparison of lipiodol chemoembolization and conservative treatment for unresectable hepatocellular carcinoma. Groupe d'Etude et de Traitement du Carcinome Hépatocellulaire. N Engl J Med 1995;332(19):1256–61.
43. Bruix J, Llovet JM, Castells A, et al. Transarterial embolization versus symptomatic treatment in patients with advanced hepatocellular carcinoma: results of a randomized, controlled trial in a single institution. Hepatology 1998;27(6): 1578–83.
44. Llovet JM, Real MI, Montaña X, et al. Arterial embolisation or chemoembolisation versus symptomatic treatment in patients with unresectable hepatocellular carcinoma: a randomised controlled trial. Lancet 2002;359(9319):1734–9.
45. Lo CM, Ngan H, Tso WK, et al. Randomized controlled trial of transarterial lipiodol chemoembolization for unresectable hepatocellular carcinoma. Hepatology 2002;35(5):1164–71.

46. Brown DB, Chapman WC, Cook RD, et al. Chemoembolization of hepatocellular carcinoma: patient status at presentation and outcome over 15 years at a single center. AJR Am J Roentgenol 2008;190(3):608–15.

47. Llovet JM, Bruix J. Systematic review of randomized trials for unresectable hepatocellular carcinoma: chemoembolization improves survival. Hepatology 2003;37(2):429–42.

48. Kasugai H, Kojima J, Tatsuta M, et al. Treatment of hepatocellular carcinoma by transcatheter arterial embolization combined with intraarterial infusion of a mixture of cisplatin and ethiodized oil. Gastroenterology 1989;97(4):965–71.

49. Kawai S, Tani M, Okamura J, et al. Prospective and randomized trial of lipiodol-transcatheter arterial chemoembolization for treatment of hepatocellular carcinoma: a comparison of epirubicin and doxorubicin (second cooperative study). The Cooperative Study Group for Liver Cancer Treatment of Japan. Semin Oncol 1997;24(2 Suppl 6). S6-38–S6-45.

50. Watanabe S, Nishioka M, Ohta Y, et al. Prospective and randomized controlled study of chemoembolization therapy in patients with advanced hepatocellular carcinoma. Cooperative Study Group for Liver Cancer Treatment in Shikoku area. Cancer Chemother Pharmacol 1994;33(Suppl):S93–6.

51. Sahara S, Kawai N, Sato M, et al. Prospective evaluation of transcatheter arterial chemoembolization (TACE) with multiple anti-cancer drugs (epirubicin, cisplatin, mitomycin c, 5-fluorouracil) compared with TACE with epirubicin for treatment of hepatocellular carcinoma. Cardiovasc Intervent Radiol 2012;35(6):1363–71.

52. Petruzzi NJ, Frangos AJ, Fenkel JM, et al. Single-center comparison of three chemoembolization regimens for hepatocellular carcinoma. J Vasc Interv Radiol 2013;24(2):266–73.

53. Poon RT, Tso WK, Pang RW, et al. A phase I/II trial of chemoembolization for hepatocellular carcinoma using a novel intra-arterial drug-eluting bead. Clin Gastroenterol Hepatol 2007;5(9):1100–8.

54. Lammer J, Malagari K, Vogl T, et al. Prospective randomized study of doxorubicin-eluting-bead embolization in the treatment of hepatocellular carcinoma: results of the PRECISION V study. Cardiovasc Intervent Radiol 2010; 33(1):41–52.

55. Burrel M, Reig M, Forner A, et al. Survival of patients with hepatocellular carcinoma treated by transarterial chemoembolisation (TACE) using drug eluting beads. Implications for clinical practice and trial design. J Hepatol 2012;56(6): 1330–5.

56. Malagari K, Pomoni M, Sotirchos VS, et al. Long term recurrence analysis post drug eluting bead (DEB) chemoembolization for hepatocellular carcinoma (HCC). Hepatogastroenterology 2013;60(126):1413–9.

57. Li X, Feng GS, Zheng CS, et al. Expression of plasma vascular endothelial growth factor in patients with hepatocellular carcinoma and effect of transcatheter arterial chemoembolization therapy on plasma vascular endothelial growth factor level. World J Gastroenterol 2004;10(19):2878–82.

58. Wang B, Xu H, Gao ZQ, et al. Increased expression of vascular endothelial growth factor in hepatocellular carcinoma after transcatheter arterial chemoembolization. Acta Radiol 2008;49(5):523–9.

59. Llovet JM, Ricci S, Mazzaferro V, et al. Sorafenib in advanced hepatocellular carcinoma. N Engl J Med 2008;359(4):378–90.

60. Pawlik TM, Reyes DK, Cosgrove D, et al. Phase II trial of sorafenib combined with concurrent transarterial chemoembolization with drug-eluting beads for hepatocellular carcinoma. J Clin Oncol 2011;29(30):3960–7.

61. Park JW, Koh YH, Kim HB, et al. Phase II study of concurrent transarterial chemoembolization and sorafenib in patients with unresectable hepatocellular carcinoma. J Hepatol 2012;56(6):1336–42.
62. Sansonno D, Lauletta G, Russi S, et al. Transarterial chemoembolization plus sorafenib: a sequential therapeutic scheme for HCV-related intermediate-stage hepatocellular carcinoma: a randomized clinical trial. Oncologist 2012;17(3): 359–66.
63. Kudo M, Imanaka K, Chida N, et al. Phase III study of sorafenib after transarterial chemoembolisation in Japanese and Korean patients with unresectable hepatocellular carcinoma. Eur J Cancer 2011;47(14):2117–27.
64. Zhao Y, Wang WJ, Guan S, et al. Sorafenib combined with transarterial chemoembolization for the treatment of advanced hepatocellular carcinoma: a large-scale multicenter study of 222 patients. Ann Oncol 2013;24(7):1786–92.
65. Liu L, Chen H, Wang M, et al. Combination therapy of sorafenib and TACE for unresectable HCC: a systematic review and meta-analysis. PLoS One 2014; 9(3):e91124.
66. Hoffmann K, Glimm H, Radeleff B, et al. Prospective, randomized, double-blind, multi-center, phase III clinical study on transarterial chemoembolization (TACE) combined with sorafenib versus TACE plus placebo in patients with hepatocellular cancer before liver transplantation - HeiLivCa [ISRCTN24081794]. BMC Cancer 2008;8:349.
67. Chung GE, Lee JH, Kim HY, et al. Transarterial chemoembolization can be safely performed in patients with hepatocellular carcinoma invading the main portal vein and may improve the overall survival. Radiology 2011;258(2): 627–34.
68. Luo J, Peng ZW, Guo RP, et al. Hepatic resection versus transarterial lipiodol chemoembolization as the initial treatment for large, multiple, and resectable hepatocellular carcinomas: a prospective nonrandomized analysis. Radiology 2011;259(1):286–95.
69. Heckman JT, Devera MB, Marsh JW, et al. Bridging locoregional therapy for hepatocellular carcinoma prior to liver transplantation. Ann Surg Oncol 2008; 15(11):3169–77.
70. Chapman WC, Majella Doyle MB, Stuart JE, et al. Outcomes of neoadjuvant transarterial chemoembolization to downstage hepatocellular carcinoma before liver transplantation. Ann Surg 2008;248(4):617–25.
71. Shaib Y, El-Serag HB. The epidemiology of cholangiocarcinoma. Semin Liver Dis 2004;24(2):115–25.
72. Yamamoto M, Ariizumi S. Surgical outcomes of intrahepatic cholangiocarcinoma. Surg Today 2011;41(7):896–902.
73. Ben-Josef E, Normolle D, Ensminger WD, et al. Phase II trial of high-dose conformal radiation therapy with concurrent hepatic artery floxuridine for unresectable intrahepatic malignancies. J Clin Oncol 2005;23(34):8739–47.
74. Valle J, Wasan H, Palmer DH, et al. Cisplatin plus gemcitabine versus gemcitabine for biliary tract cancer. N Engl J Med 2010;362(14):1273–81.
75. Maithel SK, Gamblin TC, Kamel I, et al. Multidisciplinary approaches to intrahepatic cholangiocarcinoma. Cancer 2013;119(22):3929–42.
76. Burger I, Hong K, Schulick R, et al. Transcatheter arterial chemoembolization in unresectable cholangiocarcinoma: initial experience in a single institution. J Vasc Interv Radiol 2005;16(3):353–61.
77. Vogl TJ, Naguib NN, Nour-Eldin NE, et al. Transarterial chemoembolization in the treatment of patients with unresectable cholangiocarcinoma: results and

prognostic factors governing treatment success. Int J Cancer 2012;131(3): 733–40.

78. Aliberti C, Benea G, Tilli M, et al. Chemoembolization (TACE) of unresectable intrahepatic cholangiocarcinoma with slow-release doxorubicin-eluting beads: preliminary results. Cardiovasc Intervent Radiol 2008;31(5):883–8.

79. Kuhlmann JB, Euringer W, Spangenberg HC, et al. Treatment of unresectable cholangiocarcinoma: conventional transarterial chemoembolization compared with drug eluting bead–transarterial chemoembolization and systemic chemotherapy. Eur J Gastroenterol Hepatol 2012;24(4):437–43.

80. Seo SI, Lim SB, Yoon YS, et al. Comparison of recurrence patterns between ≤5 years and >5 years after curative operations in colorectal cancer patients. J Surg Oncol 2013;108(1):9–13.

81. Geoghegan JG, Scheele J. Treatment of colorectal liver metastases. Br J Surg 1999;86(2):158–69.

82. Lang EK, Brown CL. Colorectal metastases to the liver: selective chemoembolization. Radiology 1993;189(2):417–22.

83. Martinelli DJ, Wadler S, Bakal CW, et al. Utility of embolization or chemoembolization as second-line treatment in patients with advanced or recurrent colorectal carcinoma. Cancer 1994;74(6):1706–12.

84. Abdalla EK, Bauer TW, Chun YS, et al. Locoregional surgical and interventional therapies for advanced colorectal cancer liver metastases: expert consensus statements. HPB (Oxford) 2013;15(2):119–30.

85. Vogl TJ, Gruber T, Balzer JO, et al. Repeated transarterial chemoembolization in the treatment of liver metastases of colorectal cancer: prospective study. Radiology 2009;250(1):281–9.

86. Albert M, Kiefer MV, Sun W, et al. Chemoembolization of colorectal liver metastases with cisplatin, doxorubicin, mitomycin C, ethiodol, and polyvinyl alcohol. Cancer 2011;117(2):343–52.

87. Douillard JY, Cunningham D, Roth AD, et al. Irinotecan combined with fluorouracil compared with fluorouracil alone as first-line treatment for metastatic colorectal cancer: a multicentre randomised trial. Lancet 2000;355(9209):1041–7.

88. de Gramont A, Figer A, Seymour M, et al. Leucovorin and fluorouracil with or without oxaliplatin as first-line treatment in advanced colorectal cancer. J Clin Oncol 2000;18(16):2938–47.

89. Saltz LB, Cox JV, Blanke C, et al. Irinotecan plus fluorouracil and leucovorin for metastatic colorectal cancer. Irinotecan Study Group. N Engl J Med 2000; 343(13):905–14.

90. Martin RC, Joshi J, Robbins K, et al. Hepatic intra-arterial injection of drug-eluting bead, irinotecan (DEBIRI) in unresectable colorectal liver metastases refractory to systemic chemotherapy: results of multi-institutional study. Ann Surg Oncol 2011;18(1):192–8.

91. Fiorentini G, Aliberti C, Tilli M, et al. Intra-arterial infusion of irinotecan-loaded drug-eluting beads (DEBIRI) versus intravenous therapy (FOLFIRI) for hepatic metastases from colorectal cancer: final results of a phase III study. Anticancer Res 2012;32(4):1387–95.

92. Gusani NJ, Balaa FK, Steel JL, et al. Treatment of unresectable cholangiocarcinoma with gemcitabine-based transcatheter arterial chemoembolization (TACE): a single-institution experience. J Gastrointest Surg 2008;12(1):129–37.

93. Kiefer MV, Albert M, McNally M, et al. Chemoembolization of intrahepatic cholangiocarcinoma with cisplatinum, doxorubicin, mitomycin C, ethiodol, and polyvinyl alcohol: a 2-center study. Cancer 2011;117(7):1498–505.

94. Park SY, Kim JH, Yoon HJ, et al. Transarterial chemoembolization versus supportive therapy in the palliative treatment of unresectable intrahepatic cholangiocarcinoma. Clin Radiol 2011;66(4):322–8.
95. Poggi G, Amatu A, Montagna B, et al. OEM-TACE: a new therapeutic approach in unresectable intrahepatic cholangiocarcinoma. Cardiovasc Intervent Radiol 2009;32(6):1187–92.
96. Sanz-Altamira PM, Spence LD, Huberman MS, et al. Selective chemoembolization in the management of hepatic metastases in refractory colorectal carcinoma: a phase II trial. Dis Colon Rectum 1997;40(7):770–5.
97. Tellez C, Benson AB, Lyster MT, et al. Phase II trial of chemoembolization for the treatment of metastatic colorectal carcinoma to the liver and review of the literature. Cancer 1998;82(7):1250–9.
98. Hong K, McBride JD, Georgiades CS, et al. Salvage therapy for liver-dominant colorectal metastatic adenocarcinoma: comparison between transcatheter arterial chemoembolization versus yttrium-90 radioembolization. J Vasc Interv Radiol 2009;20(3):360–7.
99. Bower M, Metzger T, Robbins K, et al. Surgical downstaging and neo-adjuvant therapy in metastatic colorectal carcinoma with irinotecan drug-eluting beads: a multi-institutional study. HPB (Oxford) 2010;12(1):31–6.
100. Narayanan G, Barbery K, Suthar R, et al. Transarterial chemoembolization using DEBIRI for treatment of hepatic metastases from colorectal cancer. Anticancer Res 2013;33(5):2077–83.

Y90 Selective Internal Radiation Therapy

Edward W. Lee, MD, PhD[a],*, Avnesh S. Thakor, MD, PhD[b], Bashir A. Tafti, MD[a],
David M. Liu, MD[b]

KEYWORDS

- Y90 • Selective internal radiation therapy • Liver • Malignancy

KEY POINTS

- Multiple prospective phase II, III, and retrospective studies have demonstrated the safety, efficacy, and tolerability of selective internal radiation therapy (SIRT) in hepatocellular cancer (HCC) and colorectal metastasis (CRM).
- SIRT could potentially be used for downsizing of an HCC lesion to allow for definitive therapies, such as liver transplantation or resection.
- SIRT has shown some survival benefit as a treatment option in patients with chemotherapy-refractory metastatic colorectal cancer.
- SIRT has its innate complications, but it seems to be better tolerated by patients than chemoembolization.

INTRODUCTION

Primary liver malignancies and liver metastases are affecting millions of individuals worldwide.[1-3] The definitive management of liver tumors (both primary and secondary) remains a challenge in the unresectable patient population.[4] Established treatment modalities including surgical resection and liver transplantation have been the only curative options offered to patients with any success but are only applicable to roughly 10% of patients.[5-8] Minimally invasive treatments, such as ablation and transarterial chemoembolization (TACE), have traditionally been used in selective patients with early disease or as a palliative option when surgery is not possible. Even when such options are made available, treatment paradigms vary; as a result, techniques, selection, and clinical outcomes (especially in the setting of embolic therapy) have been limited.

The authors have nothing to disclose.
[a] Interventional Radiology, Department of Radiology, UCLA Medical Center, David Geffen School of Medicine, Los Angeles, CA, USA; [b] Interventional Radiology, Department of Radiology, University of British Columbia Medical Center, Vancouver, British Columbia, Canada
* Corresponding author. Division of Interventional Radiology, Department of Radiology, Ronald Reagan Medical Center at UCLA, David Geffen School of Medicine at UCLA, 757 Westwood Plaza, Suite 2125, Los Angeles, CA 90095-743730.
E-mail address: EdwardLee@mednet.ucla.edu

Surg Oncol Clin N Am 24 (2015) 167–185
http://dx.doi.org/10.1016/j.soc.2014.09.011
1055-3207/15/$ – see front matter © 2015 Elsevier Inc. All rights reserved.

Hepatocellular cancer (HCC) is the sixth most common cancer in the world. Risk factors for the development of HCC include viral hepatitis (ie, hepatitis B virus and hepatitis C virus), alcohol abuse, nonalcoholic steatohepatitis, intake of aflatoxin-contaminated food, obesity, diabetes, and hereditary conditions (such as hemochromatosis).

The efficacy of lipiodol-based TACE has been established in early stage HCC[9]; however, this approach remains controversial in advanced-disease patients. Furthermore, no prospective randomized controlled comparative studies have been conducted for the use of TACE in any metastatic condition. Neuroendocrine disease, a condition notorious for variability in presentation and prognosis, represents the largest investigated population (in retrospective or single-arm prospective design trials). Drug-eluting bead has demonstrated early favorable results with the use of irinotecan in the CRM population, with limited prospective trials with moderate response (in varied clinical settings).[10]

The implementation of selective internal radiation therapy (SIRT) in the HCC and CRM setting has demonstrated a more formalized and disciplined approach, with phase III level I data demonstrated in the CRM populations and large, prospective as well as retrospective cohorts in the HCC population demonstrating safety, efficacy, and tolerability.[11–15]

History and Evolution of Radioembolization

Although radiation therapy has proven useful in the treatment of various malignancies, this by large has not been the case with hepatic malignancies. External radiation therapy has not played a major role in the treatment of HCC secondary to the relatively low tolerance of the liver to radiation.[16] The liver is only able to tolerate between 30 and 50 Gy before patients begin experiencing significant radiation-induced liver disease (RILD).[16] However, liver tumors often need radiation doses on the order of 90 to 100 Gy or greater for effective treatment.[16,17] The limitations associated with external beam radiation have been addressed with the development of radioembolization. Radioembolization or SIRT involves selectively injecting radioactive microparticles via a catheter into the hepatic artery branches feeding liver tumors, where the microparticles lodge in the tumor microvasculature.[18] With this technique, radiation doses as high as 150 Gy can be delivered to a localized region in the liver, thereby eliminating cancerous cells while sparing healthy liver and reducing the incidence of RILD.[19,20]

The theory behind radioembolization fundamentally rests on the vascular anatomy of the liver. Hepatic lesions receive most of their blood supply from the hepatic artery, whereas normal liver parenchyma receives most of its blood supply from the portal vein.[17] In addition, hepatic tumors also have neovasculature arising from the branches of the hepatic artery that is denser than that of the normal liver parenchyma.[21] Given this anatomic difference, treatment of liver tumors via a transarterial approach is clearly an attractive idea, as it would limit exposure of extremely cytotoxic medications to normal liver parenchyma.[21] In the past decade, developments have made such mechanisms safer and more efficacious in the treatment of liver disease. TACE is now a widely used treatment option for HCC and metastatic liver cancer with proven results but also with proven significant side effects, namely, hepatic toxicity.[22,23]

The mechanism of action of SIRT is fundamentally different from that of chemoembolization. During chemoembolization, blood vessels supplying the tumor are embolized/blocked to stasis, thus allowing maximum exposure of the chemotherapeutic agent to the ischemic environment created within the tumor. In contrast, blood flow and oxygen is required for SIRT to enable the generation of free radicals, via the ionization of water molecules from the emitted β-radiation. Clinical trials of yttrium-90 microsphere (Y-90) therapy for hepatic tumors date back to the early 1960s.[24] Microspheres are embedded with Yttrium-90, an isotope of yttrium and a pure beta particle emitter.[4] Y-90 has a half-life of 63 hours, a mean energy per disintegration of 0.937 MeV, and emits beta particles, which cause cell necrosis with a mean tissue penetrance of approximately 2.5 mm.[4] These characteristics make Y-90 an excellent isotope choice for internal radiation therapy.[4]

Currently, there are 2 products approved by the Food and Drug Administration (FDA) that are clinically used for radioembolization.[25] TheraSphere particles (BTG Medical, PA; FDA approved for HCC in 1999) are glass microspheres that have a high specific activity and measure 20 to 30 μm in size.[25,26] The term *specific activity* means the amount of radioactivity of Y-90 per a microsphere. Because each glass particle contains roughly 2500 Bq per sphere, only 1 to 2 million spheres (lower volume) are usually needed for each treatment.[19] SIR-Sphere particles (Sirtex, Australia; FDA approved for colorectal liver metastasis in 2002) are made of resin, have a lower specific gravity, and measure 20 to 60 μm in size.[26] Each resin microsphere contains about 50 Bq per sphere; hence, 40 to 60 million spheres are usually needed to treat an average patient. Although TheraSpheres do not have a significant embolic effect on hepatic tumors, SIRSpheres are large enough that they may have a minimal embolic effect.[19,26]

As more microparticles are administered with SIRSphere treatment, the result is in a more even distribution of particles and, hence, delivery of radiation throughout the tumor. In contrast, as TheraSphere particles are administered in lower numbers because of their higher specific activity, this predisposes them to have inhomogeneous tumoral coverage caused by the phenomenon of microclustering (particles preferentially accumulate within the periphery of the tumor). Excessive radiation exposure as a result of particle accumulation has been shown to result in parenchymal fissuring, lobar edema, or compensatory hypertrophy of nontreated liver. As each microparticle has its own dose cloud, radiation-induced treatment of tumors is the result of the collective effect of multiple microparticles that create a cumulative isodose cloud of lethal radiation exposure (via crossfire) in the range of 100 to 1000 Gy.

The amount of activity (ie, ionizing radiation) delivered with each type of microparticle can be estimated using either the body surface area (BSA) or the partition model. SIRT with resin microspheres uses the BSA model, which is supported by a recent study showing direct correlation of BSA with the volume of nontumoral liver as calculated by computed tomography (CT).[27] In contrast, SIRT with glass microspheres uses a compartmental model. Although a single compartment model is currently advocated, whereby the size of the entire liver is used irrespective of the volume of tumor burden, activity calculations previously used a 2-compartmental model incorporating both the tumor and normal background liver volume. The advantage of the latter method is that it allows more accurate optimization of the amount of radiation delivered to tumors. The compartmental model ensures that only the right amount of radiation is given to patients to cause tumor cell death and not excessive radiation placing patients at unnecessary risk of developing RILD. This point is particularly important in those patients with limited background liver reserve.[28,29] The empiric method, which is usually not recommended, incorporates only tumor size based on imaging.[30]

Radioembolization Technique

Generally, patients with a life expectancy of 3 months with unresectable primary or metastatic hepatic tumors and those with tumor burden predominantly involving the liver, which is considered a life-limiting factor, are considered for radioembolization.[31] Patients with metastatic disease not on clinical trials should either be undergoing first-line chemotherapy concurrently or have failed first-line chemotherapy.[31] Contraindications to radioembolization therapy include patients with a significant tumor burden who have a limited amount of normal liver parenchyma that would not tolerate radioembolization.[31] In addition, patients with an elevated serum total bilirubin level greater than 2 mg/dL without a reversible source are not eligible.[31] Unlike chemoembolization, portal vein thrombosis is not contraindicated, as SIRT has a minimal embolic effect.

Before undergoing radioembolization, a laboratory evaluation should be performed to assess the patients' hepatic and renal function and also to establish the baseline tumor markers (eg, alpha fetoprotein for HCC, CA 19-9 for cholangiocarcinoma, and CEA for colorectal cancer) if not already established.[31] Imaging via 3-phase contrast CT scans of the chest, abdomen, and pelvis or gadolinium-enhanced MRI is then performed to identify and characterize the hepatic tumors that will be targeted as well as the extrahepatic tumors throughout the body.[31] Using the same CT or MRI data, a 3-dimensional (3D) volumetric analysis should be done before treatment to calculate the tumor volume, total liver volume, and liver reserve (**Fig. 1**). After determining that a patient's particular tumors and clinical presentation are suitable for radioembolization, patients should undergo hepatic angiography (pre-SIRT mapping procedure) 1 to 3 weeks before the treatment (**Fig. 2**).[31] This part is vital to the pretreatment planning phase allowing for dosimetry calculations to be made before treatment administration.[31] In addition, angiography allows for the mapping of the major hepatic vessels, the superior mesenteric artery, and the celiac artery.[31] If variant anatomy is demonstrated on the angiogram that would allow for nontargeting embolization of gastroduodenal or gastric arteries, these vessels should be embolized or an antireflux catheter system should be used to avoid potential radiation injury to other organs, including radiation-induced pancreatitis or gastric ulcers.[31] In addition to vascular mapping, a hepatopulmonary shunt is assessed using 99mTc macroaggregated albumin (MAA) (**Fig. 3**).[31,32] In this nuclear medicine study, 99mTc-labelled MAA is first injected intra-arterially and then either single-photon emission CT (SPECT) or a planar study of the chest and abdomen are subsequently performed within few hours of the injection.[33] If the scan shows that the lungs and/or gastrointestinal (GI) tract are at risk for radiation exposure greater than 30 Gy, radioembolization is contraindicated given the high risk for extrahepatic toxicity, especially radiation-induced pneumonitis, which could be fatal. It is also possible to limit extrahepatic toxicity by embolizing the observed shunts or performing pre-SIRT TACE. Another 99mTc-labelled MAA scan should be done subsequently to confirm success of the embolization to decrease a shunt.

On the day of SIRT treatment, a hepatic angiogram is again performed to confirm the vascular anatomy and the optimal location of microsphere injection based on the prior mapping. After the confirmation, the vessels feeding the lobe or segment of the liver containing targeted liver tumors are accessed and microspheres are then injected based on product monograph, as each company has a unique injection apparatus and technique. Once the microspheres are injected, patients are transferred to the nuclear medicine department again for additional SPECT or a planar study of the chest and abdomen to confirm the distribution of SIRT microspheres within the desired location (**Fig. 4**). If sequential lobar treatment was planned, the other lobe should be treated about 1 month following the first treatment to give the patients and liver to recover from the treatment.

Following radioembolization, triple-phase CT or liver MRI with contrast agent is often obtained in 1, 3, and 6 months to monitor any changes in the appearance of liver

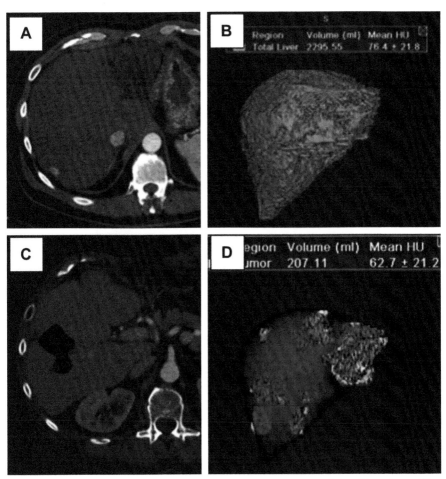

Fig. 1. A pre-SIRT treatment 2-dimensional and 3D volumetric analysis of (*A, B*) total liver volume and (*C, D*) tumor volume using CT images obtained before the treatment. These values are used for SIRT dose calculation.

and liver tumors.[34,35] The most common postprocedure initial imaging finding at 1 month is decreased attenuation or intensity in the treated regions, which represents hepatic edema, congestion, and microinfarction of tissue.[34,35] Of note, early CT findings may not represent the efficacy of the radioembolization procedure because many of these changes are reversible or partially reversible and self-limiting. Therefore, additional follow-up imaging at 3 or 6 months postprocedure is recommended to evaluate tumor response.[34,35] In addition, PET imaging may be beneficial in select patients with hypovascular tumors to track postprocedural changes and can show decreased metabolic activity of treated areas.[36]

OUTCOMES
Hepatocellular Carcinoma

Each year, more than 1.25 million new cases of HCC are diagnosed worldwide, resulting in more than 0.5 million deaths.[6,37] HCC is the sixth most common malignancy worldwide and represents the third most common cause of malignancy-related

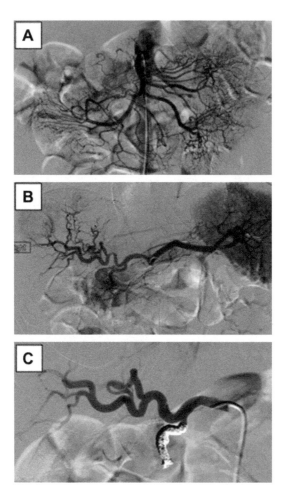

Fig. 2. A pre-SIRT treatment angiogram of (*A*) superior mesenteric artery and (*B*) celiac trunk to delineate the vascular anatomy of liver and liver tumors and to search for anatomic variants, such as replaced right or left hepatic artery. During this angiography, the gastric arteries and gastroduodenal artery are also identified; (*C*) they are prophylactically embolized to prevent any radiation-induced injury to stomach or pancreas.

morbidity.[1,6] Clearly, HCC represents a disease process that is affecting the quality of life of millions of patients worldwide. Despite new advances in medical and surgical therapies, the treatment of HCC has largely remained unsatisfactory.[4] In randomized controlled trials, locoregional therapies have been shown to improve survival in select patients. However, TACE and trans-arterial embolization (TAE) have also been associated with a high risk of inducing liver failure, particularly in patients with portal vein thrombosis that compromises blood flow to the liver and also in patients with multiple, large tumors.[38] In the past decade, extensive research has been conducted to study the effects of SIRT on HCC (**Table 1**). In their landmark study, Salem and colleagues[39] reported a cohort of 291 patients with HCC that were treated with a total of 526 SIRT sessions (mean of 1.8 per patient). The response rate and survival were the 2 principal outcomes evaluated. Response rates after treatment were 42% based on the World Health Organization (WHO) criteria and 57% based on the European Association for

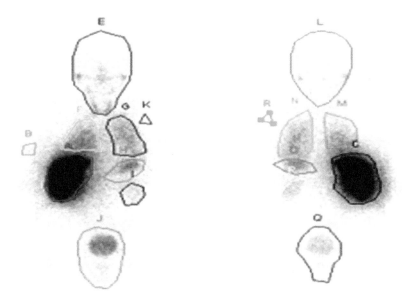

Fig. 3. A planar image of whole body after injection of 99mTc MAA. Region of interest drawn over the lung and liver to determine the lung shunt fraction.

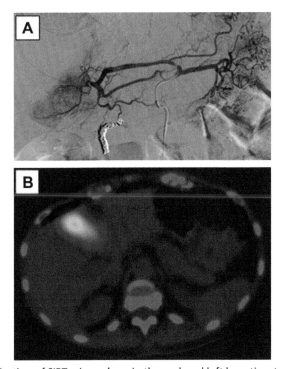

Fig. 4. (*A*) An injection of SIRT microsphere in the replaced left hepatic artery via left gastric artery. A tumor blush is noted in the angiogram, which is detected and correlated with the post-SIRT treatment SPECT CT. (*B*) This post-SIRT SPECT CT can confirm successfully concentrated and distributed SIRT microspheres within the area of treatment.

Table 1
A summary of major studies of SIRT in HCC treatment

Investigator	N	Treatment	Overall Response Rate (%)	Survival
SIRT in first- or second-line treatment of intermediate to advanced HCC				
D'Avola	35	SIRT	NR	**16 mo**
	43	Conventional Tx	NR	8 mo
Salem	291	SIRT	42 (WHO)	**17 mo (child A)**
			57 (EASL)	**8 mo (child B)**
Sangro	325	SIRT	NR	**12.8 mo**
		BCLC A		**24.4 mo**
		BCLC B		**16.9 mo**
		BCLC C		**10.0 mo**
		Child A		**14.9 mo**
		Child B		**10.3 mo**
Inarrairaegui	72	SIRT	**94**	**13 mo**
Lau	18	SIRT (>120 Gy)	**100**	**14 mo**
Chow	35	SIRT then sorafenib	**79**	**11.8 mo**
		BCLC B	**100**	**18.3 mo**
		BCLC C	**68**	**8.8 mo**
Inarrairaegui	25	SIRT in PVT	**67**	**10 mo**
Sangro	183	SIRT in PVT	NR	
		Main PVT		**10.8 mo**
		Branch PVT		**7.4 mo**

Abbreviations: BCLC, Barcelona clinic liver cancer; EASL, European Association for the Study of the Liver; PVT, Portal Vein Thrombosis; WHO, World Health Organization.

the Study of the Liver (EASL) criteria.[39] Patients with Child-Pugh class A disease survived an average of 17.2 months after the procedure, and patients with Child-Pugh class B disease survived an average of 7.7 months.[39] The procedure itself was tolerated well with a 30-day mortality rate of 3%.[39] In Europe, Sangro and Iñarrairaegui[40] studied 325 patients from 8 centers. They reported the overall median survival of 12.8 months in 325 patients (82% Child A, 18% Child B, 24% solitary, and 76% multifocal). Mazzaferro and colleagues[41] studied 52 patients undergoing radioembolization for HCC and found that a complete response was seen in 9.6% of patients, whereas an objective overall response was seen in 40.4% of patients. They also found that the procedure was fairly well tolerated with a 30- to 90-day mortality rate of 0% to 3.8%.[41]

SIRT could potentially be used for downsizing of an HCC lesion to allow for definitive therapies, such as liver transplantation or resection. Iñarrairaegui and colleagues[42] studied 21 patients who initially underwent radioembolization for palliation. However, the procedure ultimately resulted in a response significant enough for 6 patients to undergo definitive therapy. As would be expected, those responding patients demonstrated a drastic overall survival benefit.[42] Similar findings were reported by Vouche and colleagues[43] in 2013 using SIRT as a method for radiation lobectomy in 83 patients.[43] Five patients underwent curative right lobectomy, and 6 patients received liver transplant after SIRT.

Several studies have attempted to compare the effectiveness of SIRT with the conventional TACE in patients with HCC. The largest series by Salem and colleagues[44] studied 245 patients with HCC treated with either chemoembolization (122 patients) or radioembolization (123 patients). The radioembolization group had a response rate of 49%, whereas the chemoembolization group had a response rate of 36%.[44]

Time to progression was also longer for the radioembolization group at 13.3 months compared with 8.4 months for the chemoembolization group, but these differences did not result in a statistically significant difference in median survival time.[44] Lance and colleagues[45] also studied 73 patients with unresectable HCC who underwent radioembolization or chemoembolization and found that there was no statistically significant difference in median survival. However, in both studies by Salem and colleagues[44] and Lance and colleagues,[45] severe symptoms of postembolization syndrome requiring hospitalization were more prominent in the TACE group. These questions of improved quality of life after radioembolization were further investigated. Steel and colleagues[46] studied the health-related quality of life (HRQOL) in patients with HCC who received either hepatic arterial infusion of cisplatin or SIRT. Initially, the radioembolization group scored significantly higher on functional well-being and overall HRQOL.[46] Six months out from treatment, the SIRT group still scored dramatically higher in regard to functional well-being; but the overall HRQOL was not found to be significantly different.[46] Salem and colleagues[47] also studied quality of life in 29 patients undergoing SIRT and 27 patients undergoing TACE for primary HCC. They found that despite having more severe disease, the patients undergoing SIRT demonstrated a greater increase in their quality-of-life scores as compared with the patients undergoing TACE.[47]

Metastatic Tumors of the Liver

Although HCC affects a large number of individuals, the liver is also a very common site for metastatic disease from a variety of primary locations, including colon, neuroendocrine glands, breasts, and kidneys.[14,48–51] This phenomenon can largely be attributed to the fact that the liver has a large dual blood supply from the hepatic artery and the portal vein draining the GI tract.[52]

Colorectal Cancer

Colorectal cancer (CRC) represents the third most common malignancy in the United States and is the second leading cause of malignancy-related deaths,[2] and more than 100,000 new cases of colon cancer and more than 40,000 new cases of rectal cancer are diagnosed annually.[2] In patients with CRC, liver metastasis is seen in roughly 60% of patients because the liver serves as a blood filter between the hepatic venous system, the portal venous tract, and the GI tract.[50] Notably, liver metastases are regarded as the major cause of mortality and morbidity in patients with CRC.[52]

Radioembolization alone and as combined therapy with the conventional first- or second-line chemotherapy has been extensively investigated (**Table 2**). Notably, in a phase I clinical trial, Sharma and colleagues[14] studied 22 patients undergoing SIRT with systemic chemotherapy for unresectable liver metastases from colorectal cancer. Patients received oxaliplatin/fluorouracil (FU)/leucovorin (LV) for the first cycle and then just FU/LV for the second cycle followed by SIRT. Then, the patients received oxaliplatin, leucovorin, and fluorouracil (FOLFOX4) for cycles 4 through 12.[14] Partial response was seen in 18 patients, and stable disease was seen in 2 patients following treatment. The median time to progression was 12.3 months.[14] Kosmider and colleagues[53] further studied the effectiveness of SIRT coupled with systemic chemotherapy. A total of 19 patients were studied with unresectable colorectal liver metastases. Seven patients were given FU and LU in combination with radioembolization, whereas 12 patients received full FOLFOX therapy in combination with radioembolization.[53] The overall response rate for both groups was 84%, with 2 patients achieving a complete response and 14 patients receiving a partial response.[53] Chua and colleagues[54] studied 140 patients with colorectal liver metastases that were

Table 2
A summary of major studies of SIRT in CRC liver metastasis treatment

Investigator	N	Treatment	Overall Response Rate (%)	Survival
SIRT in first-line treatment of CRC liver metastasis				
Phase II/III		*FOLFOX4 alone*	*27–59*	*16.2–20.7 mo*
Gray	74	SIRT + HAC	44	39% (2 y)
		HAC alone	18	29% (2 y)
Van Hazel	21	SIRT + 5-FU/LV	91	29.4 mo
		5-FU/LV alone	0	12.8 mo
Sharma	20	SIRT + FOLFOX4	90	NR
Kosmider	19	SIRT + FOLFOX4 ± 5-FU/LV	84	29.4 mo
				37.8 mo (L)
Tie	31	SIRT + FOLFOX4 ± 5-FU/LV	91	30.7 mo (L)
SIRT in second-line treatment of CRC liver metastasis				
Phase II/III		*Irinotecan*	*4–13*	*6.4–10 mo*
		Irinotecan + cetuximab	*16–27*	*8.6–10.7 mo*
		Panitumumab	*9–14*	*6.3–9.3*
Lim	30	SIRT + 5-FU/LV (70%)	33	NR
Van Hazel	25	SIRT + irinotecan	48	12.2 mo
Cove-Smith	33	SIRT + FOLFIRI or FOLFOX-based chemo	38	17.0 mo
SIRT in salvage therapy for chemorefractory CRC liver metastasis				
Hedlisz	44	SIRT + 5-FU	86	10.0 mo
		5-FU	35	7.3 mo
Seidensticker	29	SIRT	58	8.3 mo
	29	Supportive care	0	3.5 mo
Bester	224	SIRT	NR	11.9 mo
	29	Conventional Tx		6.6 mo
Cosimelli	50	SIRT	48	12.6 mo
Sofocleous	19	SIRT	71	16 mo
Kennedy	606	SIRT	NR	9.6 mo
Coldwell	25	SIRT KRAS wt	NR	NR
		SIRT KRAS mutant	NR	7.0 mo
Leoni	51	SIRT	53	10.5 mo
Cianni	41	SIRT	82	11.8 mo
Jakobs	41	SIRT	78	10.5 mo
Nace	51	SIRT	77	10.2 mo

Abbreviations: FOLFIRI, Leucovorin + 5FU + Irinotecan; HAC, hepatic artery chemoinfusion; KRAS, name of gene; NR, not reported; Tx, treatment; wt, wild-type.

treated with radioembolization therapy and systemic chemotherapy. They found that a complete response was seen in 1% of patients, a partial response in 31%, and stable disease was seen in 31%.[54] Overall, 37% of patients experienced a progression in their disease despite radioembolization.[54] The group found that combining radioembolization with systemic chemotherapy significantly increased the efficacy of the radioembolization compared with historical data.[54]

In addition, SIRT has also been studied as a treatment option in patients with chemotherapy-refractory metastatic CRC. Cosimelli and colleagues[55] conducted a phase II clinical trial investigating the utility of radioembolization in 50 patients who previously failed systemic chemotherapy. Using RECIST (Response Evaluation Criteria In Solid Tumor) criteria, 2% of the patients experienced a complete response, 22% experienced a partial response, and 24% had stable disease.[55] Similar to the combined group noted earlier, 44% of patients were found to have progressive disease on follow-up despite radioembolization therapy.[55] The overall median survival was 12.6 months with a 2-year survival rate of 19.6%.[55] Similarly, Nace and colleagues[56] treated 51 patients with unresectable colorectal liver metastases that also failed both first- and second-line chemotherapy options with SIRT. Using RECIST criteria, 77% of patients experienced either a partial response or stable disease.[56] The overall median survival was 10.2 months after treatment.[56] In a phase III clinical trial, investigators studied 46 patients undergoing SIRT combined with chemotherapy in refractory metastatic CRC to the liver.[11] All 46 patients had previously tried first-line chemotherapy and had not responded appropriately.[11] The patients were randomized to either 5-FU alone or 5-FU combined with radioembolization.[11] Although the time to progression for liver disease was 2.1 months in the 5-FU group and 5.5 months for the group receiving 5-FU with radioembolization, the overall survival rates were not significantly different.[11] Of note, there is no consensus on which assessment criteria are best to accurately evaluate the oncologic outcome of SIRT. However, radiologic response criteria, such as WHO, RECIST, or RECIST with necrosis criteria, have been frequently used. Moreover, Keppke and colleagues (http://www.ncbi.nlm.nih.gov/pubmed/17312067) have suggested that the RECIST with necrosis criteria may provide more accurate assessment of SIRT.

SIRT has also been used as a salvage therapy. In 2011, Bester and colleagues[57] reported the outcomes of 339 patients with chemorefractory metastatic CRC treated with either SIRT or conservative palliative medical treatment. They reported that the patients who underwent SIRT treatment had an overall response rate of 63%. SIRT treatment also doubled the overall median survival to 12 months compared with 6 months in patients receiving conservative medical treatment.[57] These findings were also seen in a study reported by Seidensticker and colleagues.[58] They also reported an overall median survival of 8.3 months in patients treated with SIRT as a salvage treatment compared with a median survival of 3.5 months in the conservative treatment group.[58]

Neuroendocrine

Neuroendocrine tumors are relatively rare, with an incidence roughly between 0.002% and 0.003%.[2,59] They often arise in endocrine glands throughout the human body but are commonly found in the GI tract and lungs.[2,59] In terms of specific types, carcinoid, pancreatic islet cell, paraganglioma, pheochromocytoma, and medullary thyroid cancers are the most common.[59] These tumors often do not present with symptoms for years until the tumor size and/or hormonal hypersecretion leads to noticeable symptoms.[59] Carcinoid tumors can lead to symptoms of excess serotonin, including diarrhea, skin flushing, and bronchospasm, particularly when they metastasize to the liver.[59] In patients with metastatic neuroendocrine tumors, between 50% and 95% will ultimately have liver metastases; of those, 80% will often die within 5 years.[60] In terms of treatment options, surgical resection has been the gold standard with a goal of removing as much of the tumor as possible.[61] However, 90% of patients present with multiple large lesions that make surgical resection not an option.[61] Even with surgical resection, the 5-year survival rate has been reported as being between 60% and 80%.[61] Liver transplantation has also been tried in patients with neuroendocrine tumor liver metastases, with a modest reported 5-year survival rate of 26% to 47%.[62] For unresectable neuroendocrine metastases, proven treatment options have included medical therapies, such as somatostatin analogues; ablative therapies, such as cryotherapy or radiofrequency ablation (RFA); systemic chemotherapy; TAE; and TACE.[63–65]

SIRT has also been shown to play a potential role in the treatment of neuroendocrine metastatic disease to the liver (**Table 3**). In a prospective study by Cao and colleagues,[66] 51 patients with neuroendocrine metastases to the liver were treated with radioembolization. The results showed that 6 patients experienced a complete response, 14 patients experienced a partial response, 14 patients were found to have stable disease, and 17 patients were found to have progressed. The overall median survival was 36 months. Importantly, the 3-year survival rate was 89% at the end of the study.[66] Memon and colleagues[59] achieved similar results when treating 40 patients with neuroendocrine hepatic lesions with radioembolization. The median dose administered was 113 Gy; based on WHO criteria, 1.2% of patients achieved a complete response, whereas 62.7% achieved a partial response.[59] In addition, when using EASL criteria, the complete response rate increased to 20.5%.[59] Paprottka and colleagues[67] studied the effectiveness of SIRT in the treatment of 42 patients with refractory metastatic neuroendocrine hepatic tumors and showed positive results.[67] Three months following SIRT, the partial response rate was 22.5%, the stable disease rate was 75%, and the progressive disease rate was 2.5%. Shaheen and colleagues[68] studied 25 patients with neuroendocrine tumor liver metastasis (NETLM) treated with radioembolization using glass microspheres. They found that using the RECIST criteria, the mean percentage of necrosis following a single radioembolization session was 48%.[68] In addition, they assessed the predictors of responders and nonresponders to SIRT in NETLM. They found that the patients who had prior surgical therapies had a significantly better response to radioembolization.[68] They also found that patients with bilateral hepatic lesions or lesions involving a large percentage of the liver did not respond as favorably to the treatment.[68] In comparing glass versus resin SIRT microspheres, Rhee and colleagues[51] studied 42 patients with NETLM who were treated with radioembolization using either glass or resin microspheres. Ninety-two percent of the glass microsphere group demonstrated either a partial response or stable disease, whereas 94% of the resin microsphere group demonstrated either a partial response or stable disease.[51]

In assessing patients' symptoms caused by hyperactive/hypersecreting neuroendocrine tumors, King and colleagues[69] studied 34 patients with unresectable NETLM that underwent radioembolization. In terms of response rate using the RECIST criteria, 18% of patients demonstrated a complete response and 32% of patients

Table 3
A summary of major studies of SIRT in treatment of NETLM

Investigator	N	Treatment	Overall Response Rate (%)	Survival
SIRT in mixed cohort in chemorefractory NETLM				
Kennedy	148	SIRT	86	70 mo
King	34	SIRT + 5-FU	64.7 (symptomatic relief = 55%)	35 mo
Saxena	48	SIRT + 5-FU	77	35 mo
Cao	58	SIRT + 5-FU	66	36 mo
Rhee	42	SIRT	94	28 mo
Jakobs	25	SIRT	96 (symptomatic relief = 92%)	96% (1 y)
Coldwell	84	SIRT	100 (symptomatic relief = 80%)	NR
Ezziddin	23	SIRT	91 (symptomatic relief = 80%)	29 mo
Paprottka	42	SIRT	97 (symptomatic relief = 95%)	95% (16 mo)

demonstrated a partial response.[69] As for neuroendocrine symptomatic relief, 3 months after the procedure, 55% of patients had symptomatic improvement; 6 months after the procedure, 50% of patients had symptomatic improvement.[69] The previously mentioned study by Memon and colleagues[59] also discussed the effectiveness of SIRT embolization in improving neuroendocrine symptoms. The latter study reported clinically significant symptomatic relief in up to 84% of patients with existing symptoms.

Cholangiocarcinoma

Intrahepatic cholangiocarcinoma (IHCC) is the second most common primary hepatic malignancy.[2] Although the overall incidence is rare, it has been increasing over the past 20 years. IHCC is associated with a high mortality rate, with a median survival of 3 to 8 months.[2,70] Commonly, the patients with IHCC present with advanced disease, which is not amenable to surgical resection or liver transplantation.[70] Given IHCC's relative radiation sensitivity,[71,72] SIRT radiation embolization has been investigated to treat chemorefractory IHCC with promising results.[73,74]

Recently, 2 prospective, nonrandomized studies reported the effectiveness and feasibility of treating intrahepatic cholangiocarcinoma with SIRT.[73,74] In the study of Mouli and colleagues,[74] 46 patients with unresectable IHCC were treated with SIRT. The overall response rate was 98% using the WHO criteria (100% using EASL criteria), with 11% of the patients being downstaged enough to be eligible for liver transplant or resection.[74] Overall, the median survival was 14.6 months. The median survival of patients with peripherally located IHCC was slightly higher at 15.6 months.[74] Similar outcomes were noted by Rafi and colleagues[73] with a 79% overall response rate, with the overall median survival of 15 months in chemorefractory IHCC.

COMPLICATIONS

Although SIRT seems to be effective in the treatment of select liver tumors, there are several complications that have been associated with its use. Postradioembolization syndrome can manifest itself in the subsequent days and weeks following radioembolization therapy. The symptoms usually consist of mild abdominal pain, mild nausea, vomiting, and a low-grade fever.[26] Following SIRT therapy, postradioembolization syndrome has been seen anywhere from 20% to 55% of patients.[26] In a study by Mulcahy and colleagues,[50] fatigue was seen in 61% of patients, nausea in 21% of patients, and abdominal pain in 25% of patients. In addition, given that the radiation emitted from SIRT microspheres also affects normal liver parenchyma and the biliary system, hepatic injury and biliary dysfunction are complications that are often feared.[26] In the study published by Sangro and colleagues,[75] 20% of 25 patients developed complications stemming from hepatic damage, including jaundice and ascites, several weeks after treatment. This unusually high rate of complications is associated with patients treated in a whole-liver fashion. Otherwise, overall, the frequency of RILD after SIRT therapy has been reported as being anywhere from 0% to 4%.[75–77] In terms of biliary complications, Atassi and colleagues[78] found that 33 out of 327 post-SIRT patients had imaging findings consistent with biliary complications. Overall, it seems that the frequency of biliary complications after radioembolization therapy is no more than 10%.[78] Additional GI complications have been documented. Carretero and colleagues[79] found gastric and small bowel injury in 3 patients out of 78. Because this specific injury is anticipated with angiographic control of branches, this was likely the result of unrecognized collateral circulation to the stomach and duodenum.[79] Andrews and colleagues[4] demonstrated reversible gastritis and duodenitis in 4 patients, likely the result of deposition of microspheres near the stomach and duodenum. Another possible complication seen following radioembolization is radiation pneumonitis, which often occurs in patients with elevated shunting of blood flow to the lung on MAA scanning.[80,81] The rate of radiation pneumonitis following SIRT therapy is thought to be well less than 1%.[80,81] Radioembolization is also associated with transient lymphopenia and a 25% or greater decrease in the lymphocyte count in most patients.[82,83] However, this decrease in lymphocyte count has not been shown to lead to opportunistic infections in this patient population.[82,83]

SUMMARY

Radioembolization in select patients with unresectable liver tumors has been shown to be efficacious in decreasing tumor size and prolonging survival. Although relatively new, emerging evidence indicates that radioembolization may be as effective or even more effective in comparison with other available treatments (eg, TAE, TACE, and RFA) for this patient population and improves patients' quality of life. With both primary HCC and hepatic metastatic cancers, SIRT may provide a potential option for patients who are not surgical candidates and can offer the potential for better outcomes and improved survival. In certain patients, SIRT can also serve as a bridge to surgical resection or liver transplantation by downgrading the size and/or number of tumors so that patients who previously were not surgical candidates would now be eligible. Specifically for metastatic CRC tumors, SIRT has shown to be efficacious as an initial option when combined with chemotherapeutic agents, as a secondary option for chemotherapy resistant tumors, and as a palliative option in patients requiring salvage therapy. Lastly, SIRT has also shown favorable outcomes in the treatment of NETLM, particularly in patients who had undergone surgical therapy in the past and those patients with smaller tumors that involved a single lobe of the liver.

These advantages and efficacy of SIRT come with its innate complications as mentioned earlier. However, based on recent evidence, it is certain that SIRT will play a significant role in the treatment of selective patients with unresectable liver tumors in the coming years.

REFERENCES

1. Parkin DM, Bray F, Ferlay J, et al. Global cancer statistics, 2002. CA Cancer J Clin 2005;55:74–108.
2. Siegel R, Naishadham D, Jemal A. Cancer statistics, 2013. CA Cancer J Clin 2013;63:11–30. Available at: http://apps.who.int/bookorders/anglais/detart1.jsp?codlan=1&codcol=76&codcch=31&content=1.
3. Stewart BW, Wild CP. World Cancer Report 2014, vol. 13. World Health Organization; 2014.
4. Andrews JC, Walker SC, Ackermann RJ, et al. Hepatic radioembolization with yttrium-90 containing glass microspheres: preliminary results and clinical follow-up. J Nucl Med 1994;35:1637–44.
5. Bentrem DJ, Dematteo RP, Blumgart LH. Surgical therapy for metastatic disease to the liver. Annu Rev Med 2005;56:139–56.
6. Bosch FX, Ribes J, Borras J. Epidemiology of primary liver cancer. Semin Liver Dis 1999;19:271–85. http://dx.doi.org/10.1055/s-2007-1007117.
7. Chamberlain MN, Gray BN, Heggie JC, et al. Hepatic metastases–a physiological approach to treatment. Br J Surg 1983;70:596–8.

8. Llovet JM, Ricci S, Mazzaferro V, et al. Sorafenib in advanced hepatocellular carcinoma. N Engl J Med 2008;359:378–90. http://dx.doi.org/10.1056/NEJMoa 0708857.

9. Llovet JM, Real MI, Montana X, et al. Arterial embolisation or chemoembolisation versus symptomatic treatment in patients with unresectable hepatocellular carcinoma: a randomised controlled trial. Lancet 2002;359:1734–9. http://dx. doi.org/10.1016/S0140-6736(02)08649-X.

10. Aliberti C, Tilli M, Benea G, et al. Trans-arterial chemoembolization (TACE) of liver metastases from colorectal cancer using irinotecan-eluting beads: preliminary results. Anticancer Res 2006;26:3793–5.

11. Hendlisz A, Van den Eynde M, Peeters M, et al. Phase III trial comparing protracted intravenous fluorouracil infusion alone or with yttrium-90 resin microspheres radioembolization for liver-limited metastatic colorectal cancer refractory to standard chemotherapy. J Clin Oncol 2010;28:3687–94. http://dx.doi.org/10.1200/JCO. 2010.28.5643 JCO.2010.28.5643.

12. Kulik LM, Atassi B, van Holsbeeck L, et al. Yttrium-90 microspheres (TheraSphere) treatment of unresectable hepatocellular carcinoma: downstaging to resection, RFA and bridge to transplantation. J Surg Oncol 2006;94:572–86. http://dx.doi.org/10.1002/jso.20609.

13. Sangro B, Carpanese L, Cianni R, et al. Survival after yttrium-90 resin microsphere radioembolization of hepatocellular carcinoma across Barcelona clinic liver cancer stages: a European evaluation. Hepatology 2011;54:868–78. http://dx.doi.org/10. 1002/hep.24451.

14. Sharma RA, Van Hazel GA, Morgan B, et al. Radioembolization of liver metastases from colorectal cancer using yttrium-90 microspheres with concomitant systemic oxaliplatin, fluorouracil, and leucovorin chemotherapy. J Clin Oncol 2007; 25:1099–106. http://dx.doi.org/10.1200/jco.2006.08.7916.

15. Vouche M, Habib A, Ward TJ, et al. Unresectable solitary hepatocellular carcinoma not amenable to radiofrequency ablation: multicenter radiology-pathology correlation and survival of radiation segmentectomy. Hepatology 2014. http://dx.doi.org/10.1002/hep.27057.

16. Dawson LA, Normolle D, Balter JM, et al. Analysis of radiation-induced liver disease using the Lyman NTCP model. Int J Radiat Oncol Biol Phys 2002;58:1318–9 [author reply: 1319–20].

17. Goin JE, et al. Treatment of unresectable hepatocellular carcinoma with intrahepatic yttrium 90 microspheres: a risk-stratification analysis. J Vasc Interv Radiol 2005;16(2 Pt 1):195–203.

18. Price TJ, Townsend A. Yttrium 90 microsphere selective internal radiation treatment of hepatic colorectal metastases. Arch Surg 2007;143:675–82.

19. Kennedy AS, Nutting C, Coldwell D, et al. Pathologic response and microdosimetry of (90)Y microspheres in man: review of four explanted whole livers. Int J Radiat Oncol Biol Phys 2004;60:1552–63. http://dx.doi.org/10.1016/j.ijrobp. 2004.09.004. pii:S0360-3016(04)02563-5.

20. Yorke ED, Jackson A, Fox RA, et al. Can current models explain the lack of liver complications in Y-90 microsphere therapy? Clin Cancer Res 1999;5: 3024s–30s.

21. Sato KT, Omary Ra, Takehana C, et al. The role of tumor vascularity in predicting survival after yttrium-90 radioembolization for liver metastases. J Vasc Interv Radiol 2009;20:1564–9. http://dx.doi.org/10.1016/j.jvir.2009.08.013.

22. A comparison of lipiodol chemoembolization and conservative treatment for unresectable hepatocellular carcinoma. Groupe d'Etude et de Traitement du

Carcinome Hepatocellulaire. N Engl J Med 1995;332:1256–61. http://dx.doi.org/10.1056/NEJM199505113321903.

23. Peynircioğlu B, Cil B, Bozkurt F, et al. Radioembolization for the treatment of unresectable liver cancer: initial experience at a single center. Diagn Interv Radiol 2010;16:70–8. http://dx.doi.org/10.4261/1305-3825.DIR.2693-09.1.

24. Irving A. Radioactive isotopes for cancer therapy adjuvant. Arch Surg 1964;89:244–9.

25. Vente AD. Microspheres for radioembolization of liver malignancies. Expert Rev Med Devices 2010;7:581–3.

26. Riaz A, Lewandowski RJ, Kulik LM, et al. Complications following radioembolization with yttrium-90 microspheres: a comprehensive literature review. J Vasc Interv Radiol 2009;20:1121–30. http://dx.doi.org/10.1016/j.jvir.2009.05.030 S1051-0443(09)00578-8 [quiz: 1131].

27. Urata K, Kawasaki S, Matsunami H, et al. Calculation of child and adult standard liver volume for liver transplantation. Hepatology 1995;21:1317–21.

28. Ho S, Lau WY, Leung TW, et al. Partition model for estimating radiation doses from yttrium-90 microspheres in treating hepatic tumours. Eur J Nucl Med 1996;23:947–52.

29. Kao YH, Hock Tan AE, Burgmans MC, et al. Image-guided personalized predictive dosimetry by artery-specific SPECT/CT partition modeling for safe and effective 90Y radioembolization. J Nucl Med 2012;53:559–66. http://dx.doi.org/10.2967/jnumed.111.097469.

30. Ackerman NB, Lien WM, Kondi ES, et al. The blood supply of experimental liver metastases. I. The distribution of hepatic artery and portal vein blood to "small" and "large" tumors. Surgery 1969;66:1067–72.

31. Kennedy A, Nag S, Salem R, et al. Recommendations for radioembolization of hepatic malignancies using yttrium-90 microsphere brachytherapy: a consensus panel report from the radioembolization brachytherapy oncology consortium. Int J Radiat Oncol Biol Phys 2007;68:13–23. http://dx.doi.org/10.1016/j.ijrobp.2006.11.060.

32. Ahmadzadehfar H, Sabet A, Biermann K, et al. The significance of 99mTc-MAA SPECT/CT liver perfusion imaging in treatment planning for 90Y-microsphere selective internal radiation treatment. J Nucl Med 2010;51:1206–12. http://dx.doi.org/10.2967/jnumed.109.074559.

33. Lambert B, Mertens J, Sturm EJ, et al. 99mTc-labelled macroaggregated albumin (MAA) scintigraphy for planning treatment with 90Y microspheres. Eur J Nucl Med Mol Imaging 2010;37:2328–33. http://dx.doi.org/10.1007/s00259-010-1566-2.

34. Marn CS, Andrews JC, Francis IR, et al. Hepatic parenchymal changes after intraarterial Y-90 therapy: CT findings. Radiology 1993;187:125–8.

35. Murthy R, Xiong H, Nunez R, et al. Yttrium 90 resin microspheres for the treatment of unresectable colorectal hepatic metastases after failure of multiple chemotherapy regimens: preliminary results. J Vasc Interv Radiol 2005;16:937–45. http://dx.doi.org/10.1097/01.RVI.0000161142.12822.66. pii:16/7/937.

36. Lewandowski R, Thurston KG, Goin J, et al. 90Y microsphere (TheraSphere) treatment for unresectable colorectal cancer metastases of the liver: response to treatment at targeted doses of 135–150 gy as measured by [18F]Fluorodeoxyglucose positron emission tomography and computed tomographic imaging. J Vasc Interv Radiol 2005;16:1641–51.

37. El-Serag HB. Hepatocellular carcinoma and hepatitis C in the United States. Hepatology 2002;36:S74–83. http://dx.doi.org/10.1053/jhep.2002.36807.

38. Sangro B, Bilbao JI, Boan J, et al. Radioembolization using 90Y-resin micro-spheres for patients with advanced hepatocellular carcinoma. Int J Radiat Oncol Biol Phys 2006;66:792–800.
39. Salem R, Lewandowski RJ, Mulcahy MF, et al. Radioembolization for hepatocel-lular carcinoma using Yttrium-90 microspheres: a comprehensive report of long-term outcomes. Gastroenterology 2010;138:52–64. http://dx.doi.org/10.1053/j.gastro.2009.09.006.
40. Sangro B, Iñarrairaegui M. Radioembolization for hepatocellular carcinoma: evidence-based answers to frequently asked questions. J Nucl Med Radiat Ther 2011;01:1–6. http://dx.doi.org/10.4172/2155-9619.1000110.
41. Mazzaferro V, Sposito C, Bhoori S, et al. Yttrium-90 radioembolization for intermediate-advanced hepatocellular carcinoma: a phase 2 study. Hepatology 2013;57:1826–37. http://dx.doi.org/10.1002/hep.26014.
42. Iñarrairaegui M, Pardo F, Bilbao JI, et al. Response to radioembolization with yttrium-90 resin microspheres may allow surgical treatment with curative intent and prolonged survival in previously unresectable hepatocellular carci-noma. Eur J Surg Oncol 2012;38:594–601. http://dx.doi.org/10.1016/j.ejso.2012.02.189.
43. Vouche M, Lewandowski RJ, Atassi R, et al. Radiation lobectomy: time-dependent analysis of future liver remnant volume in unresectable liver cancer as a bridge to resection. J Hepatol 2013. http://dx.doi.org/10.1016/j.jhep.2013.06.015.
44. Salem R, Lewandowski RJ, Kulik L, et al. Radioembolization results in longer time-to-progression and reduced toxicity compared with chemoembolization in pa-tients with hepatocellular carcinoma. Gastroenterology 2011;140:497–507.e492. http://dx.doi.org/10.1053/j.gastro.2010.10.049 S0016-5085(10)01587-8.
45. Lance C, McLennan G, Obuchowski N, et al. Comparative analysis of the safety and efficacy of transcatheter arterial chemoembolization and yttrium-90 radioem-bolization in patients with unresectable hepatocellular carcinoma. J Vasc Interv Radiol 2011;22:1697–705. http://dx.doi.org/10.1016/j.jvir.2011.08.013.
46. Steel J, Baum A, Carr B. Quality of life in patients diagnosed with primary hepa-tocellular carcinoma: hepatic arterial infusion of Cisplatin versus 90-Yttrium mi-crospheres (Therasphere). Psychooncology 2004;13(2):73–9.
47. Salem R, Gilbertsen M, Butt Z, et al. Increased quality of life among hepatocellu-lar carcinoma patients treated with radioembolization, compared with chemoem-bolization. Clin Gastroenterol Hepatol 2013. http://dx.doi.org/10.1016/j.cgh.2013.04.028.
48. Abdelmaksoud MH, Louie JD, Hwang GL, et al. Yttrium-90 radioembolization of renal cell carcinoma metastatic to the liver. J Vasc Interv Radiol 2012;23:323–30.e321. http://dx.doi.org/10.1016/j.jvir.2011.11.007.
49. Jakobs TF, Hoffmann RT, Fischer T, et al. Radioembolization in patients with hepatic metastases from breast cancer. J Vasc Interv Radiol 2008;19:683–90. http://dx.doi.org/10.1016/j.jvir.2008.01.009.
50. Mulcahy MF, Lewandowski RJ, Ibrahim SM, et al. Radioembolization of colorectal hepatic metastases using yttrium-90 microspheres. Cancer 2009;115:1849–58. http://dx.doi.org/10.1002/cncr.24224.
51. Rhee TK, Lewandowski RJ, Liu DM, et al. 90Y Radioembolization for metasta-tic neuroendocrine liver tumors: preliminary results from a multi-institutional experience. Ann Surg 2008;247:1029–35. http://dx.doi.org/10.1097/SLA.0b013e3181728a45.
52. Luna-Perez P, Rodriguez-Coria DF, Arroyo B, et al. The natural history of liver me-tastases from colorectal cancer. Arch Med Res 1998;29:319–24.

53. Kosmider S, Tan TH, Yip D, et al. Radioembolization in combination with systemic chemotherapy as first-line therapy for liver metastases from colorectal cancer. J Vasc Interv Radiol 2011;22:780–6. http://dx.doi.org/10.1016/j.jvir.2011.02.023.

54. Chua TC, Bester L, Saxena A, et al. Radioembolization and systemic chemotherapy improves response and survival for unresectable colorectal liver metastases. J Cancer Res Clin Oncol 2011;137:865–73. http://dx.doi.org/10.1007/s00432-010-0948-y.

55. Cosimelli M, Golfieri R, Cagol PP, et al. Multi-centre phase II clinical trial of yttrium-90 resin microspheres alone in unresectable, chemotherapy refractory colorectal liver metastases. Br J Cancer 2010;103:324–31. http://dx.doi.org/10.1038/sj.bjc.6605770.

56. Nace GW, Steel JL, Amesur N, et al. Yttrium-90 radioembolization for colorectal cancer liver metastases: a single institution experience. Int J Surg Oncol 2011;2011:571261. http://dx.doi.org/10.1155/2011/571261.

57. Bester L, Meteling B, Pocock N, et al. Radioembolization versus standard care of hepatic metastases: comparative retrospective cohort study of survival outcomes and adverse events in salvage patients. J Vasc Interv Radiol 2012;23:96–105. http://dx.doi.org/10.1016/j.jvir.2011.09.028. pii:S1051-0443(11)01344-3.

58. Seidensticker R, Denecke T, Kraus P, et al. Matched-pair comparison of radioembolization plus best supportive care versus best supportive care alone for chemotherapy refractory liver-dominant colorectal metastases. Cardiovasc Intervent Radiol 2012;35:1066–73. http://dx.doi.org/10.1007/s00270-011-0234-7.

59. Memon K, Lewandowski RJ, Mulcahy MF, et al. Radioembolization for neuroendocrine liver metastases: safety, imaging, and long-term outcomes. Int J Radiat Oncol Biol Phys 2012;83:887–94. http://dx.doi.org/10.1016/j.ijrobp.2011.07.041.

60. Kennedy AS, Dezarn WA, McNeillie P, et al. Radioembolization for unresectable neuroendocrine hepatic metastases using resin 90Y-microspheres: early results in 148 patients. Am J Clin Oncol 2008;31:271–9.

61. Norton JA. Endocrine tumours of the gastrointestinal tract. Surgical treatment of neuroendocrine metastases. Best Pract Res Clin Gastroenterol 2005;19:577–83.

62. Florman S, Toure B, Kim L, et al. Liver transplantation for neuroendocrine tumors. J Gastrointest Surg 2004;8:208–12.

63. Berber E, Senagore A, Remzi F, et al. Laparoscopic radiofrequency ablation of liver tumors combined with colorectal procedures. Surg Laparosc Endosc Percutan Tech 2004;14:186–90.

64. Bilchik AJ, Sarantou T, Foshag LJ, et al. Cryosurgical palliation of metastatic neuroendocrine tumors resistant to conventional therapy. Surgery 1997;122:1040–7 [discussion: 1047–8]. pii:S0039-6060(97)90207-5.

65. Nijsen F, Rook D, Brandt C, et al. Targeting of liver tumour in rats by selective delivery of holmium-166 loaded microspheres: a biodistribution study. Eur J Nucl Med 2001;28:743–9.

66. Cao CQ, Yan TD, Bester L, et al. Radioembolization with yttrium microspheres for neuroendocrine tumour liver metastases. Br J Surg 2010;97:537–43. http://dx.doi.org/10.1002/bjs.6931.

67. Paprottka PM, Hoffmann R-T, Haug A, et al. Radioembolization of symptomatic, unresectable neuroendocrine hepatic metastases using yttrium-90 microspheres. Cardiovasc Intervent Radiol 2012;35:334–42. http://dx.doi.org/10.1007/s00270-011-0248-1.

68. Shaheen M, Hassanain M, Aljiffry M, et al. Predictors of response to radioembolization (TheraSphere) treatment of neuroendocrine liver metastasis. HPB (Oxford) 2012;14:60–6. http://dx.doi.org/10.1111/j.1477-2574.2011.00405.x.

69. King J, Quinn R, Glenn DM, et al. Radioembolization with selective internal radiation microspheres for neuroendocrine liver metastases. Cancer 2008;113: 921–9. http://dx.doi.org/10.1002/cncr.23685.

70. Park J, Kim MH, Kim KP, et al. Natural history and prognostic factors of advanced cholangiocarcinoma without surgery, chemotherapy, or radiotherapy: a large-scale observational study. Gut Liver 2009;3:298–305. http://dx.doi.org/10.5009/gnl.2009.3.4.298.

71. Sagawa N, Kondo S, Morikawa T, et al. Effectiveness of radiation therapy after surgery for hilar cholangiocarcinoma. Surg Today 2005;35:548–52. http://dx.doi.org/10.1007/s00595-005-2989-4.

72. Metz JM. The role of radiation therapy in intrahepatic cholangiocarcinoma. Cancer J 2006;12:102–4.

73. Rafi S, Piduru SM, El-Rayes B, et al. Yttrium-90 radioembolization for unresectable standard-chemorefractory intrahepatic cholangiocarcinoma: survival, efficacy, and safety study. Cardiovasc Intervent Radiol 2013;36:440–8. http://dx.doi.org/10.1007/s00270-012-0463-4.

74. Mouli S, Memon K, Baker T, et al. Yttrium-90 radioembolization for intrahepatic cholangiocarcinoma: safety, response, and survival analysis. J Vasc Interv Radiol 2013;24:1227–34. http://dx.doi.org/10.1016/j.jvir.2013.02.031. pii:S1051-0443(13) 00719-7.

75. Sangro B, Gil-Alzugaray B, Rodriguez J, et al. Liver disease induced by radioembolization of liver tumors: description and possible risk factors. Cancer 2008;112: 1538–46. http://dx.doi.org/10.1002/cncr.23339.

76. Kennedy AS, McNeillie P, Dezarn WA, et al. Treatment parameters and outcome in 680 treatments of internal radiation with resin 90Y-microspheres for unresectable hepatic tumors. Int J Radiat Oncol Biol Phys 2009;74:1494–500.

77. Young JY, Rhee TK, Atassi B, et al. Radiation dose limits and liver toxicities resulting from multiple yttrium-90 radioembolization treatments for hepatocellular carcinoma. J Vasc Interv Radiol 2007;18:1375–82. http://dx.doi.org/10.1016/j.jvir.2007.07.016. pii:18/11/1375.

78. Atassi B, Bangash AK, Lewandowski RJ, et al. Biliary sequelae following radioembolization with Yttrium-90 microspheres. J Vasc Interv Radiol 2008;19:691–7. http://dx.doi.org/10.1016/j.jvir.2008.01.003. pii:S1051-0443(08)00092-4.

79. Carretero C, Munoz-Navas M, Betes M, et al. Gastroduodenal injury after radioembolization of hepatic tumors. Am J Gastroenterol 2007;102:1216–20. http://dx.doi.org/10.1111/j.1572-0241.2007.01172.x. pii:AJG1172.

80. Leung TW, Lau WY, Ho SK, et al. Radiation pneumonitis after selective internal radiation treatment with intraarterial 90yttrium-microspheres for inoperable hepatic tumors. Int J Radiat Oncol Biol Phys 1995;40:583–92.

81. Salem R, Parikh P, Atassi B, et al. Incidence of radiation pneumonitis after hepatic intra-arterial radiotherapy with yttrium-90 microspheres assuming uniform lung distribution. Am J Clin Oncol 2008;31:431–8.

82. Carr BI. Hepatic arterial 90Yttrium glass microspheres (Therasphere) for unresectable hepatocellular carcinoma: interim safety and survival data on 65 patients. Liver Transpl 2004;10:S107–10. http://dx.doi.org/10.1002/lt.20036.

83. Salem R, Lewandowski RJ, Atassi B, et al. Treatment of unresectable hepatocellular carcinoma with use of 90Y microspheres (TheraSphere): safety, tumor response, and survival. J Vasc Interv Radiol 2005;16:1627–39.

Systemic Therapy for Hepatocellular Carcinoma and Cholangiocarcinoma

Vincent Chung, MD

KEYWORDS

- Hepatocellular carcinoma • Cholangiocarcinoma • Chemotherapy
- Molecular targets

KEY POINTS

- Hepatocellular carcinoma is the second most deadly cancer in the world.
- Sorafenib is the most active systemic therapy for hepatocellular carcinoma.
- Gemcitabine and cisplatin chemotherapy remains the standard treatment of cholangiocarcinoma.
- Significant progress has been made in understanding the signaling pathways that are important for carcinogenesis, leading to promising clinical trials.

SCOPE OF THE PROBLEM

The development of liver cancer is a growing problem worldwide. In the United States, the incidence rate increased by 4% from 2006 to 2010 and there will be an estimated 33,190 new cases in 2014.[1] Liver cancer can arise from hepatocytes leading to hepatocellular carcinoma or the intrahepatic bile duct leading to cholangiocarcinoma. The management of these patients requires a multidisciplinary team involving surgeons, gastroenterologists, radiologists, and oncologists in order to achieve the best outcome. This article reviews the chemotherapy treatment options.

HEPATOCELLULAR CARCINOMA

Introduction

Worldwide, hepatocellular carcinoma remains a significant problem with more than 745,000 people succumbing to the disease each year. This carcinoma is the second most deadly cancer behind lung cancer, with most cases occurring in east Asia and sub-Saharan Africa. In the United States, approximately 27,000 cases of hepatocellular carcinoma are diagnosed each year and the numbers are expected to increase.[1]

The author has nothing to disclose.
Department of Medical Oncology and Therapeutics Research, City of Hope, 1500 East Duarte Road, Duarte, CA 91010, USA
E-mail address: vchung@coh.org

The geographic variation of the disease is probably caused by the regional variation of exposure to hepatitis. In the Asian countries, hepatitis B is endemic with vertical transmission from parent to child. Aflatoxin, a mycotoxin produced by *Aspergillus flavus* and *Aspergillus parasiticus*, also plays a major role in developing countries. It commonly contaminates stored corn, peanuts, and soybeans in high-humidity areas and hepatocellular carcinoma often develops in younger individuals because of exposure at a young age. In the United States, most cases develop from hepatitis C or alcoholic cirrhosis resulting in cancer at a later age, and nonalcoholic fatty liver disease is a growing problem.[2]

Molecular Biology of Hepatocellular Carcinoma

Understanding the biology of the cancer is essential to help guide treatment. The development of cancer is a multistep process involving mutations of tumor suppressor genes or mutations leading to constitutive activation of signaling pathways. A complete discussion of the pathways is beyond the scope of this article but one of the most important pathways involved in hepatic carcinogenesis is the Ras/Raf/MAPK (mitogen-activated protein kinase) pathway.[3] Binding of epidermal growth factor, platelet-derived growth factor, or vascular endothelial growth factor (VEGF) to cell surface receptors leads to a signaling cascade activated by the Ras family of proteins (**Fig. 1**). Because of its importance in regulating cell proliferation, this pathway represents a potential target for therapy.

SORAFENIB

Sorafenib is a multikinase inhibitor that targets the serine-threonine kinase Raf-1 of the Ras/MAPK pathway in addition to having antiangiogenic properties. In the phase 1 clinical trial of sorafenib, 1 patient had an objective response by RECIST (Response

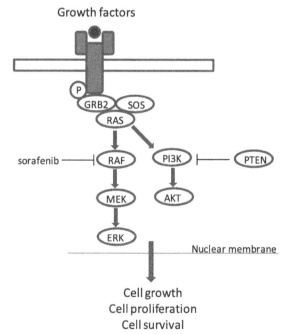

Fig. 1. RAS/RAF/MAPK signaling pathway. PI3K, phosphatidylinositol 3 kinase.

Evaluation Criteria In Solid Tumors) criteria. A follow-up phase 2 study of 137 patients with untreated hepatocellular carcinoma and Child-Pugh A or B cirrhosis were treated with sorafenib. The median overall survival of 9.2 months was encouraging compared with the historical survival of 6 months with traditional cytotoxic chemotherapy. This finding led to the international phase 3 SHARP (Sorafenib Hepatocellular Carcinoma Assessment Randomized Protocol) trial in which 602 patients with advanced hepatocellular carcinoma (defined as not eligible for or had disease progression after surgical or locoregional therapies) and preserved liver function were randomized to either sorafenib 400 mg twice per day or placebo. The trial was conducted in Europe, North America, South America, and Australia. Approximately 20% of the patients had hepatitis B, 30% hepatitis C, and 25% alcoholic cirrhosis. The primary end points were overall survival and time to symptomatic progression. This trial limited patients to Child-Pugh A cirrhosis because patients with advanced liver disease have shorter survival. The results of the SHARP trial showed a statistically significant improvement in overall survival from 7.9 months to 10.7 months in the sorafenib group. Even though the SHARP trial was not designed to assess the efficacy of sorafenib for different subgroups, analysis of the patients with hepatitis C–associated hepatocellular carcinoma showed a superior outcome of 14 months' overall survival with sorafenib compared with 7.9 months' survival with placebo. Another parallel trial was conducted called the Asia-Pacific trial. This study randomized 226 patients from China, South Korea, and Taiwan with Child-Pugh A cirrhosis and hepatocellular carcinoma to either sorafenib or placebo. Patients treated with sorafenib had a statistically significant survival benefit of 6.5 months compared with 4.2 months; however, this was much shorter than the 10.7 months observed in the SHARP trial. This difference may be caused by most of the patients in the Asia-Pacific trial having hepatitis B. The SHARP trial had a larger percentage of patients with hepatitis C. The hepatitis C core protein activating Raf-1 signaling may have conferred more sensitivity to sorafenib, a Raf-1 kinase inhibitor. On November 16, 2007, the US Food and Drug Administration (FDA) approved sorafenib for the treatment of patients with unresectable hepatocellular carcinoma.[4]

Management of Sorafenib Toxicities

Diarrhea

In the SHARP trial, the incidence of treatment-related adverse events was 80% in the sorafenib group compared with 52% in the placebo group but the discontinuation rate was similar between the two groups. Gastrointestinal toxicities were the most common side effect, with most patients experiencing diarrhea. One proposed mechanism of tyrosine kinase inhibitor–induced diarrhea was pancreatic insufficiency. In a small study, fecal fat was measured and found to be increased, supporting the pancreatic exocrine deficiency hypothesis. The malabsorption of fats led to rapid transit times, vitamin D deficiency, and secondary hyperparathyroidism. Patients observed that fatty meals exacerbated the frequency of stools and, in this subset of patients, the use of pancreatic enzymes was helpful in decreasing the frequency of bowel movements.[5] However, most patients can be managed with antimotility drugs such as loperamide, which slows transit by decreasing the tone of the longitudinal smooth muscles, allowing a longer time for water to be absorbed.

Hand-Foot Syndrome

Another common side effect of sorafenib is hand-foot skin reaction and rash, which can be disabling enough to stop therapy. This side effect typically presents as dry skin and a macular/papular rash. Erythema of the palms and soles can develop and serious cases can lead to blisters and desquamation. Early skin care is essential to maintain patients on therapy, otherwise chemotherapy holidays or dose reductions are required. Patients initiating sorafenib should begin frequent application of moisturizing lotions, especially to the hands and feet. Urea-based creams work well and prevent the skin cracking, which can lead to infections. Harsh chemicals such as household cleaning products that irritate the skin need to be discontinued and wearing shoes that minimize friction is helpful. **Table 1** provides dosing guidelines for sorafenib depending on the grade of toxicity. Most patients are able to tolerate sorafenib following these guidelines. Holding therapy or reducing the dose should prevent patients from having to discontinue therapy. In the SHARP trial, 11% of the patients discontinued therapy because of an adverse event.

Hypertension

Hypertension is a common problem with sorafenib treatment and is considered a pharmacodynamic effect of therapy because of the inhibition of VEGF. Decreased nitric oxide production leads to increased vascular tone soon after starting therapy. This increase is usually reversible but permanent endothelial damage may occur and hypertension can persist despite stopping therapy. Occurrences are usually early in the course of therapy and most patients can be managed with standard antihypertensive therapy. All patients initiating treatment should be monitored on a weekly basis for the first 6 weeks. For systolic blood pressure greater than 140 mm Hg and diastolic

Table 1
Management of hand-foot syndrome

Skin Toxicity Grade	Occurrence	Suggested Dose Modification
Grade 1: numbness, dysesthesia, paresthesia, tingling, painless swelling, erythema, or discomfort of the hands or feet which does not disrupt the patient's normal activities	Any occurrence	Continue treatment with sorafenib and consider topical therapy for symptomatic relief
Grade 2: painful erythema and swelling of the hands or feet and/or discomfort affecting the patient's normal activities	First occurrence	Continue treatment with sorafenib and consider topical therapy for symptomatic relief. If no improvement within 7 d, see below
	No improvement within 7 d or second or third occurrence	Interrupt sorafenib treatment until toxicity resolves to grade 0–1 When resuming treatment, decrease sorafenib dose by 1 dose level (400 mg daily or 400 mg every other day)
	Fourth occurrence	Discontinue sorafenib treatment
Grade 3: moist desquamation, ulceration, blistering or severe pain of the hands or feet, or severe discomfort that causes the patient to be unable to work or perform activities of daily living	First or second occurrence	Interrupt sorafenib treatment until toxicity resolves to grade 0–1. When resuming treatment, decrease sorafenib dose by 1 dose level (400 mg daily or 400 mg every other day)
	Third occurrence	Discontinue sorafenib treatment

(*Data from* Nexavar® (sorafenib) [package insert]. West Haven, CT: Bayer Healthcare; 2005.)

blood pressure greater than 90 mm Hg, medication should be initiated. Persistent hypertension despite medical management necessitates holding therapy or even permanently discontinuing it.[6]

CHALLENGES WITH TREATMENT

The difficulty in treating patients with advanced hepatocellular carcinoma is that they not have cancer but also liver disease. Most patients develop hepatocellular carcinoma in the setting of cirrhosis, and thus their hepatic reserves are limited. The Child-Pugh score was originally developed to predict mortality from surgery but is now used as a prognostic marker that aids in the determination of systemic therapy (**Table 2**). Because of the hepatotoxicity of chemotherapy, treatment potentially leads to more risk than benefit, which should always be taken into consideration when deciding on treatment options.

Ultimately, surgery is the only curative approach but many patients are poor surgical candidates due to impaired liver function. For those patients who have advanced liver disease and hepatocellular carcinoma fitting the highly selective Milan criteria (1 lesion $\leq$ 5 cm or 3 lesions each $\leq$ 3 cm), liver transplant is potentially curative, with more than 75% of patients being cured.[7,8] University of California, San Francisco, has expanded the criteria to allow patients with larger lesions up to 6.5 cm to be eligible for transplant. In their series of patients, survival was similar to patients fitting the Milan criteria. Unfortunately, donor livers are a scarce resource and many patients are left with palliative liver directed therapies or systemic therapy.

Sorafenib is a standard treatment of patients not candidates for surgery or liver-directed therapy and is a category 1 recommendation in the National Comprehensive Cancer Network guidelines for Child-Pugh A patients. For Child-Pugh B patients, this is a category 2A recommendation and, for Child-Pugh C patients, sorafenib is not recommended. Metabolism of sorafenib depends on the cytochrome P-450 system and UDP-glucuronosyltransferase. Note that the pharmacokinetic profile is similar between Child-Pugh A and B patients. In order to learn more about the toxicities of sorafenib, the GIDEON (Global Investigation of Therapeutics Decision in Hepatocellular Carcinoma and of its Treatment with Sorafenib) trial was initiated. This was a noninterventional study to evaluate the safety of sorafenib under real-life conditions, especially for Child-Pugh B patients. More than 3000 patients were enrolled and, as expected, there were more serious drug-related adverse events in the Child-Pugh B patients

Table 2 Child-Pugh classification			
Points	1	2	3
Bilirubin (mg/dL)	<2	2 to 3	>3
Albumin (g/dL)	>3.5	2.8–3.5	<2.8
INR	<1.7	1.7–2.3	>2.3
Encephalopathy	None	Grade 1–2	Grade 3–4
Ascites	Absent	Slight	Moderate
Class A, 5–6 points (1-y survival, 100%; 2-y survival, 85%)			
Class B, 7–9 points (1-y survival, 81%; 2-y survival, 57%)			
Class C, 10–15 points (1-y survival, 45%; 2-y survival, 35%)			

From Child CG, Turcotte JG. Surgery and portal hypertension. In: Child CG, editor. The liver and portal hypertension. Philadelphia: Saunders; 1964. p. 50–64; with permission.

(14.1% vs 8.8%) and the discontinuation rate was higher (40% vs 25%) but the overall safety profile was similar to Child-Pugh A patients. Because worsening of hepatic function occurs in more than 50% of patients treated with sorafenib, there is the potential for more harm in Child-Pugh C patients. These patients have limited survival because of the liver disease alone and the impact of systemic therapy on survival is small. Also, tolerance to systemic therapy in this group of patients is not good and should not be recommended.

FAILURE OF CLINICAL TRIALS

During this time, multiple small-molecule tyrosine kinase inhibitors or monoclonal antibodies to VEGF were being developed but the standard had been set with sorafenib being the first molecularly targeted therapy to show a survival benefit in a phase 3 clinical trial. Drugs such as bevacizumab, sunitinib, and brivanib showed promising activity in smaller phase 2 clinical trials but none of the therapies proved to be better than sorafenib in the phase 3 setting (**Table 3**). This article discusses some of the important molecular pathways and the challenges of conducting clinical trials.

Sunitinib, an oral multikinase inhibitor targeting vascular endothelial growth factor receptor 1 (VEGFR1), VEGFR2, platelet derived growth factor receptor (PDGFR)-alpha/beta, c-kit, Fms-like tyrosine kinase 3, and RET (rearranged during transfection) showed activity in earlier trials but toxicity was limiting. Survival was worse with sunitinib treatment but the non-Asian patients fared particularly poorly compared with those on sorafenib. This finding may be caused by hepatitis B being the most common cause of hepatocellular carcinoma in Asian countries, compared with hepatitis C in Western countries. Infection of tissues with hepatitis C leads to activation of the Raf-1/MEK and extracellular-signal-regulated kinases pathway resulting in cell proliferation. Because sorafenib and not sunitinib inhibits the Raf-1 kinase, sorafenib has a

Table 3		
Pivotal phase 3 clinical trials in hepatocellular carcinoma		
Trial	**n**	**Overall Survival**
Sorafenib vs Placebo		
SHARP[4]	602	10.7 vs 7.9 mo HR = 0.69; P = .00058
Asia-Pacific[11]	226	6.5 vs 4.2 mo HR = 0.68; P = .014
Sorafenib vs Brivanib		
BRISK-FL[10]	1150	9.5 vs 9.9 mo HR = 1.06; P = .31
Sorafenib vs Sunitinib		
SUN[9]	1074	10.2 vs 7.2 mo HR = 1.3; P = .001
Sorafenib vs Linifanib		
LIGHT[12]	1035	9.8 vs 9.1 mo HR = 1.05; P = NS
Sorafenib vs Sorafenib + Erlotinib		
SEARCH[13]	720	8.5 vs 9.5 mo HR = 1.13; P = .91

Abbreviations: HR, hazard ratio; NS, nonsignificant.

comparative advantage in patients with hepatitis C.[9] The phase 3 sorafenib versus sunitinib trial was terminated early because of futility.

Fibroblast growth factor receptor (FGF) has also been found to be an important driver of angiogenesis, and brivanib is a small-molecule inhibitor of VEGF and FGF. The BRISK-FL study randomized patients with advanced unresectable hepatocellular carcinoma to either brivanib or sorafenib and the primary end point was overall survival noninferiority. Even though both agents had similar antitumor activity, the primary end point was not met and brivanib was not as well tolerated as sorafenib. The discontinuation rate because of adverse events was 33% for sorafenib and 43% for brivanib.[10] Many new drugs have been tested with varying degrees of activity but, so far, none have been able to surpass sorafenib.

Hepatocyte growth factor (HGF) plays a central role in angiogenesis and tumorigenesis by regulating cell growth and motility. Binding to the c-met receptor activates a signaling cascade affecting multiple signal transduction pathways. In a normal liver, HGF/c-met promotes hepatocyte proliferation and regeneration but, in hepatocellular carcinoma, there seems to be amplification of c-met leading to activation of the RAS, phosphatidylinositol 3 kinase (PI3K), signal transducers and activators of transcription, wnt, and Notch pathways. Because of the importance of this pathway in cell proliferation and metastasis, many companies have produced small-molecule inhibitors such as cabozantinib, tivantinib, and foretinib. In phase 2 clinical trials of unselected patients, modest activity was seen. In subgroup analysis, positive c-met expression by immunohistochemistry was associated with an improvement in overall survival from 3.8 to 7.2 months ($P = .01$). There is an on-going phase 3 clinical trial randomizing c-met–positive hepatocellular carcinoma to either tivantinib or placebo.

LIVER-DIRECTED THERAPY AND SORAFENIB

Hepatocellular carcinoma receives most of its blood supply from the hepatic artery, making liver-directed therapy an attractive treatment option for patients with localized disease. Selective localization of blood vessels feeding the tumor allows delivery of chemotherapy directly to the tumor while interrupting blood flow. This treatment helps to preserve normal hepatocytes. Previous studies have shown 1-year and 2-year survivals of 82% and 63% respectively with a median overall survival of more than 30 months. Because transarterial chemoembolization (TACE) only helps to slow down the growth of cancer, several trials have been conducted combining TACE with systemic sorafenib. In the Japanese and Korean trial, 458 patients with unresectable hepatocellular carcinoma were randomized to 400 mg twice a day of sorafenib or placebo after 1 or 2 TACE sessions. The primary end point of time to progression was not met in this study, possibly because 73% of the patients required dose reductions, which was much higher than that observed in the SHARP trial. In addition, most patients randomized to the sorafenib arm did not start therapy for at least 2 months. There are on-going studies giving sorafenib at the time of the procedure to try to prevent the increase in VEGF levels that occurs as a result of hypoxia from the TACE. Additional combinations with sorafenib and liver-directed therapy are being tested in clinical trials (**Table 4**).

Cytotoxic Chemotherapy

Doxorubicin has been the most extensively studied chemotherapy in this disease. At doses of 75 mg/m^2 every 3 weeks, tumor shrinkage of at least 25% was reported in 8% of the patients and there was a small survival benefit compared with best supportive care. In the past this has been a standard treatment of unresectable hepatocellular

Table 4
Trials combining sorafenib with liver-directed therapy

Trial	Trial Number
Sorafenib with radiation therapy	NCT00892658
Sorafenib + SBRT	NCT01801163
Sorafenib ± proton beam radiotherapy	NCT01141478
Sorafenib before RFA	NCT00813293
Sorafenib combined with TACE	NCT01556815, NCT00768937
—	NCT00855218, NCT01829035

Abbreviations: RFA, radiofrequency ablation; SBRT, stereotactic body radiation therapy.

carcinoma; however, the toxicities limit its use. In clinical practice, cumulative doses of more than 400 mg/m^2 significantly increase the risk of cardiac damage and cardiomyopathy. Neutropenia also occurs, which can lead to sepsis in the setting of biliary obstruction. Doxorubicin can be used after sorafenib failure and there is an on-going clinical trial randomizing patients to sorafenib with or without doxorubicin (NCT01015833).

5-Fluorouracil has a broad range of activity and can be given in the setting of hepatic dysfunction. Usage is not recommended for bilirubin levels greater than 5 mg/dL but a 50% dose reduction can be given for a bilirubin level less than 5 mg/dL. Because response rates were around 20% and survival was only 4 months,[14] combinations with oxaliplatin were tested to try to increase activity. In an Asian trial, 371 patients were randomized between FOLFOX (5-fluorouracil, leucovorin, oxaliplatin) versus doxorubicin and results showed a trend toward improved survival of 6.4 months compared with 5 months ($P = .07$).[15] Oxaliplatin was previously tested in an organ dysfunction study and standard doses could be given at all levels of liver dysfunction without any alteration of clearance.[16] Given the limited systemic therapies for hepatocellular carcinoma, 5-fluorouracil or FOLFOX is commonly used in the refractory setting. In order to advance the care of patients, consideration should be given to enrolling all patients on clinical trials. Current directions include targeting the c-met and VEGF pathways, as well as immune therapies (**Table 5**).

Table 5
Second-line clinical trials after sorafenib failure

Trial #	Trial	Mechanism of Action
NCT01908426, NCT01737827	Cabozantinib (XL184), INC280	c-met
NCT01774344	Regorafenib	VEGF, Ret, Kit, PDGFR, Raf
NCT01752933	SGI-110	DNA methyltransferase inhibitor
NCT01375569	TRC105	Endoglin (CD105)
NCT01777594	G-202	Thapsigargin prodrug
NCT01628640	Intratumoral Injection of Vesicular Stomatitis Virus Expressing Human Interferon Beta Modified Vaccinia Virus	Oncolytic virus
NCT02089763	Pegylated Recombinant Human Arginase 1	Arginine depletion

CHOLANGIOCARCINOMA
Introduction

Cholangiocarcinomas are rare cancers that arise from the epithelial cells of the liver bile ducts and only account for about 3% of all gastrointestinal malignancies. In the United States, there are about 6600 new cases of intrahepatic cholangiocarcinomas each year, with the incidence increasing.[1] However, most patients are diagnosed with advanced disease and systemic therapy is the treatment of choice.

Cytotoxic Chemotherapy

Gemcitabine is a nucleoside analogue with a broad range of activity in many malignancies. By incorporating into DNA during replication, chain termination and apoptosis results. It also functions as a ribonucleotide reductase inhibitor, preventing the production of the deoxyribonucleotides required for DNA replication. Gemcitabine has a favorable toxicity profile, with bone marrow suppression being the most common side effect. Nausea and vomiting are easily controlled with medications and fatigue is usually mild. As a single agent in biliary cancers the response has been modest, ranging for 7% to 24%. Overall survival ranged from 8 to 13 months in small phase 2 studies. Future studies are based on combinations using gemcitabine as the backbone of therapy.

One trial conducted in Europe combined gemcitabine plus cisplatin chemotherapy (ABC-01). Eighty-six patients were randomized to either gemcitabine 1000 mg/m^2 on days 1, 8, and 15 every 28 days or gemcitabine 1000 mg/m^2 plus cisplatin 25 mg/m^2 on days 1 and 8 every 21 days. The combination arm had a higher incidence of lethargy (28.6% vs 9.1%) but this did not result in increased withdrawal from treatment. There were no complete responses but only partial responses, and rates of stable disease were higher in the combination arm.[17] Because of the promising results, the study was extended into the phase 3 ABC-02 trial, which was powered to determine an improvement in overall survival. A total of 410 patients with locally advanced or metastatic cholangiocarcinoma, gallbladder, or ampullary cancer were randomized between the two arms. The median overall survival was 11.7 months in the gemcitabine and cisplatin arm compared with 8.1 months in the gemcitabine alone arm (hazard ratio, 0.64; 95% confidence interval, 0.52–0.80; P<.001).[18] Based on this large phase 3 clinical trial, gemcitabine and cisplatin became the standard of care and the new backbone for the design of future clinical trials.

5-Fluorouracil has been the mainstay chemotherapy for many gastrointestinal malignancies. As a single agent, there is limited activity in biliary cancers but one phase 2 clinical trial combining gemcitabine 1000 mg/m^2 on days 1 and 8 and capecitabine 650 mg/m^2 twice per day for 14 days had 3 complete responses. A total of 22 of 75 patients responded and the overall survival was 12.7 months.[19] However, there is no head-to-head comparison with gemcitabine and cisplatin chemotherapy.

Oxaliplatin is widely used in gastrointestinal malignancies and tolerability is good except for the neuropathy. Several phase 2 trials have been done combining gemcitabine and oxaliplatin at varying schedules. Gemcitabine has been given on days 1, 8, and 15 with oxaliplatin given on day 1 and 15. The largest trial gave gemcitabine on day 1 at 1000 mg/m^2 and oxaliplatin at 100 mg/m^2 on day 2 every 2 weeks. This international phase 2 trial accrued 70 patients, with 73% having metastatic disease. The objective response rate was 20.5% in nongallbladder cancer and only 4.3% in patients with gallbladder cancer. Thirty-six percent of the patients had stable disease and the median overall survival was 8.8 months.[20] Additional phase 2 clinical trials have shown activity with oxaliplatin chemotherapy but the current standard is still

Table 6
Clinical trials for cholangiocarcinoma

Trial	Mechanism of Action
Cabozantinib (XL184)	c-met
Regorafenib	VEGF, Ret, Kit, PDGFR, Raf
Sunitinib	VEGF
Trametinib	MEK1/2
Pazopanib + GSK1120212	VEGF and MEK1/2
Gem/Cis + panitumumab	EGFR
Gem/Cis + bevacizumab	VEGF

gemcitabine plus cisplatin chemotherapy. Decisions to alter this combination should be based on the toxicity profile of the drug.

Molecular Biology of Cholangiocarcinoma

The epidermal growth factor receptor (EGFR) is important for intracellular downstream signaling leading to cell proliferation, angiogenesis, invasion, and metastasis. There are 4 receptor tyrosine kinases: EGFR (ErbB-1), HER2/c-neu (ErbB-2), Her 3 (ErbB-3), and Her 4 (ErbB-4). Binding of the ligand to the receptor leads to dimerization and subsequent phosphorylation of the receptor tyrosine kinase. Because 50% of cholangiocarcinomas overexpress EGFR, clinical trials with erlotinib were conducted.[21] However, a randomized trial of GEMOX plus or minus erlotinib did not meet its primary end point of improving progression-free survival. There was a higher response rate with erlotinib but further research is needed to identify biomarkers of response.[22] Another pathway currently being studied is c-Met. c-Met is a proto-oncogene that encodes for HGF receptor, which is essential for embryonic development. However, aberrant activation of the receptor leads to tumor growth, angiogenesis, and metastasis.[23,24] A phase 2 study of cabozantinib in patients with advanced cholangiocarcinomas is in progress (**Table 6**).

SUMMARY

Understanding core signaling pathways in hepatic carcinogenesis has brought about a new era in the management of hepatocellular carcinoma. Sorafenib was the first molecular targeted therapy to be approved for advanced hepatocellular carcinoma and is the benchmark for all other therapies. So far, no drugs have been able to surpass sorafenib. For cholangiocarcinoma, cytotoxic chemotherapy remains the mainstay treatment of advanced disease and currently there are no FDA-approved molecular targeted therapies. With the hope of more personalized medicine, clinical trials are being designed to try to match mutations to drugs blocking that pathway. If clinicians are able to minimize the toxicity of therapy by targeting the driving mechanism of cell proliferation, they will be able to significantly improve the survival and quality of life of patients.

REFERENCES

1. American Cancer Society. Cancer facts & figures 2014. Atlanta(GA): American Cancer Society; 2014.

2. White DL, Kanwal F, El-Serag HB. Association between nonalcoholic fatty liver disease and risk for hepatocellular cancer, based on systematic review. Clin Gastroenterol Hepatol 2012;10(12):1342–59.e2.
3. Llovet JM, Bruix J. Molecular targeted therapies in hepatocellular carcinoma. Hepatology 2008;48(4):1312–27.
4. Llovet JM, Ricci S, Mazzaferro V, et al. Sorafenib in advanced hepatocellular carcinoma. N Engl J Med 2008;359(4):378–90.
5. Mir O, Coriat R, Boudou-Rouquette P, et al. Sorafenib-induced diarrhea and hypophosphatemia: mechanisms and therapeutic implications. Ann Oncol 2012; 23(1):280–1.
6. Maitland ML, Kasza KE, Karrison T, et al. Ambulatory monitoring detects sorafenib-induced blood pressure elevations on the first day of treatment. Clin Cancer Res 2009;15(19):6250–7.
7. Mazzaferro V, Bhoori S, Sposito C, et al. Milan criteria in liver transplantation for hepatocellular carcinoma: an evidence-based analysis of 15 years of experience. Liver Transpl 2011;17(Suppl 2):S44–57.
8. Lim KC, Chow PK, Allen JC, et al. Systematic review of outcomes of liver resection for early hepatocellular carcinoma within the Milan criteria. Br J Surg 2012; 99(12):1622–9.
9. Cheng AL, Kang YK, Lin DY, et al. Sunitinib versus sorafenib in advanced hepatocellular cancer: results of a randomized phase III trial. J Clin Oncol 2013;31(32): 4067–75.
10. Johnson PJ, Qin S, Park JW, et al. Brivanib versus sorafenib as first-line therapy in patients with unresectable, advanced hepatocellular carcinoma: results from the randomized phase III BRISK-FL study. J Clin Oncol 2013;31(28):3517–24.
11. Cheng AL, Kang YK, Chen Z, et al. Efficacy and safety of sorafenib in patients in the Asia-Pacific region with advanced hepatocellular carcinoma: a phase III randomised, double-blind, placebo-controlled trial. Lancet Oncol 2009;10(1):25–34.
12. Cainap C, Qin S, Huang W-T, et al. Phase III trial of linifanib versus sorafenib in patients with advanced hepatocellular carcinoma (HCC) [abstract 249]. J Clin Oncol 2013;30(suppl 34).
13. Zhu A, Rosmorduc O, Evans J, et al. Search: a phase III, randomized, double-blind, placebo-controlled trial of sorafenib plus erlotinib in patients with hepatocellular carcinoma (HCC). ESMO, [abstract 917].
14. Tetef M, Doroshow J, Akman S, et al. 5-Fluorouracil and high-dose calcium leucovorin for hepatocellular carcinoma: a phase II trial. Cancer Invest 1995;13(5): 460–3.
15. Qin S, Bai Y, Lim HY, et al. Randomized, multicenter, open-label study of oxaliplatin plus fluorouracil/leucovorin versus doxorubicin as palliative chemotherapy in patients with advanced hepatocellular carcinoma from Asia. J Clin Oncol 2013;31(28):3501–8.
16. Doroshow JH, Synold TW, Gandara D, et al. Pharmacology of oxaliplatin in solid tumor patients with hepatic dysfunction: a preliminary report of the National Cancer Institute Organ Dysfunction Working Group. Semin Oncol 2003;30(4 Suppl 15):14–9.
17. Valle JW, Wasan H, Johnson P, et al. Gemcitabine alone or in combination with cisplatin in patients with advanced or metastatic cholangiocarcinomas or other biliary tract tumours: a multicentre randomised phase II study - The UK ABC-01 Study. Br J Cancer 2009;101(4):621–7.
18. Valle J, Wasan H, Palmer DH, et al. Cisplatin plus gemcitabine versus gemcitabine for biliary tract cancer. N Engl J Med 2010;362(14):1273–81.

19. Knox JJ, Hedley D, Oza A, et al. Combining gemcitabine and capecitabine in patients with advanced biliary cancer: a phase II trial. J Clin Oncol 2005;23(10): 2332–8.
20. Andre T, Reyes-Vidal JM, Fartoux L, et al. Gemcitabine and oxaliplatin in advanced biliary tract carcinoma: a phase II study. Br J Cancer 2008;99(6): 862–7.
21. Philip PA, Mahoney MR, Allmer C, et al. Phase II study of erlotinib in patients with advanced biliary cancer. J Clin Oncol 2006;24(19):3069–74.
22. Lee J, Park SH, Chang HM, et al. Gemcitabine and oxaliplatin with or without erlotinib in advanced biliary-tract cancer: a multicentre, open-label, randomised, phase 3 study. Lancet Oncol 2012;13(2):181–8.
23. Socoteanu MP, Mott F, Alpini G, et al. c-Met targeted therapy of cholangiocarcinoma. World J Gastroenterol 2008;14(19):2990–4.
24. Nakazawa K, Dobashi Y, Suzuki S, et al. Amplification and overexpression of c-erbB-2, epidermal growth factor receptor, and c-met in biliary tract cancers. J Pathol 2005;206(3):356–65.

Integrating Systemic and Surgical Approaches to Treating Metastatic Colorectal Cancer

CrossMark

Kaihong Mi, MD, PhD[a], Matthew F. Kalady, MD[a,b],
Cristiano Quintini, MD[c], Alok A. Khorana, MD[a,*]

KEYWORDS

- Colorectal cancer • Liver metastases • Liver-directed therapy
- Antiangiogenic therapy • Antineoplastic therapy

KEY POINTS

- Median survival has increased substantially in recent years to nearly 30 months in patients with metastatic colorectal cancer treated with contemporary regimens.
- All patients with metastatic disease should undergo evaluation for potential resectability and/or liver-directed therapy, which can significantly improve outcomes and potentially cure a minority of patients.
- Chemotherapy regimens in initial and subsequent settings should be accompanied by a targeted agent, unless specific contraindications exist.
- RAS status should be checked in all patients with metastatic colorectal cancer. Anti–epidermal growth factor receptor antibodies should be only used in patients with "extended" RAS wild-type tumors.

INTRODUCTION

Metastatic colorectal cancer is an important contributor to the public health burden of cancer-related mortality. An estimated 136,830 people in the United States will be diagnosed with colorectal cancer in 2014. Approximately one-fifth of these patients will have distant metastatic disease at the time of presentation.[1] The spread of primary colorectal cancer can occur by lymphatic and hematogenous dissemination, as well as by contiguous and transperitoneal routes. The presence of right upper quadrant

Dr Khorana discloses consulting honoraria from Genentech, Inc.
[a] Taussig Cancer Institute, Department of Hematology and Oncology, Cleveland Clinic, 9500 Euclid Avenue, Cleveland, OH 44195, USA; [b] Digestive Disease Institute, Department of Colorectal Surgery, Cleveland Clinic, 9500 Euclid Avenue, Cleveland, OH 44195, USA; [c] Digestive Disease Institute, HPB and Liver Transplant Program, Cleveland Clinic, 9500 Euclid Avenue, Cleveland, OH 44195, USA
* Corresponding author. 9500 Euclid Avenue, R35, Cleveland, OH 44195.
E-mail address: Khorana@ccf.org

pain, abdominal distension, early satiety, supraclavicular adenopathy, or periumbilical nodules usually signals advanced metastatic disease. However, given extensive staging and surveillance protocols, it is also common to identify metastatic disease based on imaging studies. The first site of hematogenous dissemination is usually the liver, followed by the lungs and bone. An exception is rectal cancer, which may metastasize initially to the lung because the inferior rectal vein drains into the inferior vena cava rather than into the portal venous system.

Although the prognosis for patients with metastatic disease without specific treatment remains limited, multiple new treatment options developed during the past 2 decades are now available for the treatment of metastatic disease. As a result, median survival has increased to nearly 30 months in the latest large randomized study,[2] from approximately 6 months in the 1990s.[3] This improvement in survival has been driven not by a single "magic bullet" but by the sequential deployment of a variety of chemotherapy and so-called targeted therapy agents. This latter class includes monoclonal antibodies to vascular endothelial growth factor (VEGF) (bevacizumab) and epidermal growth factor receptor (EGFR) (cetuximab and panitumumab), aflibercept, a recombinant fusion protein also directed against VEGF, and regorafenib, an active inhibitor of multiple tyrosine kinases. Finally, a small but substantial minority of patients with isolated sites of metastases may potentially be curable with surgery and liver-directed therapies.

The availability of multiple therapeutic agents for the treatment of metastatic colorectal cancer therefore requires a strategic approach to maximize patient benefit, in terms of both life expectancy and quality of life. When determining initial treatment, the first step is to evaluate whether the patient is potentially curable by a surgical resection of metastases either at the time of diagnosis or after conversion therapy. This approach will guide the choice and timing of chemotherapy. Treatments with the potential highest response rates and the greatest potential to downsize metastasis are the most appropriate for potentially curable patients. If the patient does not seem curable, treatment regimens that offer the longest progression-free survival (PFS) and overall survival (OS) and that maintain quality of life as long as possible are to be preferred. This review focuses on describing systemic approaches to the treatment of patients with metastatic colorectal cancer, with notes on the incorporation of liver-directed and primary resection modalities in the appropriate context.

SYSTEMIC REGIMENS FOR METASTATIC COLORECTAL CANCER

In patients with unresectable metastatic colorectal cancer, who comprise most cases, systemic treatment is focused on tumor control, which is occasionally symptom-directed (palliative) and not curative. The treatment goals are to increase life expectancy while maintaining quality of life for as long as possible. In this context, the model of distinct lines of chemotherapy is being abandoned in favor of a continuum-of-care approach similar to that taken in other chronic illnesses.[4] Using currently available data, the authors propose an algorithm for treatment selection based on emerging clinical and molecular data (**Fig. 1**).

The 3 active conventional chemotherapy agents for metastatic colorectal cancer are fluoropyrimidines (including intravenous 5-fluorouracil or its oral prodrug equivalent, capecitabine), irinotecan, and oxaliplatin (**Table 1**). Patients clearly benefit from access to all active agents.[4,5] A variety of targeted therapy agents are also available (**Table 2**), which are incorporated into conventional chemotherapy regimens at various time points across the continuum of care.

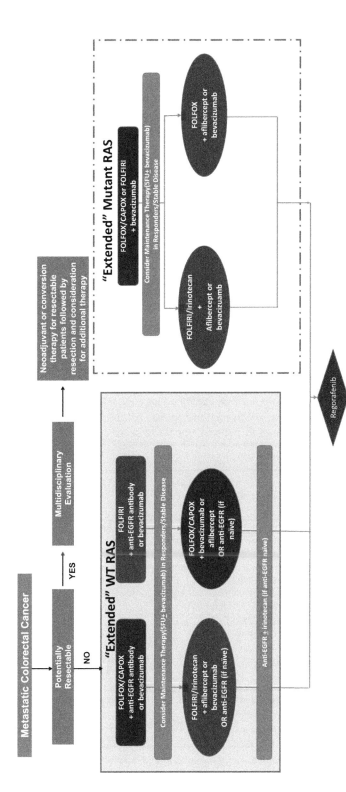

Fig. 1. A proposed algorithm for selection of systemic treatment and integration with surgical resection in patients with metastatic colorectal carcinoma, based on available clinical and molecular data. 5FU, 5-fluorouracil; CAPOX, capecitabine and oxaliplatin; FOLFIRI, irinotecan, 5-fluorouracil, and leucovorin; FOLFOX, oxaliplatin, 5-fluorouracil, and leucovorin; WT, wild-type.

Table 1
Conventional chemotherapy agents

Category	Mechanism	Major Adverse Effects
Fluoropyrimidines (5-fluorouracil/capecitabine)	Thymidylate synthase inhibitors; the accumulated deoxyuridine monophosphate misincorporates into DNA, resulting in inhibition of DNA synthesis and function	Myelosuppression Mucositis and/or diarrhea Hand-foot syndrome
Irinotecan	Converted by carboxylesterase to SN38, which prevents the relegation of DNA and further results in double-strand DNA breaks and cellular death	Diarrhea Myelosuppression Alopecia
Oxaliplatin	A third-generation platinum compound, covalently binding to DNA, which results in inhibition of DNA synthesis and transcription	Neurotoxicity Acute cold-triggered sensory neuropathy Chronic cumulative sensory neuropathy

Initial Treatment: The Chemotherapy Backbone

Data from head-to-head comparisons suggest that outcomes with first-line oxaliplatin, 5-fluorouracil, and leucovorin (FOLFOX) and irinotecan, 5-fluorouracil, and leucovorin (FOLFIRI) are similar.[6] Studies have evaluated the substitution of the oral fluoropyrimidine capecitabine for intravenous 5-fluorouracil, with either irinotecan (CAPIRI) or oxaliplatin (CAPOX). CAPIRI has been associated with excessive toxicity,[7] and is not recommended. Data also suggest that CAPOX has similar antitumor efficacy but potentially more toxicity, especially thrombocytopenia, hand-foot syndrome, and diarrhea,[8,9] but may be considered in patients unable to receive ambulatory infusional

Table 2
Targeted therapy agents

Category	Mechanism	Major Side Effects
VEGF inhibitors (bevacizumab, aflibercept)	Bevacizumab: a recombinant humanized monoclonal antibody to VEGF-A receptors Aflibercept: a VEGF receptor decoy fusion protein consisting of extracellular domain components of VEGF-R1 and VEGF-R2 fused with the Fc region of IgG1	Hypertension Bleeding Gastrointestinal perforation Arterial thromboembolism (including stroke and myocardial infarction)
Anti-EGFR antibodies (cetuximab, panitumumab)	Monoclonal antibodies against EGFR	Infusion reactions Hypomagnesemia Pruritus/dry skin Pulmonary toxicity Diarrhea
Kinase inhibitor (regorafenib)	A small-molecule inhibitor of multiple cell-signaling kinases	Hand-foot syndrome Fatigue Diarrhea Hypertension

Abbreviations: EGFR, epidermal growth factor receptor; IgG1, immunoglobulin G1; VEGF, vascular endothelial growth factor.

therapy. Irinotecan and oxaliplatin (IROX) may be considered in a small proportion of patients who are intolerant of 5-fluorouracil.[10]

The choice between initial FOLFIRI and FOLFOX or CAPOX should be based on expected treatment-related toxicity in the context of coexisting comorbidities for any given patients. For instance, a patient with long-standing diabetes mellitus or pre-existing neuropathy may be recommended FOLFIRI rather than the neuropathy-inducing FOLFOX regimen. For patients who are not candidates for an intensive oxaliplatin-based or irinotecan-based regimen because of comorbidities, performance status, or personal preference, fluoropyrimidine therapy alone (with or without a targeted therapy agent) can be considered. In early studies, high rates of successful resection and favorable long-term survival rates for patients with initially unresectable liver metastases have been reported for a triplet regimen that combines all 3 classes of conventional chemotherapy (FOLFOXIRI),[11,12] and this regimen may be considered in highly select patients until additional randomized data are available.

For patients receiving a FOLFIRI-like regimen after progression on FOLFOX, expected response rates are between 4% and 20%, and PFS of 2.5 to 7.1 months, respectively.[13,14] On the other hand, studies of oxaliplatin-based therapy in patients failing an initial irinotecan-based regimen describe response rates around 10%, and median time to progression (TTP) of 4 to 5 months.[14,15] The current standard approach to metastatic colorectal cancer includes either oxaliplatin-based therapy after progression on a FOLFIRI-like regimen, or irinotecan-based therapy after progression on a FOLFOX-like regimen; most clinicians, including the authors, prefer an oxaliplatin-based regimen first, based on perceived higher response rate and slightly better toxicity profile, although neither of these perceptions has been substantially proved in head-to-head studies. FOLFIRI is preferred in patients with a history of adjuvant FOLFOX in the preceding 12 months.

The Chemotherapy Backbone: Bottom Line

- Either FOLFOX or FOLFIRI can be used in the first-line setting, depending on patient preferences and concerns about specific toxicities.
- Single-agent fluoropyrimidine may be used in settings where patients are unable or unwilling to receive combination therapy.
- FOLFOXIRI may be considered in highly select patients in whom a high response rate and aggressive approach are warranted.
- Targeted agents should be added to all chemotherapy backbones when possible.

Incorporating Anti–Vascular Endothelial Growth Factor Agents

The anti-VEGF monoclonal antibody, bevacizumab, does not have significant single-agent activity in metastatic colorectal cancer.[16] However, multiple clinical trials have shown that it adds benefits to first-line fluoropyrimidine-, oxaliplatin- and irinotecan-based regimens given across the continuum of care in patients with metastatic disease.[17–19] In the randomized TREE-2 trial, for instance, adding bevacizumab to oxaliplatin and 5-fluorouracil-containing regimens in previously untreated patients resulted in a median OS of 23.7 months versus 18.2 months for the combined non–bevacizumab-treated groups.[20] The addition of bevacizumab to oxaliplatin-based regimen in previously treated patients with metastatic colorectal cancer (with 5-fluorouracil or irinotecan) also led to improved PFS (7.3 vs 4.7 months) and median OS (12.9 vs 10.8 months) compared with FOLFOX alone in the ECOG 3200 trial conducted in the second-line setting.[16] Thus, the accepted consensus in the management of metastatic colorectal cancer is to add bevacizumab to the chemotherapy backbone chosen for the individual patient for initial or subsequent treatments. Bevacizumab is associated with increased rates of grade 3 or 4 hypertension, bowel perforation, impaired wound healing, arterial thromboembolism, and bleeding events.[21] Careful patient selection and monitoring for toxicity is important, as is timing of discontinuation of treatment if surgical intervention is to be considered. Given that the half-life of bevacizumab is approximately 3 weeks, the authors' general recommendation is to hold bevacizumab for a period of 4 to 6 weeks before and after surgery to avoid post-surgical complications such as wound dehiscence.

Traditional teaching with conventional treatments has been to discontinue all classes of drugs when patients progress. It is unclear, however, whether a similar strategy should be adopted with biological agents, particularly those with antiangiogenic activity. The efficacy of continuing bevacizumab beyond progression was tested in the ML18147 phase III trial, which demonstrated a significant improvement in PFS (5.7 vs 4.1 months) and OS (11.2 vs 9.8 months). Bevacizumab-related adverse events were not increased in comparison with historical data of first-line bevacizumab treatment.[22]

Aflibercept is a recombinant fusion protein that binds with higher affinity to VEGF-A than does bevacizumab in a cell-free system.[23] In the United States, aflibercept is approved for use in combination with FOLFIRI for the treatment of patients with metastatic colorectal cancer that is resistant to or has progressed following an oxaliplatin-containing regimen, based on the placebo-controlled VELOUR trial.[24] The median OS was significantly longer in patients treated with aflibercept (13.5 vs 12.1 months) as was median PFS (6.9 vs 4.7 months). Treatment benefit was similar regardless of prior bevacizumab exposure (about 30% of patients in the trial).[25] However, there are no head-to-head trials comparing continuation of bevacizumab beyond progression with switching to aflibercept in this setting; hence, either strategy is considered appropriate.

Incorporating Anti–Epidermal Growth Factor Receptor Agents: Role of Precision Therapy

Anti-EGFR agents can improve outcomes in metastatic disease, both as single agents and in combination regimens. Biomarker analysis is critical to patient selection for therapy with an EGFR inhibitor, a form of so-called precision or personalized medicine whereby tumor mutations in individual specimens are used to select systemic therapy. Activating mutations in KRAS, which result in constitutive activation of the RAS-RAF-ERK pathway, lead to resistance to anti-EGFR therapy.[26] In 2009, the American Society of Clinical Oncology recommended that all patients being considered for anti-EGFR therapy undergo KRAS mutation testing of their tumors, and that treatment with these agents be restricted to those with wild-type (WT) KRAS,[27] defined as an absence of mutations in exon 2 of KRAS gene by qualitative real-time polymerase chain reaction. Emerging data suggest that resistance to anti-EGFR therapies can also be mediated by lower-frequency mutations in KRAS outside of exon 2 and in NRAS.[28–31] In 2013, the PRIME study demonstrated that within the so-called classic WT KRAS population (without mutations in exon 2), patients with mutations in other KRAS exons (exons 3 and 4) or in NRAS (exons 2 and 3) did not benefit from the addition of panitumumab to FOLFOX. Of concern, such patients had a nonsignificantly worse PFS (7.3 vs 8.0 months, $P = .33$) and OS (hazard ratio 1.39, $P = .12$) with the addition of anti-EGFR therapy.[28] Furthermore, the addition of panitumumab to chemotherapy increased OS significantly in patients with so-called extended WT RAS (no mutations in exons 2, 3, and 4 of KRAS and NRAS).[28] Other analyses have confirmed these findings. The emerging consensus is that all patients with metastatic colorectal cancer should be tested for extended RAS mutations and that those with such muta-tions should not be recommended anti-EGFR therapy.

First-line cetuximab was explored in the CRYSTAL trial in previously untreated met-astatic colorectal cancer; patients were randomly assigned to FOLFIRI with or without cetuximab. Among patients with WT KRAS, response rates were significantly higher in those who received cetuximab (57% vs 40%), as was median PFS and OS (23.5 vs 20 months).[32] The EPIC trial randomly assigned 1298 oxaliplatin-refractory patients to irinotecan with or without cetuximab. PFS was significantly higher with combined therapy (4 vs 2.6 months), as were rates of objective response (16% vs 4%) and overall disease control (61% vs 46%).[33] Increasing data also support the efficacy of first-, second-, and third-line panitumumab in combination with oxaliplatin-based or irinotecan-based regimens in patients with WT RAS tumors.[28,34-39] Cetuximab and panitumumab appear to have comparable efficacy when used as single agents for salvage therapy in patients with chemotherapy-refractory metastatic colorectal can-cer,[40,41] and when used for initial or subsequent therapy for metastatic colorectal can-cer in conjunction with an irinotecan-based chemotherapy regimen. The choice of anti-EGFR agent largely depends on provider comfort with specific agents, concerns regarding infusional reactions, and logistics (cetuximab is a weekly regimen whereas panitumumab is every other week).

Although response rates in individual studies were higher with the addition of cetux-imab to chemotherapy than by adding bevacizumab in patients with WT KRAS status, the median survival benefit is similar.[16,20,32,33] Where there is likelihood of converting patients to resectable metastatic disease, the improved response rates support using anti-EGFR therapy in the first-line setting. Dual antibody therapy targeting both VEGF and EGFR has been tested and found to lead to worsened outcomes, and is therefore not recommended.[42,43]

Among patients with WT RAS, an important issue is whether to add bevacizumab or anti-EGFR therapy to the chemotherapy backbone as initial therapy. Two initial trials with small sample sizes suggested benefit for an "anti-EGFR first" approach.[30,31] However, definitive results from the largest such study, C80405, a US Intergroup study, were presented in 2014 and showed no survival difference for either cetuximab or bevacizumab when combined with a chemotherapy backbone in the initial treat-ment setting (29.9 vs 29 months, $P = .34$).[2] Therefore, either antibody can be used in the initial therapy setting, with choice driven again by toxicity, patient preference, and logistics. It should be noted that C80405 did include patients who may have had extended RAS mutations (only classic KRAS mutants were excluded); results of this subgroup analysis may alter the final conclusions in the future.

Regorafenib

Regorafenib targets a variety of kinases implicated in angiogenic and tumor growth-promoting pathways. Its activity in refractory metastatic colorectal cancer was demonstrated in the CORRECT trial.[44] Patients who had progressed after multiple standard therapies assigned to regorafenib had a modest though statistically signifi-cant improvement in median OS (6.4 vs 5 months), and PFS (1.9 months vs 1.7 months).[44] At present, regorafenib is reserved for patients whose cancers have progressed on the other standard chemotherapeutic and targeted therapy agents.

Targeted Therapy: Bottom Line

- All chemotherapy backbones in initial and subsequent settings should be accompanied by one targeted agent, unless specific contraindications exist.

- Anti-EGFR approaches should be used only in patients with extended RAS WT tumors.
- Bevacizumab or anti-EGFR therapy may be used in the initial setting in such extended RAS WT patients.
- Bevacizumab may be continued beyond progression with a change in chemotherapy backbone.
- Dual antibody therapy should be avoided.

MAINTENANCE REGIMENS

Approximately 75% of patients discontinue first-line chemotherapy in trials for reasons other than progressive disease, and face the question of whether to consider maintenance chemotherapy or take a chemotherapy break. The OPTIMOX trials showed that oxaliplatin can be safely stopped after 6 cycles in a FOLFOX regimen, and that complete discontinuation of chemotherapy had a negative impact on PFS compared with maintenance therapy with 5-fluorouracil.[45,46] Results from CAIRO-3 showed that maintenance therapy with bevacizumab plus capecitabine after 6 cycles of CAPOX plus bevacizumab was associated with a significant longer PFS (8.5 vs 4.1 months).[47] Decisions regarding maintenance therapy versus treatment breaks must also take into account patient preferences and cost.

POTENTIALLY CURABLE ADVANCED COLORECTAL CANCER

The liver is the first site of hematogenous dissemination in most patients with colorectal cancer. Approximately 10% of patients can live past 5 years even with metastatic disease.[48] The definition of resectable metastatic disease is evolving, and there is not an accepted standard: even bilobar metastases and extrahepatic disease are no longer considered contraindications. Decision-making in this setting requires multidisciplinary collaboration: a practical approach requires that patients should be medically fit for surgery, existing liver disease should be resectable with adequate liver remnant, and extrahepatic disease should be controlled. Surgical resection is the preferred treatment in patients with oligometastatic disease primarily in the liver, with 5-year survival rates of approximately 50% to 60% in patients with favorable prognostic features.[49,50] Approximately one-fifth of such patients survive beyond 10 years in some series,[51] and this applies also to nonhepatic disease in certain series. When the primary tumor site is controlled and the metastatic disease is limited in lungs without extrapulmonary location (except for resectable or resected hepatic lesion), resection of isolated pulmonary metastases can increase survival rates up to 40% at 5 years.[25,52]

Select patients with initially unresectable liver metastases may become eligible for resection if the response to chemotherapy is sufficient. This approach has been termed conversion therapy to distinguish it from neoadjuvant therapy. Conversion therapy allows 12% to 33% of initially unresectable or borderline resectable metastases to become eligible for metastasectomy.[11,12,53] Five-year survival rates average 30% to 35%, which is substantially better than expected with chemotherapy alone.

A regimen with a high likelihood of objective response is typically chosen because of the strong correlation with subsequent resection rates. However, the choice of regimen is not well established. The triplet chemotherapy regimen FOLFOXIRI with bevacizumab was associated with significantly higher response rates (65% vs 53%) and PFS (median 12.2 vs 9 months) in comparison with FOLFIRI plus bevacizumab in the phase III TRIBE trial.[11] However, FOLFOXIRI did not result in a significantly higher secondary complete (R0) liver resection rate (15% vs 12%), and was associated with greater adverse effects.[54] Combination of anti-EGFR inhibitor with either irinotecan-based or oxaliplatin-based regimens has shown modestly improved resection rates in patients with WT KRAS status.[55,56] The German multicenter randomized phase II trial (CELM study), by using FOLFOX plus cetuximab or FOLFIRI plus cetuximab, showed 62% tumor response in all patients with 70% in WT KRAS patients, but no OS and PFS improvement.[55] A promising recent phase II study reported a surgical R0 resection conversion rate of approximately 70% (14 of 20 patients) with FOLFOX with dose-escalating cetuximab in initially unresectable patients with WT KRAS status.[57] Hepatic intra-arterial chemotherapy either alone or in addition to systemic therapy also has the potential to downstage hepatic metastases.[58,59] However, there are no randomized trials comparing hepatic pumps with contemporary systemic chemotherapy alone, and this approach is not currently widely used in the United States.

For patients with initially resectable liver metastases, a common sequence (particularly for patients with synchronous metastatic disease) is initial systemic chemotherapy, mainly to obtain prognostic information, treat potentially disseminated micrometastases as early as possible, evaluate for emerging additional metastases, and test the chemosensitivity of the tumor. Upfront surgery is an appropriate option for patients with metachronous presentation of hepatic metastases. The European Organization for Research and Treatment of Cancer Intergroup trial 40983 enrolled 364 resectable patients with up to 4 metastases without prior exposure to oxaliplatin who were randomly assigned to liver resection with or without perioperative FOLFOX chemotherapy.[60] Initial chemotherapy improved patient selection for hepatic resection. The postoperative complication rate was significantly higher in the chemotherapy group (25% vs 16%). However, the postoperative mortality was not higher than surgery alone (1 vs 2 deaths). In the latest update, at a median follow-up of 8.5 years, there was a nonstatistically significant trend in 5-year PFS favoring chemotherapy (38% vs 33%), but 5-year OS was not significantly better in the chemotherapy group (51% vs 48%).[61] A recent retrospective study suggested that neoadjuvant therapy only benefits high-risk patients.[62] In patients with more than 2 risk factors, those who received neoadjuvant chemotherapy had improved median survival (38.9 vs 28.4 months). By contrast, for low-risk patients, survival outcomes were similar with or without neoadjuvant chemotherapy, median survival (60.0 vs 60.0 months) and 5-year OS (64% vs 57%, $P>.05$).[62]

Liver metastases recur in up to 80% of patients after liver resection, with approximately half being confined to the liver. In these patients, provided that the aforementioned resectability criteria are fulfilled, repeat liver resection is safe and can lead to survival rates that are equivalent to those reported for first hepatectomy.[63,64] It is therefore important to monitor patients carefully to detect hepatic recurrence at a resectable stage. Only limited evidence is available regarding the optimal follow-up strategy after liver resection for metastatic colorectal cancer.[65,66] The following surveillance strategy for patients with metastatic disease rendered disease-free is reasonable: carcinoembryonic antigen, liver function tests, and computed tomography scan of the chest, abdomen, and pelvis every 3 to 6 months for 2 years, then every 6 to 12 months for up to 5 years.

Other Liver-Directed Treatments

Several other regional therapies, including local tumor ablation, regional hepatic intra-arterial chemotherapy or chemoembolization, and stereotactic body radiation therapy, are options for patients with liver-isolated colorectal cancer metastases who are not candidates for surgery.[67,68] These therapies are often incorporated with initial hepatic resection or used as alternatives in patients who are not medically fit enough to undergo surgical resection. Although these methods can provide excellent local control, long-term survival outcomes are not well studied.

ROLE FOR RESECTION OF PRIMARY TUMOR

There are 2 broad indications for resection of the primary tumor in metastatic colorectal cancer: palliation of symptoms and intention cure. The approach therefore can be categorized according to symptoms of the primary tumor and resectability of the metastatic disease.

Symptomatic Primary Tumor with Unresectable Metastatic Disease

The most common symptoms requiring intervention of the primary tumor are obstruction, bleeding/anemia, and perforation. There is generally not time nor a role for neoadjuvant chemotherapy in this setting. The goal is to palliate symptoms and improve the quality of life. Although surgical oncology principles are encouraged, diffuse disease or carcinomatosis may not allow a proper oncologic operation. For example, a diverting stoma or bypass of an obstructing tumor may be performed to limit morbidity and facilitate quicker transition to systemic therapy.

Symptomatic Primary with Resectable Metastatic Disease

As already mentioned, treatment of symptomatic tumors requires timely intervention. However, if the metastatic disease is treatable surgically, a decision must be made as regards timing. The primary objective is to relieve the symptoms and approach the primary tumor with surgical oncologic principles such as high ligation of vessels, adequate lymph node harvest, minimal manipulation of the tumor, and achievement of adequate margins. If the symptom is acute obstruction or perforation and the patient requires emergent surgery, only the primary tumor should be approached. In the setting of an elective operation, the decision to resect liver metastases depends on the extent of disease and magnitude of surgery required. In general, if a simple wedge resection/metastasectomy is all that is required, the liver may be addressed at the same time as the colon resection. If more extensive liver resection is required, the primary tumor alone should be addressed with a plan for chemotherapy and staged liver resection.

Asymptomatic Primary Tumor with Unresectable Metastatic Disease

The role for resection of an asymptomatic primary tumor in the setting of unresectable distant disease is controversial. Although retrospective data suggest a survival benefit of resection and a prospective study showed that an unresected primary led to major morbidity in a subgroup of patients (n = 12 of 86),[69] the evidence is not definitive. Proponents of resection argue that patients may achieve a better response to chemotherapy with a lower tumor burden, and that it eliminates the risk of complications developing during chemotherapy such as obstruction or perforation. The argument against resection is based on the potential for postoperative complications that may delay or even prevent chemotherapy.[70] Factors associated with improved survival include age less than 70 years, no extrahepatic disease, good functional status, and liver burden less than 50%.[70]

Asymptomatic Primary Tumor with Resectable Metastatic Disease

Resecting the primary tumor remains the essential cornerstone of treatment in resectable metastatic disease. The timing of resection of the primary in relation to liver resection and chemotherapy remains an issue of debate, and multiple approaches show equipoise. The classic approach involves resection of the primary tumor, followed by adjuvant chemotherapy, then metastasectomy. Some groups champion neoadjuvant therapy to attack the systemic disease first, as distant diseases determine survival. This approach allows the tumor biology to declare itself through response to therapy. Patients who progress and become unresectable are saved from the morbidity of surgery on the primary. Patients who respond will go on to resection of the primary and liver lesions. Both synchronous resections and staged resections have been described. Some groups prefer a staged resection with a liver-first approach, but the success is variable.[71] Management of these cases is best served by discussion with a multidisciplinary team involving hepatobiliary surgeons, colorectal surgeons, and oncologists.

SUMMARY AND FUTURE DIRECTIONS

The past decade has seen an impressive improvement in outcomes for patients with metastatic colorectal cancer. Patients seen in the clinic today can have discussions about expected survival outcomes ranging in "years." Even the term "cure" is not out of place in a discussion in the metastatic setting. This remarkable improvement in outcomes has resulted not from a "magic bullet" but from a convergence of forces: new drugs and regimens that can be used sequentially to allow quality of life and extended life expectancy, improvement in surgical techniques, and data demonstrating the value of surgical resection and liver-directed therapy.

Integrating personalized medicine into the care of patients with colorectal cancer will be the next step forward. The development of biomarkers that predict response to anti-EGFR therapy is an example of how molecular profiling can significantly improve outcomes in patients with RAS WT tumors, and can spare patients with RAS mutant tumors both toxicity and cost. Commercial vendors are already offering next-generation genomic sequencing at the bedside. The authors and others are participating in novel trials that offer targeted agents based on mutations identified using genomic sequencing. As additional data become available, it is anticipated that far greater individualization of treatment will be possible. In a recent analysis of 1290 colorectal cancers using gene-expression profiling, 6 clinically different subtypes were identified, each showing different degrees of activation of Wnt signaling and "stemness," response to anti-EGFR and irinotecan-based therapy, and survival in the adjuvant and metastatic settings.[72] Further such research will accelerate novel drug development and testing, and allow clinicians to continually refine and individualize treatment. The successes of the past decade have raised hopes and expectations that the conversion of metastatic colorectal cancer from a lethal to a chronic illness, with durable remissions and even cures, can be a reality for most patients.

ACKNOWLEDGMENTS

Dr A.A. Khorana would like to acknowledge research support from the Sondra and Stephen Hardis Chair in Oncology Research and the Scott Hamilton CARES Initiative. Dr M.F. Kalady is the Krause-Lieberman Chair in Colorectal Surgery.

REFERENCES

1. Siegel R, Ma J, Zou Z, et al. Cancer statistics, 2014. CA Cancer J Clin 2014;64(1): 9–29.
2. Venook AP, Niedzwiecki D, Lenz HJ, et al. CALGB/SWOG 80405: phase III trial of irinotecan/5-FU/leucovorin (FOLFIRI) or oxaliplatin/5-FU/leucovorin (mFOLFOX6)

with bevacizumab (BV) or cetuximab (CET) for patients (pts) with KRAS wild-type (wt) untreated metastatic adenocarcinoma of the colon or rectum (MCRC). J Clin Oncol 2014;32:5s.

3. Scheithauer W, Rosen H, Kornek GV, et al. Randomised comparison of combination chemotherapy plus supportive care with supportive care alone in patients with metastatic colorectal cancer. BMJ 1993;306(6880):752–5.

4. Goldberg RM, Rothenberg ML, Van Cutsem E, et al. The continuum of care: a paradigm for the management of metastatic colorectal cancer. Oncologist 2007;12(1):38–50.

5. Grothey A, Sargent D. Overall survival of patients with advanced colorectal cancer correlates with availability of fluorouracil, irinotecan, and oxaliplatin regardless of whether doublet or single-agent therapy is used first line. J Clin Oncol 2005;23(36):9441–2.

6. Colucci G, Gebbia V, Paoletti G, et al. Phase III randomized trial of FOLFIRI versus FOLFOX4 in the treatment of advanced colorectal cancer: a multicenter study of the Gruppo Oncologico Dell'Italia Meridionale. J Clin Oncol 2005; 23(22):4866–75.

7. Patt YZ, Lee FC, Liebmann JE, et al. Capecitabine plus 3-weekly irinotecan (XELIRI regimen) as first-line chemotherapy for metastatic colorectal cancer: phase II trial results. Am J Clin Oncol 2007;30(4):350–7.

8. Diaz-Rubio E, Tabernero J, Gomez-Espana A, et al. Phase III study of capecitabine plus oxaliplatin compared with continuous-infusion fluorouracil plus oxaliplatin as first-line therapy in metastatic colorectal cancer: final report of the Spanish Cooperative Group for the treatment of digestive tumors trial. J Clin Oncol 2007; 25(27):4224–30.

9. Porschen R, Arkenau HT, Kubicka S, et al. Phase III study of capecitabine plus oxaliplatin compared with fluorouracil and leucovorin plus oxaliplatin in metastatic colorectal cancer: a final report of the AIO Colorectal Study Group. J Clin Oncol 2007;25(27):4217–23.

10. Sanoff HK, Sargent DJ, Campbell ME, et al. Five-year data and prognostic factor analysis of oxaliplatin and irinotecan combinations for advanced colorectal cancer: N9741. J Clin Oncol 2008;26(35):5721–7.

11. Falcone A, Ricci S, Brunetti I, et al. Phase III trial of infusional fluorouracil, leucovorin, oxaliplatin, and irinotecan (FOLFOXIRI) compared with infusional fluorouracil, leucovorin, and irinotecan (FOLFIRI) as first-line treatment for metastatic colorectal cancer: the Gruppo Oncologico Nord Ovest. J Clin Oncol 2007;25(13):1670–6.

12. Masi G, Loupakis F, Pollina L, et al. Long-term outcome of initially unresectable metastatic colorectal cancer patients treated with 5-fluorouracil/leucovorin, oxaliplatin, and irinotecan (FOLFOXIRI) followed by radical surgery of metastases. Ann Surg 2009;249(3):420–5.

13. Bidard FC, Tournigand C, Andre T, et al. Efficacy of FOLFIRI-3 (irinotecan D1,D3 combined with LV5-FU) or other irinotecan-based regimens in oxaliplatin-pretreated metastatic colorectal cancer in the GERCOR OPTIMOX1 study. Ann Oncol 2009;20(6):1042–7.

14. Tournigand C, Andre T, Achille E, et al. FOLFIRI followed by FOLFOX6 or the reverse sequence in advanced colorectal cancer: a randomized GERCOR study. J Clin Oncol 2004;22(2):229–37.

15. Rothenberg ML, Oza AM, Bigelow RH, et al. Superiority of oxaliplatin and fluorouracil-leucovorin compared with either therapy alone in patients with progressive colorectal cancer after irinotecan and fluorouracil-leucovorin: interim results of a phase III trial. J Clin Oncol 2003;21(11):2059–69.

16. Giantonio BJ, Catalano PJ, Meropol NJ, et al. Bevacizumab in combination with oxaliplatin, fluorouracil, and leucovorin (FOLFOX4) for previously treated metastatic colorectal cancer: results from the Eastern Cooperative Oncology Group Study E3200. J Clin Oncol 2007;25(12):1539–44.
17. Hurwitz HI, Fehrenbacher L, Hainsworth JD, et al. Bevacizumab in combination with fluorouracil and leucovorin: an active regimen for first-line metastatic colorectal cancer. J Clin Oncol 2005;23(15):3502–8.
18. Kabbinavar FF, Hambleton J, Mass RD, et al. Combined analysis of efficacy: the addition of bevacizumab to fluorouracil/leucovorin improves survival for patients with metastatic colorectal cancer. J Clin Oncol 2005;23(16):3706–12.
19. Vincenzi B, Santini D, Russo A, et al. Bevacizumab in association with de Gramont 5-fluorouracil/folinic acid in patients with oxaliplatin-, irinotecan-, and cetuximab-refractory colorectal cancer: a single-center phase 2 trial. Cancer 2009;115(20):4849–56.
20. Hochster HS, Hart LL, Ramanathan RK, et al. Safety and efficacy of oxaliplatin and fluoropyrimidine regimens with or without bevacizumab as first-line treatment of metastatic colorectal cancer: results of the TREE Study. J Clin Oncol 2008; 26(21):3523–9.
21. Scappaticci FA, Skillings JR, Holden SN, et al. Arterial thromboembolic events in patients with metastatic carcinoma treated with chemotherapy and bevacizumab. J Natl Cancer Inst 2007;99(16):1232–9.
22. Bennouna J, Sastre J, Arnold D, et al. Continuation of bevacizumab after first progression in metastatic colorectal cancer (ML18147): a randomised phase 3 trial. Lancet Oncol 2013;14(1):29–37.
23. Holash J, Davis S, Papadopoulos N, et al. VEGF-Trap: a VEGF blocker with potent antitumor effects. Proc Natl Acad Sci U S A 2002;99(17):11393–8.
24. Joulain F, Van Cutsem E, Iqbal SU, et al. Aflibercept versus placebo in combination with FOLFIRI in previously treated metastatic colorectal cancer (mCRC): mean overall survival (OS) estimation from a phase III trial (VELOUR). J Clin Oncol 2012;30(15). Abstract: 3602.
25. Allegra CJ, Lakomy R, Tabernero J, et al. Effects of prior bevacizumab (B) use on outcomes from the VELOUR study: a phase III study of aflibercept (Afl) and FOLFIRI in patients (pts) with metastatic colorectal cancer (mCRC) after failure of an oxaliplatin regimen. J Clin Oncol 2012;30(15). Abstract: 3505.
26. Dahabreh IJ, Terasawa T, Castaldi PJ, et al. Systematic review: anti-epidermal growth factor receptor treatment effect modification by KRAS mutations in advanced colorectal cancer. Ann Intern Med 2011;154(1):37–49.
27. Allegra CJ, Jessup JM, Somerfield MR, et al. American Society of Clinical Oncology provisional clinical opinion: testing for KRAS gene mutations in patients with metastatic colorectal carcinoma to predict response to anti-epidermal growth factor receptor monoclonal antibody therapy. J Clin Oncol 2009;27(12): 2091–6.
28. Douillard JY, Oliner KS, Siena S, et al. Panitumumab-FOLFOX4 treatment and RAS mutations in colorectal cancer. N Engl J Med 2013;369(11):1023–34.
29. Loupakis F, Ruzzo A, Cremolini C, et al. KRAS codon 61, 146 and BRAF mutations predict resistance to cetuximab plus irinotecan in KRAS codon 12 and 13 wild-type metastatic colorectal cancer. Br J Cancer 2009;101(4):715–21.
30. Schwartzberg LS, Rivera F, Karthaus M, et al. Analysis of KRAS/NRAS mutations in PEAK: A randomized phase II study of FOLFOX6 plus panitumumab (pmab) or bevacizumab (bev) as first-line treatment (tx) for wild-type (WT) KRAS (exon 2) metastatic colorectal cancer (mCRC). J Clin Oncol 2013;31(15). Abstract: 3631.

31. Stintzing S, Jung A, Rossius L, et al. Analysis of KRAS/NRAS and BRAF mutations in FIRE-3: a randomized phase III study of FOLFIRI plus cetuximab or bevacizumab as first-line treatment for wild-type (WT) KRAS (exon 2) metastatic colorectal cancer (mCRC) patients. Data presented at the 13th annual European Cancer Congress (ECC), Amsterdam, The Netherlands. September 28, 2013.
32. Van Cutsem E, Kohne CH, Lang I, et al. Cetuximab plus irinotecan, fluorouracil, and leucovorin as first-line treatment for metastatic colorectal cancer: updated analysis of overall survival according to tumor KRAS and BRAF mutation status. J Clin Oncol 2011;29(15):2011–9.
33. Sobrero AF, Maurel J, Fehrenbacher L, et al. EPIC: phase III trial of cetuximab plus irinotecan after fluoropyrimidine and oxaliplatin failure in patients with metastatic colorectal cancer. J Clin Oncol 2008;26(14):2311–9.
34. Andre T, Blons H, Mabro M, et al. Panitumumab combined with irinotecan for patients with KRAS wild-type metastatic colorectal cancer refractory to standard chemotherapy: a GERCOR efficacy, tolerance, and translational molecular study. Ann Oncol 2013;24(2):412–9.
35. Cohn AL, Shumaker GC, Khandelwal P, et al. An open-label, single-arm, phase 2 trial of panitumumab plus FOLFIRI as second-line therapy in patients with metastatic colorectal cancer. Clin Colorectal Cancer 2011;10(3):171–7.
36. Douillard JY, Siena S, Cassidy J, et al. Randomized, phase III trial of panitumumab with infusional fluorouracil, leucovorin, and oxaliplatin (FOLFOX4) versus FOLFOX4 alone as first-line treatment in patients with previously untreated metastatic colorectal cancer: the PRIME study. J Clin Oncol 2010;28(31):4697–705.
37. Kohne CH, Hofheinz R, Mineur L, et al. First-line panitumumab plus irinotecan/5-fluorouracil/leucovorin treatment in patients with metastatic colorectal cancer. J Cancer Res Clin Oncol 2012;138(1):65–72.
38. Peeters M, Price TJ, Cervantes A, et al. Final results from a randomized phase 3 study of FOLFIRI {+/-} panitumumab for second-line treatment of metastatic colorectal cancer. Ann Oncol 2014;25(1):107–16.
39. Seymour MT, Brown SR, Middleton G, et al. Panitumumab and irinotecan versus irinotecan alone for patients with KRAS wild-type, fluorouracil-resistant advanced colorectal cancer (PICCOLO): a prospectively stratified randomised trial. Lancet Oncol 2013;14(8):749–59.
40. Price T, Peeters M, Kim TW, et al. ASPECCT: a randomized, multicenter, open-label, phase 3 study of panitumumab (pmab) vs cetuximab (cmab) for previously treated wild-type (WT) KRAS metastatic colorectal cancer (mCRC). Data presented at the 2013 annual European Cancer Congress (ECC), Amsterdam, The Netherlands. September 29, 2013.
41. Van Cutsem E, Peeters M, Siena S, et al. Open-label phase III trial of panitumumab plus best supportive care compared with best supportive care alone in patients with chemotherapy-refractory metastatic colorectal cancer. J Clin Oncol 2007;25(13):1658–64.
42. Hecht JR, Mitchell E, Chidiac T, et al. A randomized phase IIIB trial of chemotherapy, bevacizumab, and panitumumab compared with chemotherapy and bevacizumab alone for metastatic colorectal cancer. J Clin Oncol 2009;27(5):672–80.
43. Tol J, Koopman M, Cats A, et al. Chemotherapy, bevacizumab, and cetuximab in metastatic colorectal cancer. N Engl J Med 2009;360(6):563–72.
44. Grothey A, Van Cutsem E, Sobrero A, et al. Regorafenib monotherapy for previously treated metastatic colorectal cancer (CORRECT): an international, multicentre, randomised, placebo-controlled, phase 3 trial. Lancet 2013;381(9863):303–12.

45. Chibaudel B, Maindrault-Goebel F, Lledo G, et al. Can chemotherapy be discontinued in unresectable metastatic colorectal cancer? The GERCOR OPTIMOX2 Study. J Clin Oncol 2009;27(34):5727–33.
46. Tournigand C, Cervantes A, Figer A, et al. OPTIMOX1: a randomized study of FOLFOX4 or FOLFOX7 with oxaliplatin in a stop-and-go fashion in advanced colorectal cancer–a GERCOR study. J Clin Oncol 2006;24(3):394–400.
47. Koopman M, Simkens L, May A, et al. Final results and subgroup analyses of the phase 3 CAIRO3 study: maintenance treatment with capecitabine and bevacizumab versus observation after induction treatment with chemotherapy and bevacizumab in metastatic colorectal cancer (mCRC). J Clin Oncol 2014;32(3). Abstract: LBA388.
48. Ferrarotto R, Pathak P, Maru D, et al. Durable complete responses in metastatic colorectal cancer treated with chemotherapy alone. Clin Colorectal Cancer 2011; 10(3):178–82.
49. Rees M, Tekkis PP, Welsh FK, et al. Evaluation of long-term survival after hepatic resection for metastatic colorectal cancer: a multifactorial model of 929 patients. Ann Surg 2008;247(1):125–35.
50. Fong Y, Fortner J, Sun RL, et al. Clinical score for predicting recurrence after hepatic resection for metastatic colorectal cancer: analysis of 1001 consecutive cases. Ann Surg 1999;230(3):309–18 [discussion: 318–21].
51. Tomlinson JS, Jarnagin WR, DeMatteo RP, et al. Actual 10-year survival after resection of colorectal liver metastases defines cure. J Clin Oncol 2007;25(29):4575–80.
52. Pfannschmidt J, Dienemann H, Hoffmann H. Surgical resection of pulmonary metastases from colorectal cancer: a systematic review of published series. Ann Thorac Surg 2007;84(1):324–38.
53. Adam R, Wicherts DA, de Haas RJ, et al. Patients with initially unresectable colorectal liver metastases: is there a possibility of cure? J Clin Oncol 2009;27(11): 1829–35.
54. Falcone A, Cremolini C, Masi G, et al. FOLFOXIRI/bevacizumab (bev) versus FOLFIRI/bev as first-line treatment in unresectable metastatic colorectal cancer (mCRC) patients (pts): results of the phase III TRIBE trial by GONO group. J Clin Oncol 2013;31(15). Abstract: 3505.
55. Folprecht G, Gruenberger T, Bechstein W, et al. Survival of patients with initially unresectable colorectal liver metastases treated with FOLFOX/cetuximab or FOLFIRI/cetuximab in a multidisciplinary concept (CELIM study). Ann Oncol 2014; 25(5):1018–25.
56. Ye LC, Liu TS, Ren L, et al. Randomized controlled trial of cetuximab plus chemotherapy for patients with KRAS wild-type unresectable colorectal liver-limited metastases. J Clin Oncol 2013;31(16):1931–8.
57. Wagman LD, Geller DA, Jacobs SA, et al. NSABP FC-6: phase II study to determine surgical conversion rate in patients (pts) receiving neoadjuvant (NA) mFOLFOX7 plus dose-escalating cetuximab (C) for unresectable K-RAS wild-type (WT) colorectal cancer with metastases (mCRC) confined to the liver. Ann Surg Oncol 2014;21:S13.
58. Goere D, Deshaies I, de Baere T, et al. Prolonged survival of initially unresectable hepatic colorectal cancer patients treated with hepatic arterial infusion of oxaliplatin followed by radical surgery of metastases. Ann Surg 2010;251(4):686–91.
59. Kemeny NE, Melendez FD, Capanu M, et al. Conversion to resectability using hepatic artery infusion plus systemic chemotherapy for the treatment of unresectable liver metastases from colorectal carcinoma. J Clin Oncol 2009;27(21): 3465–71.

60. Nordlinger B, Sorbye H, Glimelius B, et al. Perioperative chemotherapy with FOL-FOX4 and surgery versus surgery alone for resectable liver metastases from colorectal cancer (EORTC Intergroup trial 40983): a randomised controlled trial. Lancet 2008;371(9617):1007–16.

61. Nordlinger B, Sorbye H, Glimelius B, et al. Perioperative FOLFOX4 chemotherapy and surgery versus surgery alone for resectable liver metastases from colorectal cancer (EORTC 40983): long-term results of a randomised, controlled, phase 3 trial. Lancet Oncol 2013;14(12):1208–15.

62. Zhu D, Zhong Y, Wei Y, et al. Effect of neoadjuvant chemotherapy in patients with resectable colorectal liver metastases. PLoS One 2014;9(1):e86543.

63. Adam R, Bismuth H, Castaing D, et al. Repeat hepatectomy for colorectal liver metastases. Ann Surg 1997;225(1):51–60 [discussion: 60–2].

64. Kulik U, Bektas H, Klempnauer J, et al. Repeat liver resection for colorectal metastases. Br J Surg 2013;100(7):926–32.

65. Jones RP, Jackson R, Dunne DF, et al. Systematic review and meta-analysis of follow-up after hepatectomy for colorectal liver metastases. Br J Surg 2012; 99(4):477–86.

66. Verberne CJ, Wiggers T, Vermeulen KM, et al. Detection of recurrences during follow-up after liver surgery for colorectal metastases: both carcinoembryonic antigen (CEA) and imaging are important. Ann Surg Oncol 2013;20(2):457–63.

67. Fiorentini G, Aliberti C, Tilli M, et al. Intra-arterial infusion of irinotecan-loaded drug-eluting beads (DEBIRI) versus intravenous therapy (FOLFIRI) for hepatic metastases from colorectal cancer: final results of a phase III study. Anticancer Res 2012;32(4):1387–95.

68. Wong SL, Mangu PB, Choti MA, et al. American Society of Clinical Oncology 2009 clinical evidence review on radiofrequency ablation of hepatic metastases from colorectal cancer. J Clin Oncol 2010;28(3):493–508.

69. McCahill LE, Yothers G, Sharif S, et al. Primary mFOLFOX6 plus bevacizumab without resection of the primary tumor for patients presenting with surgically unresectable metastatic colon cancer and an intact asymptomatic colon cancer: definitive analysis of NSABP trial C-10. J Clin Oncol 2012;30(26):3223–8.

70. de Mestier L, Manceau G, Neuzillet C, et al. Primary tumor resection in colorectal cancer with unresectable synchronous metastases: a review. World J Gastrointest Oncol 2014;6(6):156–69.

71. Jegatheeswaran S, Mason JM, Hancock HC, et al. The liver-first approach to the management of colorectal cancer with synchronous hepatic metastases: a systematic review. JAMA Surg 2013;148(4):385–91.

72. Sadanandam A, Lyssiotis CA, Homicsko K, et al. A colorectal cancer classification system that associates cellular phenotype and responses to therapy. Nat Med 2013;19(5):619–25.

United States Postal Service

Statement of Ownership, Management, and Circulation
(All Periodicals Publications Except Requestor Publications)

1. Publication Title	2. Publication Number	3. Filing Date
Surgical Oncology Clinics of North America	0 1 2 - 5 6 5	9/14/14

4. Issue Frequency	5. Number of Issues Published Annually	6. Annual Subscription Price
Jan, Apr, Jul, Oct	4	$290.00

7. Complete Mailing Address of Known Office of Publication (Not printer) (Street, city, county, state, and ZIP+4®)

Elsevier Inc.
360 Park Avenue South
New York, NY 10010-1710

Contact Person: Stephen R. Bushing

Telephone (Include area code): 215-239-3688

8. Complete Mailing Address of Headquarters or General Business Office of Publisher (Not printer)

Elsevier Inc., 360 Park Avenue South, New York, NY 10010-1710

9. Full Names and Complete Mailing Addresses of Publisher, Editor, and Managing Editor (Do not leave blank)

Publisher (Name and complete mailing address)

Linda Belfus, Elsevier, Inc., 1600 John F. Kennedy Blvd. Suite 1800, Philadelphia, PA 19103-2899

Editor (Name and complete mailing address)

Jessica McCool, Elsevier, Inc., 1600 John F. Kennedy Blvd. Suite 1800, Philadelphia, PA 19103-2899

Managing Editor (Name and complete mailing address)

Adrianne Brigido, Inc., 1600 John F. Kennedy Blvd. Suite 1800, Philadelphia, PA 19103-2899

10. Owner (Do not leave blank. If the publication is owned by a corporation, give the name and address of the corporation immediately followed by the names and addresses of all stockholders owning or holding 1 percent or more of the total amount of stock. If not owned by a corporation, give the names and addresses of the individual owners. If owned by a partnership or other unincorporated firm, give its name and address as well as those of each individual owner. If the publication is published by a nonprofit organization, give its name and address.)

Full Name	Complete Mailing Address
Wholly owned subsidiary of	1600 John F. Kennedy Blvd, Ste. 1800
Reed/Elsevier, US holdings	Philadelphia, PA 19103-2899

11. Known Bondholders, Mortgagees, and Other Security Holders Owning or Holding 1 Percent or More of Total Amount of Bonds, Mortgages, or Other Securities. If none, check box → None

Full Name	Complete Mailing Address
N/A	

12. Tax Status (For completion by nonprofit organizations authorized to mail at nonprofit rates) (Check one)
The purpose, function, and nonprofit status of this organization and the exempt status for federal income tax purposes:

- ☐ Has Not Changed During Preceding 12 Months
- ☐ Has Changed During Preceding 12 Months (Publisher must submit explanation of change with this statement)

PS Form 3526, August 2012 (Page 1 of 3 (Instructions Page 3)) PSN 7530-01-000-9931 PRIVACY NOTICE: See our Privacy policy in www.usps.com

---

13. Publication Title	14. Issue Date for Circulation Data Below
Surgical Oncology Clinics of North America	July 2014

15. Extent and Nature of Circulation			Average No. Copies Each Issue During Preceding 12 Months	No. Copies of Single Issue Published Nearest to Filing Date
a. Total Number of Copies (Net press run)			454	482
b. Paid Circulation (By Mail and Outside the Mail)	(1)	Mailed Outside-County Paid Subscriptions Stated on PS Form 3541. (Include paid distribution above nominal rate, advertiser's proof copies, and exchange copies)	194	241
	(2)	Mailed In-County Paid Subscriptions Stated on PS Form 3541 (Include paid distribution above nominal rate, advertiser's proof copies, and exchange copies)		
	(3)	Paid Distribution Outside the Mails Including Sales Through Dealers and Carriers, Street Vendors, Counter Sales, and Other Paid Distribution Outside USPS®	73	85
	(4)	Paid Distribution by Other Classes Mailed Through the USPS (e.g. First-Class Mail®)		
c. Total Paid Distribution (Sum of 15b (1), (2), (3), and (4))			267	326
d. Free or Nominal Rate Distribution (By Mail and Outside the Mail)	(1)	Free or Nominal Rate Outside-County Copies Included on PS Form 3541	33	11
	(2)	Free or Nominal Rate In-County Copies Included on PS Form 3541		
	(3)	Free or Nominal Rate Copies Mailed at Other Classes Through the USPS (e.g. First-Class Mail)		
	(4)	Free or Nominal Rate Distribution Outside the Mail (Carriers or other means)		
e. Total Free or Nominal Rate Distribution (Sum of 15d (1), (2), (3) and (4))			33	11
f. Total Distribution (Sum of 15c and 15e)			300	337
g. Copies not Distributed (See instructions to publishers #4 (page #3))			154	145
h. Total (Sum of 15f and g)			454	482
i. Percent Paid (15c divided by 15f times 100)			89.00%	46.74%

16. Total circulation includes electronic copies. Report circulation on PS Form 3526-X worksheet.

17. Publication of Statement of Ownership
If the publication is a general publication, publication of this statement is required. Will be printed in the October 2014 issue of this publication.

18. Signature and Title of Editor, Publisher, Business Manager, or Owner

[signature] Stephen R. Bushing – Inventory Distribution Coordinator

Date: September 14, 2014

I certify that all information furnished on this form is true and complete. I understand that anyone who furnishes false or misleading information on this form or who omits material or information requested on the form may be subject to criminal sanctions (including fines and imprisonment) and/or civil sanctions (including civil penalties).

PS Form 3526, August 2012 (Page 2 of 3)

Moving?

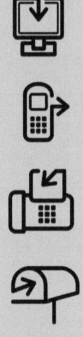

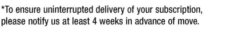

Printed and bound by CPI Group (UK) Ltd, Croydon, CR0 4YY

07/10/2024

01040498-0003